# Acute and Chronic Pancreatitis

# Acute and Chronic Pancreatitis

Editor: Sylvia Harlow

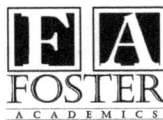

**FA FOSTER** ACADEMICS

www.fosteracademics.com

www.fosteracademics.com

**FA**
**FOSTER**
ACADEMICS

Cataloging-in-Publication Data

Acute and chronic pancreatitis / edited by Sylvia Harlow.
p. cm.
Includes bibliographical references and index.
ISBN 978-1-63242-677-2
1. Pancreatitis. 2. Pancreas--Diseases. 3. Inflammation. I. Harlow, Sylvia.
RC858.P35 A28 2019
616.37--dc23

Foster Academics,
118-35 Queens Blvd., Suite 400,
Forest Hills, NY 11375, USA

ISBN 978-1-63242-677-2 (Hardback)

# Contents

# Preface

This book has been an outcome of determined endeavour from a group of educationists in the field. The primary objective was to involve a broad spectrum of professionals from diverse cultural background involved in the field for developing new researches. The book not only targets students but also scholars pursuing higher research for further enhancement of the theoretical and practical applications of the subject.

The medical condition characterized by the inflammation of the pancreas is known as pancreatitis. There are two principal categories of pancreatitis - acute and chronic pancreatitis. Symptoms of pancreatitis are abdominal pain, nausea and vomiting. In acute pancreatitis, the pancreas undergoes sudden inflammation. It is caused by a gallstone blocking the common bile duct, systemic diseases, trauma, heavy alcohol use and mumps. It can be recurrent or it may progress into chronic pancreatitis. It can be treated through intravenous nutritional support, pain control and intravenous fluid rehydration. Chronic pancreatitis is a long-term inflammation of the pancreas in which the structure and function of the pancreas is irreversibly changed. It is generally caused by idiopathic pancreatitis, tumors, intraductal obstruction, calcific stones, ischemia, etc. Chronic pancreatitis can be treated through therapeutic endoscopy and surgery. This book brings forth some of the most innovative concepts and elucidates the unexplored aspects of acute and chronic pancreatitis. It strives to provide a fair idea about these medical conditions to help develop a better understanding of the latest diagnostic and therapeutic advances in this field. Coherent flow of topics, student-friendly language and extensive use of examples make this book an invaluable source of knowledge.

It was an honour to edit such a profound book and also a challenging task to compile and examine all the relevant data for accuracy and originality. I wish to acknowledge the efforts of the contributors for submitting such brilliant and diverse chapters in the field and for endlessly working for the completion of the book. Last, but not the least; I thank my family for being a constant source of support in all my research endeavours.

**Editor**

# Do Elderly Patients with Acute Pancreatitis Need a Special Treatment Strategy?

Marcel Cerqueira César Machado , Fabiano Pinheiro da Silva and Ana Maria Mendonça Coelho

## 1. Introduction

Acute pancreatitis(AP) in spite of thousands of experimental and clinical studies remains a disease with significant impact in many countries being one of the most common gastrointestinal diseases requiring hospital admission in the United States[1]. Although the overall mortality in AP patients is about 5% in severe AP is increasing up to 25 [2] mainly in elderly people [3]

The aging process is believed to influence the course and outcome of AP. Indeed, AP in elderly patients is associated with high morbidity and mortality [4]. Although Frey at al [5] have related the presence of comorbidities in elderly patients to their increased mortality, others consider advanced age to be an independent prognostic factor in AP [6].

The mechanisms underlying the increased severity of AP in elderly patients are not completely understood. Possibilities include the presence of a proinflammatory status in older people [7] or organ-specific alterations that may contribute to increased systemic inflammation in AP. The lungs are particularly affected in AP, releasing a second wave of inflammatory mediators that may increase systemic inflammation in older patients [8].

## 2. Aging and systemic inflammation

Cytokine production in elderly patients with sepsis is higher than in young people [9]. We have observed that old people sometimes have a smooth initial postoperative course, followed by an increased inflammatory response that may have catastrophic outcomes. Delayed explosive levels of interleukin (IL)-6 have been observed in elderly patients after surgery [10].

A recent report also demonstrated that the production of tumor necrosis factor (TNF)-$\alpha$, IL-1$\beta$ or IL-6 in the lung cells of older subjects after exposure to lipopolysaccharide occurs relatively late, but remain sustained when compared to lung cells from young subjects [11]. Monocyte activation and hypercytokinemia have also been observed in elderly patients after surgical procedures [12] and *in vitro* studies have demonstrated that mitogen-stimulated peripheral mononuclear cells from the elderly produce higher levels of TNF-$\alpha$, IL-6, and IL-1 when compared to young subjects [13]. All these findings support the concept that aging affects the immune system and promotes inflammation that is also associated with metabolic dysfunctions [14].

# 3. Molecular mechanisms of the proinflammatory status related to aging

The molecular mechanisms involved in the proinflammatory condition of aged people are still poorly understood, but inflammatory genes dysregulation may be involved in the process.

The potential role of the poly(ADPribose) polymerase-1 gene in inflammation and in the aging process has been reported [15].

Higher splenic expression of toll-like receptor-4 and CD14 were also demonstrated in older animals with sepsis when compared with young animals [16]. In this report, an increased 2A adrenergic receptor and phosphodiesterase in older animals was also found. It was concluded that in old animals the proinflammatory status is related to the innate immune response and to the upregulation of the adrenergic autonomic nervous system that also may contribute to the increased proinflammatory cytokine production [16].

Besides the proinflammatory condition in aging animals with acute pancreatitis, an increase in plasma concentration of plasminogen activator inhibitor-1, a primary inhibitor of the fibrinolytic system, has been shown in experimental pancreatitis resulting in increased extra pancreatic thrombosis [17].

We are currently evaluating the differential gene expression in older patients with sepsis compared to young patients. Recently, the important role of adipose triglyceride lipase (ATGL) activity in the increased inflammatory status related to the aging process has been reported [18]. Reduction of ATGL in aging animals is related to the increased inflammatory status in these animals [18]. However, the mechanism by which ATGL modulates the production of inflammatory mediators is still unknown.

# 4. Acute pancreatitis in the elderly population

The mortality rate in elderly patients is significantly higher than in younger patients(21.3 % vs 5.9%) [6].Recent clinical study also reported that elderly patients with severe acute pancreatitis have significant higher mortality rates than younger patients (17.0% vs 5.3%) [20].We have observed similar findings in our own experience. Although no differences in local complications in acute pancreatitis between young and elderly people have been observed, the increased mortality that occurs with aging is related to increased rates of organ failure [19–21].

The mechanisms underlying this increased distant organ failure and mortality associated with aging is not completely understood. However, possible explanations include the increased inflammatory response, worsened organ response to injury, or increased bacterial translocation with increased systemic injury.

Recently, it was reported that there is a loss of pancreatitis-associated proteins with aging. These are a group of innate pancreatic proteins with a protective effect, that are induced in the process of AP and that are related to the increased severity of acute pancreatitis in the aging population [22].

However in elderly patients with AP, there is a similar occurrence of local complications associated with a significant increase in multiple organ failure when compared to young patients [20].

It is well established that older patients are more susceptible to infections in surgical procedures, probably related to an exaggerated inflammatory response after surgery that can be attributed to the proinflammatory status of older people [23].

It is conceivable that in surgical procedures and in acute pancreatitis, bacterial translocations due to increased intestinal damage may be the underlying process that increases distant organ failure. Intestinal fatty acid binding protein (IFABP) is a 15-kd protein located at the tips of intestinal mucosal villi usually undetected in plasma circulation. Recently it has been shown that IFABP is a specific marker of gut epithelial dysfunction in clinical cases of acute pancreatitis and a useful marker of the severity of the disease [24]. In our laboratory we also demonstrated in an experimental model of acute pancreatitis that plasma levels of IFABP are correlated with bacterial translocation (unpublished data).

In fact we have demonstrated increased intestinal damage, evaluated by plasma levels of ileal fatty acid binding protein in an experimental model of acute pancreatitis in aging animals when compared to young animals. This increased intestinal damage was followed by increased bacterial translocation and pancreatic infection in old animals (unpublished data; Figs 1, 2 and 3).

This increased bacterial translocation in older animals when compared to young ones was associated with an increased systemic damage characterized by increased pulmonary myeloperoxidase, and increased serum levels of liver enzymes, creatinine and glucose.

We also demonstrated that expression of intestinal proinflammatory cytokines genes is increased in aging animals with acute experimental pancreatitis. This increased intestinal inflammatory process may be related to the intestinal damage observed in the elderly animals.

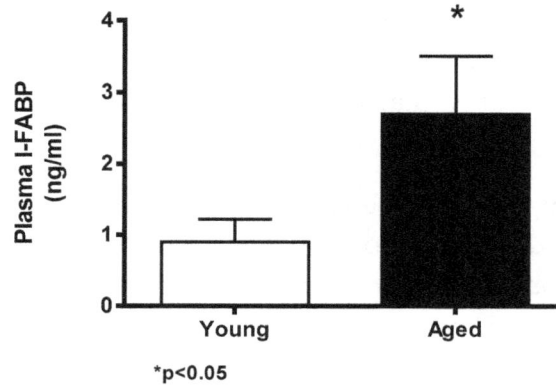

**Figure 1.** Plasma ileal fat acid binding protein levels.

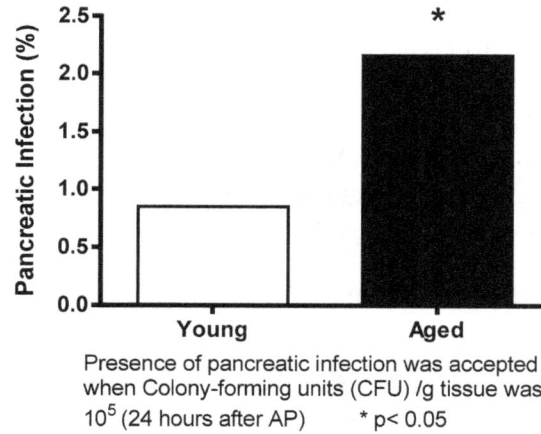

**Figure 2.** Pancreatic infection.

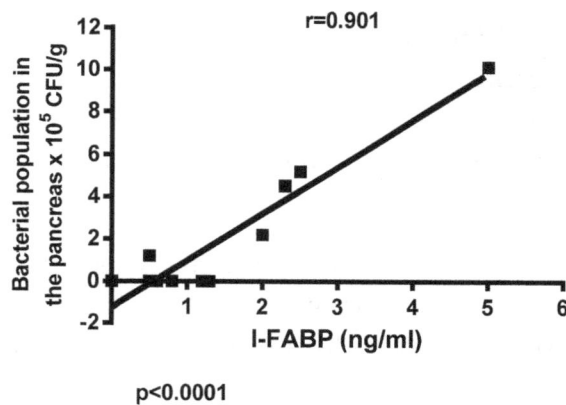

**Figure 3.** Correlation between plasma fat acid binding protein levels and bacterial translocation.

This concept is supported by the observation that administration of anti-platelet-activating factor reduces the bacterial translocation in a model of acute pancreatitis [25]. It is therefore possible that the reduction in the increased intestinal inflammatory process may decrease bacterial translocation and the systemic damage observed in aged patients.

Finally, we have been studying the role of antimicrobial peptides in aging. Surprisingly, we found that the production of alpha-defensin-5 is increased in the ileum of old rats when compared to young rats in an experimental model of acute pancreatitis (manuscript in preparation). This finding goes against the prevalent hypothesis that the elderly are immuno-suppressed compared to the young. Antimicrobial peptides are ancient weapons of innate immunity. Despite their killing properties, a wide variety of cellular responses is affected by these molecules. Antimicrobial peptides are largely distributed in nature, being found in protozoa, prokaryotes, invertebrates, vertebrates and plants. Further research is necessary to understand the molecular pathways triggered by antimicrobial peptides during AP– whether they are produced to attack bacteria that invade the bloodstream, as a result of bacterial translocation, or are merely coordinating the innate immune response during sterile systemic inflammation.

## 5. Special treatment strategy

Our current knowledge indicates that we need new strategies to reduce the exaggerated inflammatory response in elderly patients with AP.

Previous reports from our group have shown that in experimental AP, peritoneal lavage [26], administration of hypertonic saline solution [27], use of platelet-activating factor antagonists [25], and administration of pentoxifylline [28] reduce the inflammatory response in acute pancreatitis in young animals. We are now investigating if these strategies are also effective in old animals.

Since bacterial translocation is increased in acute pancreatitis in aging animals with increased distant organ damage it is conceivable that different therapeutic strategies should be used in aged patients with acute pancreatitis. More liberal utilization of hemofiltration or even peritoneal lavage [26,29] may decrease the plasma level of cytokines and therefore minimize the systemic damage induced by these substances.

We agree with recent guidelines [30] that do not recommend the use of prophylactic antibiotics in patients with severe acute pancreatitis. However, in elderly patients antibiotics may not be prophylactic.

Recent experimental studies including ours (Fig 1) have demonstrated an increased bacterial infiltration in pancreatic tissues in acute pancreatitis in old animals [22].

Early antibiotic treatment in these patients may reduce the effect of increased bacterial translocation and the systemic inflammatory response may therefore decrease the age-related mortality in acute pancreatitis.

## Author details

Marcel Cerqueira César Machado , Fabiano Pinheiro da Silva and
Ana Maria Mendonça Coelho

Emergency Medicine Department, University of São Paulo, Brazil

## References

[1] Russo MW, Wei JT, Thiny MT, Gangarosa LM, Brown A, Ringel Y et al. Digestive and liver diseases statistics Gastroenterology.2004;126(5):1448-53

[2] Tonsi AF, Bacchion M, Crippa S, Malleo G, Bassi C..Acute pancreatitis at the beginning of the 21st century: the state of the art. World J Gastroenterol. 2009;15(24): 2945-59.

[3] Akshintala VS1, Hutfless SM, Yadav D, Khashab MA, Lennon AM, Makary MA, Hirose K, Andersen DK, Kalloo AN, Singh VK A population-based study of severity in patients with acute on chronic pancreatitis Pancreas. 2013; 42(8):1245-50.

[4] Fagenholz PJ, Castillo CF, Harris NS, Pelletier AJ, Camargo CA Jr. Increasing United States hospital admissions for acute pancreatitis, 1988-2003. Ann Epidemiol. 2007;17:491–7.

[5] Frey C, Zhou H, Harvey D, White RH. Co-morbidity is a strong predictor of early death and multi-organ system failure among patients with acute pancreatitis. J Gastrointest Surg. 2007;11:733–42.

[6] Fan ST, Choi TK, Lai CS, Wong J. Influence of age on the mortality from acute pancreatitis. Br J Surg. 1988;75:463–6.

[7] Miki C, Kusunoki M, Inoue Y, Uchida K, Mohri Y, Buckels JA, et al. Remodeling of the immunoinflammatory network system in elderly cancer patients: implications of inflamm-aging and tumor-specific hyperinflammation. Surg Today. 2008;38:873–8.

[8] Starr M E, Ueda J, Yamamoto S, Evers, B M, Saito H. The effects of aging on pulmonary oxidative damage, protein nitration, and extracellular superoxide dismutase down-regulation during systemic inflammation. Free Radic Biol Med. 2011;50:371–80.

[9] Turnbull I R, Clark A,Stromberg PE, Dixon DJ, Woolsey CA, Davis CG, et al. Effects of aging on the immunopathologic response to sepsis. Crit Care Med. 2009;37:1018–23.

[10] Kudoh A, Katagai H, Takazawa T. Matsuki A. Plasma proinflammatory cytokine response to surgical stress in elderly patients. Cytokine. 2001; 15:270–3.

[11] Ren X, Du H, Li Y, Yao X, Huang J, Li Z, et al. Age-related activation of MKK/p38/NF-κB signaling pathway in lung: From mouse to human. Exp Gerontol. 2014; 57C:29–40.

[12] Ono S, Aosasa S, Tsujimoto H, Ueno C, Mochizuki H. Increased monocyte activation in elderly patients after surgical stress. Eur Surg Res. 2001;33:33–8.

[13] Fagiolo U, Cossarizza A, Scala E, Fanales-Belasio E, Ortolani C, Cozzi E, et al. Increased cytokine production in mononuclear cells of healthy elderly people. Eur J Immunol. 1993;23:2375–8.

[14] Mathis D, Shoelson SE. Immunometabolism: an emerging frontier. Nat Rev Immunol. 2011; 11:81–3.

[15] Walston J. D, Matteini M, Nievergelt C, Lange LA, Fallin DM, Barzilai N, et al. Inflammation and stress-related candidate genes, plasma interleukin-6 levels, and longevity in older adults. Exp Gerontol. 2009;44:350–5.

[16] Leong J, Zhou M, Jacob A, Wang P. Aging-related hyperinflammation in endotoxemia is mediated by the α2Aadrenoceptor and CD14/TLR4 pathways. Life Sci. 2010; 86:740–6.

[17] Okamura D, Starr ME, Lee EY, Stromberg AJ, Evers BM, Saito H. Age-dependent vulnerability to experimental acute pancreatitis is associated with increased systemic inflammation and thrombosis. Aging Cell. 2012;11:760-9.

[18] Lettieri Barbato D, Tatulli G, Aquilano K, Ciriolo MR. Inhibition of age-related cytokines production by ATGL: a mechanism linked to the anti-inflammatory effect of resveratrol. Mediators Inflamm. 2014;2014:917698.

[19] Lankisch PG, Burchard-Reckert S, Petersen M, Lehnick D, Schirren CA, Stöckmann F, et al. Etiology and age have only a limited influence on the course of acute pancreatitis. Pancreas. 1996;13:344–9.

[20] Xin MJ, Chen H, Luo B, Sun JB. Severe acute pancreatitis in the elderly: etiology and clinical characteristics. World J Gastroenterol. 2008;14:2517–21.

[21] Gardner TB. Vege SS, Chari ST, Pearson RK, Clain JE, Topazian MD, et al. The effect of age on hospital outcomes in severe acute pancreatitis. Pancreatology. 2008;8:265–70.

[22] Fu S, Stanek A, Mueller CM, Brown NA, Huan C, Bluth MH, et al. Acute pancreatitis in aging animals: loss of pancreatitis-associated protein protection? World J Gastroenterol. 2012;18:3379–88.

[23] Simmonds PD, Best L, George S et al. Surgery for colorectal cancer in elderly patients: a systematic review. Colorectal Cancer Collaborative Group. Lancet 2000;356:968–74.

[24] Pan L, Wang X, Li W, Li N, Li J. The intestinal fatty acid binding protein diagnosing gut dysfunction in acute pancreatitis: a pilot study. Pancreas. 2010;3:633–8.

[25] de Souza LJ, Sampietre SN, Assis RS, Knowles CH, Leite KR, Jancar S, et al. Effect of platelet-activating factor antagonists (BN-52021, WEB-2170, and BB-882) on bacterial translocation in acute pancreatitis. J Gastrointest Surg. 2001;5:364–70.

[26] Souza LJ, Coelho AM, Sampietre SN, Martins JO, Cunha JE, Machado MC. Anti-inflammatory effects of peritoneal lavage in acute pancreatitis. Pancreas. 2010;39:1180–4.

[27] Machado MC, Coelho AM, Pontieri V, Sampietre SN, Molan NA, Soriano F, et al. Local and systemic effects of hypertonic solution (NaCl 7.5%) in experimental acute pancreatitis. Pancreas. 2006;32:80–6.

[28] Matheus AS, Coelho A, Sampietre S, Jukemura J, Patzina RA, Cunha JE, et al. Do the effects of pentoxifylline on the inflammatory process and pancreatic infection justify its use in acute pancreatitis? Pancreatology. 2009; 9:687–93.

[29] Matsumoto K, Miyake Y, Nakatsu M, Toyokawa T, Ando M, Hirohata M, et al. Usefulness of early-phase peritoneal lavage for treating severe acute pancreatitis. Intern Med. 2014;53:1–6.

[30] Tenner S, Baillie J, DeWitt J, Vege S; American College of Gastroenterology. American College of Gastroenterology guideline: management of acute pancreatitis. Am J Gastroenterol. 2013;108:1400–15; 1416

# 2

# Stem Cell Therapies on Pancreatitis

Mukaddes Esrefoglu

## 1. Introduction

Pancreatitis is an inflammatory acute or chronic disease of the pancreas. Although etiology of acute and chronic pancreatitis remains poorly defined, so far a variety of environmental, hereditary and immunological factors and bile duct obstructions have been described. Treatment of patients suffering from severe acute pancreatitis (AP) remains challenging, and despite improved strategies, mortality is still between 30 and 50 % [1]. The prognosis of patients with acute pancreatitis is largely determined by the presence of organ failure and infected pancreatic necrosis with associated mortality rates of 15%-30% [2].

AP is an inflammatory disease of the pancreas characterized by edema, acinar cell necrosis, hemorrhage and severe inflammation of the pancreas [3,4] and some of the other organs including liver [3,5]. Some inflammatory factors including interleukin (IL)-1, IL-6, IL-8, C-reactive protein, tumor necrosis factor (TNF), nitric oxide (NO) and endothelin are suggested to be involved in the genesis and progression of AP as well as in the progression from slight AP to severe AP [6]. By electron microscopic observation, dilatation of irregularly arranged cisternae of rough endoplasmic reticulum and of some of the cisternae of Golgi apparatus are prominent. The mitochondria with increased translucence of the matrix, partial destruction or loss of the cristae are edematous. Sometimes myelin figures are observed within the mitochondrial matrix. Numerous, large autophagosomes containing amorphous, membranous or granular masses and zymogen granules are present within the cytoplasm (Figure 1,2). Nuclear chromatin clumping and margination indicating apoptosis are present [4] (Figure 2).

Chronic pancreatitis (CP) characterized by fibrosis, and pain is a long-standing inflammation of the pancreas that alters its normal structure and functions. Regions of the pancreas are transformed from glandular tissue to a mass of almost complete fibrosis. The secretory parenchyma is destroyed by processes such as necrosis/ apoptosis, inflammation or duct obstruction. Pancreatic stallate cells present in the periacinar space and

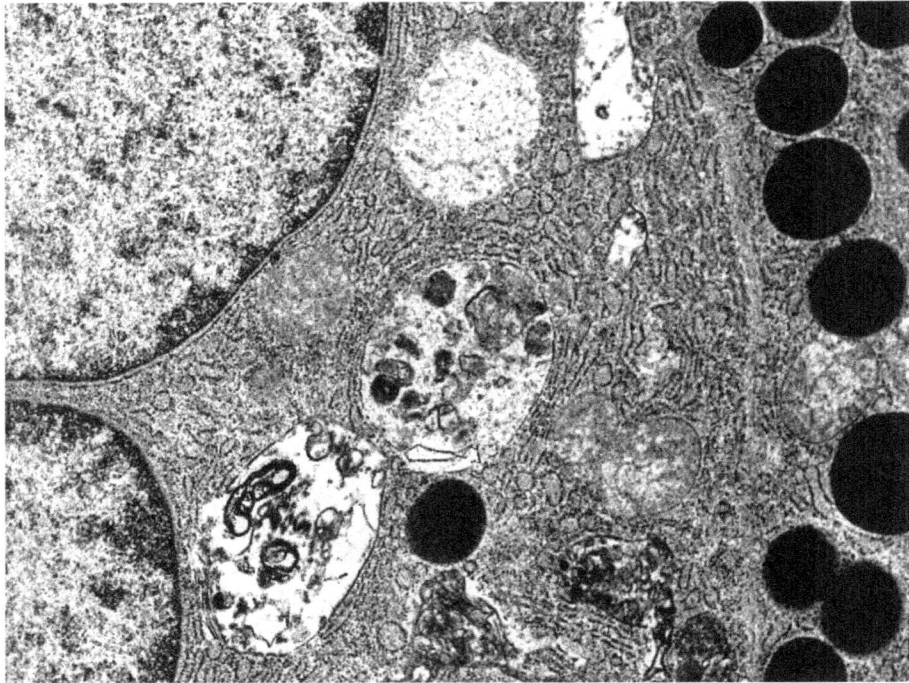

**Figure 1.** Mitochondral edema and degeneration, and accumulation lysosomes containing identifiable cytoplasmic elements, amorphous, membranous or granular masses are observed in the cytoplasm of an acinar cell in cerulein-induced experimental acute pancreatitis. X 10.000

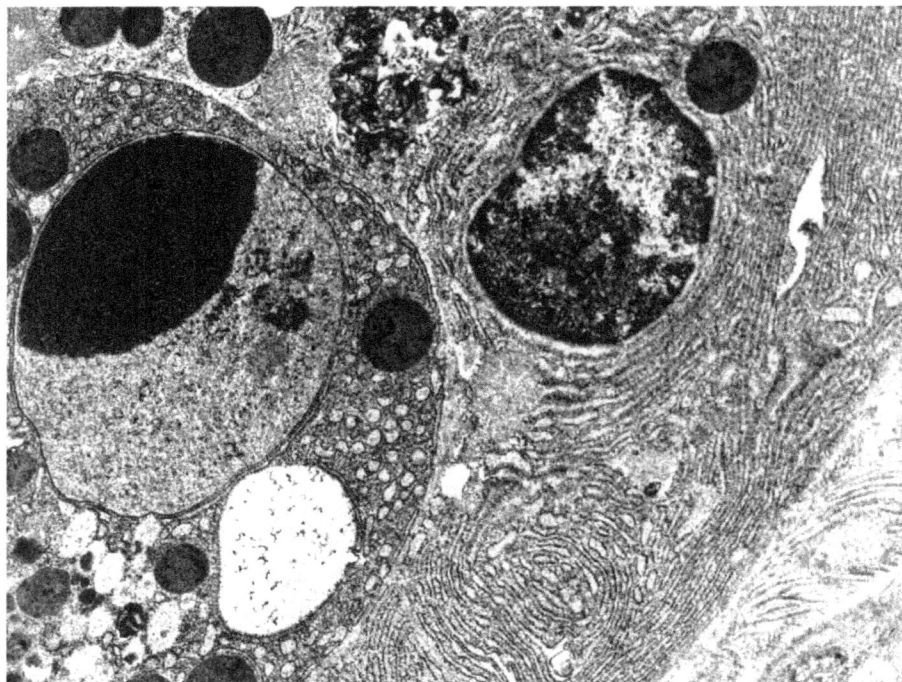

**Figure 2.** Nuclear chromatin clumping and margination indicating apoptosis, and organelle degeneration as well as lysosome accumulation are observed in the cytoplasm of acinar cells in cerulean-induced experimental acute pancreatitis. Note that apoptotic cell is engulfed by a neighboring acinar cell. X 8.000

have long cytoplasmic processes that encircle the base of the acinus are strongly involved not only in the pathogenesis of CP but also in pancreatic cancer. They are located in the periacinar, perivascular and periductal regions of the pancreas [7, 8].

Over the past decades, our understanding of the pathogenesis of pancreatitis has significantly improved. Animal models including caerulein, taurocholate, L-arginine studies are important in order to understand the pathogenesis of pancreatitis, however none of them are fully satisfactory. It is now widely accepted that AP is triggered by premature activation of proenzymes within pancreatic acinar cells, thereby leading to autodigestion of the pancreas. Esrefoglu *et al* [3,4,9] emphasized the role of oxidative stress on the pathogenesis of careulein-induced pancreatitis. They showed potent therapeutic effects of some antioxidant agents including melatonin, ascorbic acid and N-acetyl cysteine on AP in rats. In fact, in recent years, valuable data on the efficiency of antioxidants against oxidative damage have been obtained from experimental studies with rodents. With the inspiration of the results of these experiments, efficiency of some of these antioxidants has been tried on the patients with AP and found beneficial. However, at present there is insufficient clinical data to support the benefits of antioxidants, alone or in combination with conventional therapy, in the management of AP in humans [10]. The effects of stem cells transplantation on tissue oxidative stress level have been studied lately. In fact, stem cell transplantation helps to maintain tissue regeneration by replacing the degenerated cells as well as by regulating oxidative stress production. Stem cells have been shown to be able to scavenge reactive oxygene and nitrogen species, and to limit oxidative stress-induced tissue damage [11]. Recently, mesenchymal stem cells have been found beneficial in a traumatic brain injury in vitro model and myocardial ischemia/reperfusion model decreasing oxidative stress levels by their paracrine effects [12,13]. Mesenchymal stem cells have been shown to increase tissue SOD, activity but decrease tissue MDA level on AP in rats [14].

Development of evidence based therapies for pancreatitis has lagged behind advances in understanding of the pathophysiology of the disease. Herein, no pharmacologic therapy has been shown to affect disease progression. Several potential reasons for the lack of progress in development of treatments for pancreatitis includes a lack of sustained effort to transition basic science findings into clinical trials and a lack of appropriate preclinical models for testing potential therapeutic agents. In recent years, the efficacy of stem cell transplantation applications is widely investigated in the course of several diseases in experimental animals and also in humans. In pancreatitis, stem cells might recover the damaged pancreatic tissue by their excessive proliferating and differentiating capabilities and regulatory functions on oxidative stress levels under the regulatory control of the microenviroment. Unfortunately, the results obtained from rodents studies might not be similiar to those obtained from human studies. Herein I tried to review the results of stem cell transplantation therapies obtained from rodent and human studies on AP and CP. However, I realize that although researchers agree about the therapeutic potency of transplanted progenitor and stem cells on acute and chronic pancreatitis, any clinical trial has been performed so far.

## 2. Catagorization of stem cells

Stem cells are different from the other cell types since they are unspecialized cells that are capable of changing themselves into various types of specialized cells. The main features of stem cells are the capability to divide, proliferate, and self-renewal; to differentiate to one or several cell types and to survive in an undifferentiated stage for a while. In fact, they may remain in such an undifferentiated state for long time periods. When the morphological as well as functional differentiation begins, these cells differentiate into multiple specialized cell lineages. One stem cell may divide into two identical stem cells by symmetrical division or it may divide into one stem cell and one progenitor cell by asymmetrical division. One progenitor cell also may divide into identical progenitor cells by symmetrical division. The committed progenitor cells exhibit a capacity to give rise to terminally differentiated cells under favorable influences which are not fully known yet.

Stem cells are classified depending on the potential for differentiation into specialized cell types. The most capable stem cells which are totipotent cells of the zygote within first 4 days of the intrauterine life are able to form a full organism in appropriate microenvironment. However, pluripotent cells, known as 'embryonic stem cells'(ESCs), principally derived from the inner cell mass of the embryo can form virtually any cell type derived from any of three embryonic germ layers; ectoderm, mesoderm or endoderm. Thus, an embryonic stem cell can form enterocyte (endodermal in origin), cardiomyocyte (mesodermal in origin), and keratinocyte (ectodermal in origin). Surplus embryos obtained from in-vitro fertilization laboratories are the main sources of the ESCs. However, some disadvantages including high immune reaction risk and some ethical concerns limit their applications. The third type of stem cells is multipotent stem cells which are also known as 'adult stem cells'. These cells with a relatively limited differentiation potential can form several cell types of the tissue. These cells reside together with the specialized cell types of the adult tissues and they are thought to be responsible for the tissue maintenance and repair. The exact mechanisms that affect them to stay in undifferentiated stage for a period of time and force them to differentiate into a specialized cell type are not fully known yet. The two major populations of adult stem cells are bone marrow mesenchymal and hematopoietic stem cells (HSCs). Hematopoietic stem cells have a predetermined fate to form all types of the mature blood cells. Mesenchymal stem cells can differentiate into multiple cell lineages, including tendon cells, muscle cells, osteocytes, fat cells etc. The term 'multipotent stromal cell' implies the multipotent stem cells of both bone morrow and of none-morrow tissues such as umbilical cord blood, adipose tissue, muscle tissue, dental pulp etc. Important data obtained from mainly cell culture studies have provided clues about the ability of adult stem cells to differentiate into various cell types from different germ layers. For instance; the HSCs which are derived from mesoderm can transform into hepatocytes which are derived from endoderm or brain stem cells which are derived from ectoderm can form skeletal muscle fibers which are derived from mesoderm. Multipotent cells are genetically identical to their hosts, thus they don't cause any immune reaction. However, these cells are restricted in their ability to form different cell types in comparison with ESCs. Moreover, they have some disadvantages including slow rate of cell division and difficulties to isolate in sufficient numbers for application because of their sparsity within the tissues. The last type of stem cells is unipotent stem cells that have a very limited capacity for differentiation and can give rise to only one type of cell under normal conditions. For instance; unipotent stem cells of colony forming unit of erythrocytes (CFU-E) can only give rise to mature erythrocytes of blood.

In recent years stem cells are widely studied for their promising potential therapeutic use in both rodents and humans. However, some of the human studies failed to be successful. Researchers agree that as well as isolation of adequate numbers of healthy stem cells, selection of most convenient transporting route, regulation of stem cell differentiation into a special cell type, and obtainment of the usual functions of the differentiated cells are very important regarding the benefit of stem cell applications. The most important risk of the transplanted stem cells is generation of tumors if cell division continues in an uncontrolled manner. Unfortunately, the stem cell transplantation therapy may be considered as a sort of two-edged sword.

## 2.1. Stem cells in exocrine pancreas

Identification of stem and/or progenitor cells in the adult pancreas has been an area of intense investigation in the past decades, but the results remain controversial [15]. Determined stem cells for pancreatic cell therapies have not been considered an option based on evidence that there are no or only rare pancreatic stem cells in postnatal tissues [16]. Rare stem cell populations have been identified within the pancreas and that express pluripotency genes (OCT4, SOX2) [17-19]. The few studies in which OCT4 and SOX21 multipotent stem cells have been identified in adult pancreas have indicated also their rarity [19]. Smukler *et al* [17] described pancreas-derived multipotent cells, which are rare (1/5000 pancreas cells) and form spheres in vitro. They can differentiate into multiple lineages, including several endocrine cell types and neurons. Gong *et al* [20], using stem cell marker nestin, reported experimental clues supporting the lack of primary stem cells in adult pancreas tissue. They suggested that the so-called pancreatic stem cells may actually originate from bone marrow stem cells. When pancreatic tissue is injured, bone marrow stem cells may participate in the repair.

The location of stem cells in each organ has been widely investigating. Wang *et al* [21] provide evidence that the biliary tree is a reservoir of stem cells for the pancreas. They present evidence to suggest the biliary tree and pancreatic networks are connected anatomically and functionally to comprise maturational lineages relevant to pancreatic organogenesis. They showed that determined stem cell populations, present throughout life, are precursors for pancreatic committed progenitors in the pancreatic duct glands (a novel ductal compartment that is gathered in gland-like outpouches), and are present in the ramifying, continuous network of ducts and associated glands of the biliary tree.

The postnatal pancreas has long been thought to contain only committed progenitors, found in pancreatic ducts [22,23] and, in the pancreatic duct glands [24]. These precursors are reported to be limited in their proliferative and self-renewal potential. A recent study of Stanger *et al* [25] suggested that the final size of the pancreas is also determined by the number of embryonic progenitor cells, each with an autonomous restriction on the amount of tissue it was capable of generating. Centroacinar cells and terminal duct cells lie at the junction between peripheral acinar cells and the adjacent ductal epithelium. Both of these cell types are supposed to be candidate pancreatic progenitors. Specifically, these cells express high levels of Ptf1a, Sox9, Sca-1, SDF-1, c-Met, and Nestin [26]. Magliano et al [27] have reported that although Sox9 is expressed throughout the pancreas epithelium, pancreatic ductal cells in the adult pancreas, excluding acinar and centroacinar cells, it is reactivated in acinar cells that undergo de-differentiation after induction of pancreatitis with cerulein. The findings suggest that at least a subset of cells residing in a centroacinar/terminal ductal location is capable of progenitor function. The finding that this population undergoes dramatic expansion during an epithelial injury suggests that these cells are involved in pancreatic epithelial regeneration. Together with their location at the junction between peripheral secretory cells and more central ductal epithelium, these features suggest similarity between centroacinar/terminal ductal cells and hepatic oval cells which are progenitor cell type capable of multilineage differentiation in the event of any injury [28].

In the primary transition pancreas, primary stem cell type is multipotent stem cells, capable of contributing to all epithelial cell lineages of the pancreas parenchyma. These cells coexpress important transcription factors including Pdx1, Ptf1a, Nkx6.1, Hnf1$\beta$, and Sox9 [29-31]. During the secondary transition period, pancreatic epithelium forms finger-like projections into the surrounding mesenchyme generating a tree-like epithelial structure with recognizable 'tip' and 'trunk' segments [32,33]. The bipotential progenitor cell population within the trunk segment seems to be progenitors of both endocrine and duct lineages [31,34,35]. Solar et al [34] provided clues on the potency of these cells to contribute to the endocrine and ductal lineages by genetic lineage tracing of Hnf1$\beta$ positivity. Following their specification, endocrine precursor cells leave the trunk compartment to form mature islets [36-38] whereas the remaining cells that remain within the trunk contribute to the pancreatic duct [39]. Recently we investigated prenatal and postnatal development of the rat pancreas as well as the other organs of the digestive system (Unpublished data). At prenatal 10th day pancreas premordium was composed of a few tubes lined with a simple epithelium and surrounding mesenchymal tissue rich in vessels. Many mitotic figures were observed within the epithelium (Figure 3A). At prenatal 14th day, branching of the tubes was prominent. The tips of the branhcing trunk were formed as primitive acini (Figure 3B). The epithelium was still rich in mitosis. At prenatal 17th day, further branches gave rise to increased number of acini (Figure 3C). Endocrine cell islets were observed at prenatal 17th day for the first time. However, at postnatal 15th day, it was so clear that the same trunk gave rise to both exocrine and endocrine compartments of the pancreas (Figure 3D).

Pancreatic regeneration involves two pathways; proliferation and differentiation of pancreatic progenitor cells, and replication of preexisting differentiated acinar, islet, and ductal epithelial cells [40]. Expression of transcription factors and cell differentiation are under the control of some regulating signalling factors either secreted from neighbouring tissues or pancreatic mesenchymal cells (e.g. fibroblast growth factors) [41,42] or are expressed on the surface of differentiating pancreatic cells (e.g. Notch) [43]. Mammalian pancreas displays a significant capacity for regeneration following injury. A variety of cell types have been proposed as possible pancreatic progenitors, including cells associated with ductal epithelium [19],

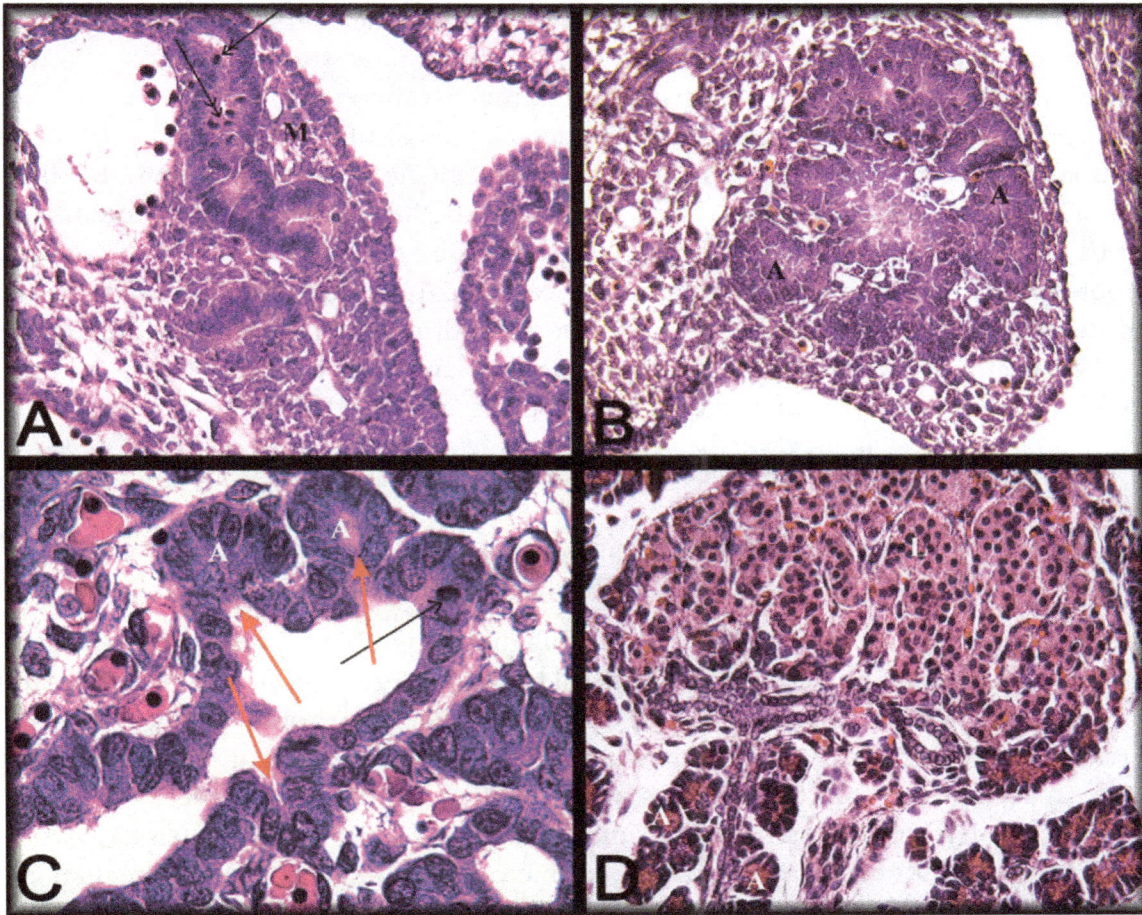

**Figure 3.** The histological features of the pancreas during development. A. Prenatal 10th day. Pancreas premordium is composed of a few tubes lined with a simple epithelium and surrounding mesenchymal tissue rich in vessels. Many mitotic figures are observed within the epithelium. B. Prenatal 14th day. Branching of the tubes is prominent. The tips of the branhcing trunk form primitive acini. C. Prenatal 17th day. Increased number of acini was formed by further branches (red arrows). Many figures of mitosis are present within the epithelium (black arrows). D. Postnatal 15th day. The same trunk gives rise to both exocrine and endocrine compartments of the pancreas.

mesenchymal-like nestin expressing cells [44] and preexisting acinar cells [45]. Centroacinar cells and terminal duct cells are frequently supposed to be candidate pancreatic progenitors. These cells are markedly enriched for transcripts encoding Sca1, Sdf1, c-Met, Nestin, and Sox9 markers which were previously associated with progenitor populations in embryonic pancreas. Fluorescent Activated Cell-Sorted centroacinar/terminal duct cells are shown to be able to form self-renewing "pancreatospheres" in suspension culture. The progenitor cells of the spheres have capacity for spontaneous endocrine and exocrine differentiation; additionally they have ability to glucose-responsive insulin secretion. Moreover, when injected into cultured embryonic dorsal pancreatic buds, these adult cells display capacity to contribute to the embryonic endocrine and exocrine lineages. Finally, the number of these cells is shown to be significantly increased in the setting of chronic epithelial injury [26].

Taguchi *et al* [40] observed newly formed acinar cells on day 7 following the induction of acute necrotizing pancreatitis in rats. They reported that proliferation started in the main and large ducts at 24 h; marked mitotic activity was evident in small ductal epithelial cells and tubular complexes on day 3, and in acinar cells on day 7. The lobular structure returned to normal appearance on day 28. These results suggest that regeneration after necrotizing pancreatitis involves proliferation and differentiation of pancreatic progenitor cells. Ductal epithelial cells with duodenum homeobox protein 1 (PDX-1)-positive nuclei may contribute to the differentiation of the stem cells in the main duct of pancreas.PDX-1-positive cells in the main duct might be quiescent pancreatic stem cells. PDX-1 might be a marker of cells that regain their multipotency to differentiate into any pancreatic cell types [46], and is thought to be an intrinsic signal determining the region of gut endoderm that ultimately becomes the pancreas [47]. PDX-1 has an important role in the determination of pancreatic progenitors [48] and neurogenin-3 is required for determination of endocrine precursor [49].

# 3. Stem cell transplantation therapies

The use of stem cells for the treatment of various diseases in both humans and animals has been the focus of considerable interest. Stem cell technology gives hope of effective treatment for a variety of diseases through the rapid developing field that combines the efforts of cell researchers and clinicians. However; it seems to be early to carry out a Bench-to-Bedside program applying stem cell therapeutics in the clinical setting yet. Detailed researches are necessary to understand the optimal transplantation routes and doses as well as the mechanisms of stem cell interaction with the injured microenvironment as clues for realizing stem cell behavior.Stem cell therapy offers the possibility of repairing acutely or chronically injured tissue and has the potential to regulate immune function and reduce inflammatory changes.

Recently, I reviewed the role of stem cells in repair of liver injury and experimental and clinical benefit of transferred stem cells on liver failure [50]. I was suprised to recognize of how many fundemantal and clinical trial on stem cell transplantation have been performed on acute and chronic liver failure. In this chapter, I review cell types involved in pancreas regeneration and cell transplantation therapies for both acute and chronic pancreatitis, with an emphasis on regeneration. However, I realise that even fundamental studies are very limited. Adipose-derived, bone marrow-derived and umblical cord-derived mesenchymal stem cells (MSCs) have been subjected to the basic stem cell trials. To my knowledge any clinical trial has been performed so far.

## 3.1. Mesenchymal stem cells

The MSCs, belong to a class of mesodermal adult stem cells population are found in numerous living tissues including bone marrow, adipose tissue, amniotic fluid, liver, lung, skeletal muscle and kidney. It has been reported that among MSCs obtained from bone marrow, adipose tissue, umbilical cord blood and placenta could be expanded extensively in vitro. The studies have confirmed that MSCs could differentiate into a range of cell types. For instance; bone marrow derived MSCs could differentiate into a range of cell types such as adipocytes, osteoblasts, nerve cells, and liver cells under different conditions [51-53]. Additionally, the experimental and clinical studies have shown that the MSCs could reduce the expression of a variety of inflammatory factors [54,55], inhibit immune responses [56,57], and promote the regeneration of various tissues and organs [58,59] including lung, kidney, liver and heart [60-63]. Imunomodulatory functions of MCSs include suppression of T cell and B cell proliferation, and suppression of terminal differentiation of B cells, and immune modulation of other cell of the immune system including NK cells and macrophages [64]. Here are the results obtained from various trials related with stem cell transplantations on acute and chronic pancreatitis.

### 3.1.1. Bone morrow derived MSCs

Bone marrow-derived MSCs harbor a biological basis which can be used as a candidate for severe AP therapy. Cui *et al* [65] found transplanted and mobilized bone marrow stem cells beneficial on mice with severe AP. They mobilized bone marrow stem cells by injection of granulocyte colony stimulating factor. The mortality rate and serum level of amylase were found to be significantly decreased in the mice pretreated with bone marrow-derived MSCs' transplantation or G-CSF injection. Chen *et* al [66] injected $1 \times 10^6$ mL MSC via tail vein at 0th, 0th and 6th, 0th, 6th and 12th hours after AP induction by 5% sodium taurocholate injection to biliopancreatic duct. After treatment with MSCs, the damage was less severe than that in the untreated AP groups. Besides, MSCs therapy could improve renal injury in rats with severe AP, probably by reducing the damage to renal interstitial capillary endothelial barrier, and up-expression of AQP1 in kidney. Tu *et al* [14] reported that MSCs can effectively relieve injury to pancreatic acinar cells and small intestinal epithelium. MSCs were shown to be able to promote the proliferation of enteric epithelium and repair of the mucosa as well as to attenuate systemic inflammation in rats with severe AP. Serum malondialdehyde (MDA) level was reduced while superoxide dismutase (SOD) activity was increased the rats from AP + MSCs group. They concluded that MSCs transplantation could reduce pancreatitis-related oxidative injury by inhibiting lipid peroxidation, by protecting the stability of the membranes, and by improving the scavenging ability of oxygen-derived free radicals. Recently, Sun *et al* [67] intraperitoneally injected the third-generation bone marrow-derived MSC at a dose of 5×10(6) once daily for 3 days. All rats were sacrificed after 72 h. Compared with severe AP group, histomorphological alternations of small intestine were significantly lower in MSC injected group. The relative expression quantity of TNF-$\alpha$ mRNA and IL-1$\beta$ mRNA in small intestine was both significantly higher in severe AP and MSC groups than those in control group. Compared with AP group, the expression quantity of TNF-$\alpha$ mRNA and IL-1$\beta$ mRNA in pancreas was significantly lower in MSC group. The relative expression quantity of TNF-$\alpha$ mRNA and IL-1$\beta$ mRNA in small intestine were both significant higher in severe AP and MSC groups than those in control group. The expressions of TNF-$\alpha$ mRNA and IL-1$\beta$ mRNA in MSC group were lower than those in severe AP group. The beneficial effects of MSCs seem to be primarily mediated via indirect actions but not by their differentiation into target cells. Wang *et al* [68] showed beneficial effects of bone marrow-derived MSCs on AP-associated lung injury in rats. Results showed that serum amylase activity was decreased and pulmonary edema and the expression of TNF-$\alpha$ was significantly diminished in MSC transplanted group.

It has also been reported that autologous bone marrow MSCs can be used for the treatment of CP.

It has been suggested that bone marrow-derived MSCs has a role in pancreatic tissue repair by contribute to the pancreatic stellate cell population. In the absence of preneoplastic lesions, these cells contribute at a very low level to the ductal epithelium of the chronically inflamed pancreas [69]. MSCs are thought to alleviate pancreatic edema and inflammatory infiltration by regenerating pancreatic cells. Jung *et al* [55] proposed that MSCs alleviate AP through specific accumulation in injured pancreatic tissue rather than through cell regeneration. In this study, inflammation was inhibited by promoting apoptosis of CD4+ T cells. Bone marrow-derived MSCs reduced expression of inflammation mediators and cytokines in rats with mild and severe AP. MSCs suppressed the mixed lymphocyte reaction and increased expression of Foxp3(+) (a marker of regulatory T cells) in cultured rat lymph node cells. Rats with mild or severe AP that were given infusions of hcMSCs had reduced numbers of CD3(+) T cells and increased expression of Foxp3(+) in pancreas tissues. MSCs might alleviate pancreatitis by regulating immune function rather than by regeneration of pancreatic tissue.

### 3.1.2. Adipose-derived MSCs

After in vivo administration, human adipose-derived stem cells (hADSCs) migrate into injured tissue, where they inhibit the release of pro-inflammatory cytokines, promote the survival of injured cells, and finally inhibit inflammation [70]. Baek *et al* [71] have shown that the migration of hADSCs into injured/inflamed sites in vivo is mediated by various factors including growth factors and chemokines. hADSCs would be a potential therapeutic strategy for AP, based on its properties that control inflammation, immune response, and tissue repair. Further research should focus on the interaction between hADSCs and pancreatic acinar cells, immune cells, pancreatic stellate cells, and fibroblasts [72]. Although reserachers agree about the potency of adipose-derived MSCs on tissue repair, to my knowledge, any related experimental and clinical study has been reported so far.

### 3.1.3. Umblical cord-derived MSCs

The studies about the umblical-cord derived stem cells (UCMSCs) are also limited. Yang *et al* [73] injected $5 \times 10^4$, $5 \times 10^5$ $5 \times 10^6$ or $1 \times 10^7$ cells/kg of umblical cord stem cell suspension into the tail vein at 0 h, 1 h, 6 h and 12 h after the induction of severe AP by sodium taurocholate in rats. Mortality in rats receiving $5 \times 10^6$ cells/kg of UCMSCs at 0 h was 10% compared with 58% in the severe AP group. Ascites, serum amylase and wet-dry pancreatic weight significantly decreased. Pathologic injuries of pancreatic and pulmonary tissues were markedly alleviated. Administration of umblical cord-derived MSCs at the doses of $5 \times 10^5$, $5 \times 10^6$ and $1 \times 10^7$ cells/kg at 1 h or $5 \times 10^6$ cells/kg at 6 h significantly reduced the severity of AP. The data of the study of Yang *et al* [73] showed that UCMSCs cannot differentiate into other cells in 24 hours. The authors conclude that the prevention of damage has nothing to do with a differentiation of cells and that it seems to be a paracrine effect that can modulate immune function.

UCMSCs may also be a promising therapeutic intervention for human CP in the future. In the study of Zhou *et al* [74] a rat model of CP induced by dibutyltin dichloride (DB) was used. UCMSCs were administered intravenously on day 5 after the administration of DB. UCMSCs were detected in inflamed pancreatic tissues on days 14 and 28. Umbilical cord mesenchymal stem cell treatment reduced the histological scores of pancreas samples and improved the fibrosis. The expression of cytokines in the DB group was significantly higher than that of DB + UCMSC group. Pancreatic stellate cell activation was also inhibited by UCMSC treatment.

Stem cell types, dosages, application routes, main benefits and adverse reactions of stem cell therapies on acute and chronic pancreatitis are summarized in Table 1.

| Source (Country) | Pancreatitis type | Experimental design | Species | Stem cell type | Dosage | Route | Sacrification time | Examined organ/organs | Main benefits | Adverse effects |
|---|---|---|---|---|---|---|---|---|---|---|
| Cui et al; 2003 China (Ref. no: 65) | Severe AP | L-arginin-induced | Female Balb/c mice | Bone marrow-derived MSC | $2\times10^7$; 4 days prior to SAP induction | Tail vein | 24th., 48th. and 72th.after induction of SAP | Pancreas | Mortality rate Amylase level Pathological changes | ☺ |
| Chen et al; 2013 China (Ref. no: 66) | Severe AP | 5% sodium taurocholate-induced | Male Sprague-Dawley rats | Bone marrow-derived MSC | 1ml ($1\times10^6$/mL) at 0. hour of SAP induction | Tail vein | 6th.- 12th. 24th. hours after induction of SAP | Pancreas Kidney | Amylase level Creatine level BUN level Pathological changes US changes | ☺ |
| Tu et al; 2012 China (Ref. no: 14) | Severe AP | Sodium deoxycholate-induced | Male Sprague-Dawley rats | Bone marrow-derived MSC | 2ml ($1\times10^6$ cells/mL) 2 min after SAP induction | Caudal vein | 6th. 24th. 72th. hours after induction of SAP | Pancreas cells (in culture) Small intestines | Amylase LD level MDA content Pathological changes SOD activity | ☺ |
| Sun et al; 2013 China (Ref. no: 67) | Severe AP | L-arginin-induced | Male Sprague-Dawley rats | Bone marrow-derived MSC | $5\times10^6$, once daily for 3 days | Peritoneal | 72th. hour after induction of SAP | Pancreas Small intestines | TNF-α mRNA IL-1β mRNA Pathological changes | ☺ |
| Wang et al; 2012 China (Ref. no: 68) | Severe AP | 5% sodium taurocholate-induced | Male Sprague-Dawley rats | Bone marrow-derived MSC | 1 ml ($1\times10^6$/mL), 2 hours after SAP induction | Injection | 1th., 3th., 6th., 12th. and 24th. hours after induction of SAP | Lung | Amylase level MPO level TNF-α Substance P Pathological changes | ☺ |
| Marrache et al; 2008 USA (Ref. no: 69) | Severe CP | Cerulein-induced | Female C57BL/6 rats | Bone marrow-derived progenitor cells | Total $5\times10^6$ bone marrow cells, 4 weeks before CP induction | Tail vein | 0, 6, 20, 30, 45 weeks after CP induction | Pancreas | Pathological changes | Eosinophilic metaplasia (a reactive change to BMT) |
| Yang et al; 2013 China (Ref. no: 73) | Severe AP | Sodium taurocholate-induced | Male Sprague-Dawley rats | Umbilical cord-derived MSC | $5\times10^4$- $5\times10^6$, $1\times10^7$ cells/kg of UCMSC suspension | Tail vein | 48 hours after AP induction | Pancreas Lung | Mortality rate Amylase level Ascite TNF-α Interferon-γ Pathological changes | ☺ |
| Zhou et al; 2013 China (Ref. no: 74) | Severe CP | Dibutyltin dichloride-induced | Male Sprague-Dawley rats | Umbilical cord-derived MSC | $2\times10^6$ UCMSCs in 100 µL of PBS on day 5 after CP induction | Jugular vein | On days 14th and 28th after CP induction | Pancreas | Amylase level Pathological changes Fibrosis | ☺ |

AP: Acute pancreatitis, BMT: Bone marrow transplantation, BUN: Blood urea nitrogen, CP: Chronic pancreatitis, IL: Interleukin, LD: Lactate dehydrogenase, MDA: Malondialdehyde, MPO: Myeloperoxidase, MSC: Mesenchymal stem cell, SAP: Severe acute pancreatitis, SOD: Superoxide dismutase, TNF: Tumor necrosis factor, UCMSC: Umblical cord mesenchymal stem cell, US: Ultrastructural

**Table 1.** A brief summary of characteristics of included studies

As a conclusion, although stem cell transplantation to patients with acute or chronic pancreatitis has not been performed so far, it is clear that stem cell transplantation might be a promising therapeutic approach for acute and chronic pancreatitis in the very near future.

## Acknowledgements

The pictures are obtained from previous studies of the author on her various studies related with pancreas.

## Author details

Mukaddes Esrefoglu*

Address all correspondence to: drmukaddes@hotmail.com, mdrmukaddes@yahoo.com

Bezmialem Vakif University, Medical Faculty, Dept. of Histology and Embryology, Fatih, Istanbul, Turkey

Esrefoglu M solely contributed to this chapter.

## References

[1] Nathens AB, Curtis JR, Beale RJ, Cook DJ, Moreno RP, Romand JA, Skerrett SJ, Stapleton RD, Ware LB, Waldmann CS. Management of the critically ill patient with severe acute pancreatitis. *Crit Care Med* 2004; 32: 2524–2536 [PMID: 15599161]

[2] Petrov MS, Shanbhag S, Chakraborty M, Phillips AR, Windsor JA. Organ failure and infection of pancreatic necrosis as determinants of mortality in patients with acute pancreatitis. *Gastroenterology* 2010; 139: 813-820 [PMID:0540942 DOI: 10.1053/j.gastro.2010.06.010]

[3] Eşrefoğlu M, Gül M, Ates B, Batçioğlu K, Selimoğlu MA. Antioxidative effect of melatonin, ascorbic acid and N-acetylcysteine on caerulein-induced pancreatitis and associated liver injury in rats. *World J Gastroenterol* 2006; 12: 259-64 [PMID: 16482627]

[4] Eşrefoğlu M, Gül M, Ateş B, Selimoğlu MA. Ultrastructural clues for the protective effect of melatonin against oxidative damage in cerulein-induced pancreatitis. *J Pineal Res* 2006; 40: 92-7 [PMID: 16313504]

[5] Eşrefoğlu M, Gül M, Turan F. Comparative effects of several therapatic agents on hepatic damage induced by acute experimental pancreatitis. *Dig Dis Sci* 2008; 53: 1303-10 [PMID: 17934852]

[6] Cappell MS. Acute pancreatitis: etiology, clinical presentation, diagnosis, and therapy. *Med Clin North Am* 2008; 92: 889-923 [PMID:18570947 DOI: 10.1016/j.mcna.2008.04.013]

[7]  Omary MB, Lugea A, Lowe AW, Pandol SJ. The pancreatic stellate cell: a star on the rise in pancreatic diseases. *J Clin Invest* 2007; 117: 50-9 [PMID: 17200706]

[8]  Madro A, Slomka M, Celinski K. Can we expect progress in the treatment of fibrosis in the course of chronic pancreatitis? *Adv Med Sci* 2011; 56: 132-7 [PMID:21940269 DOI: 10.2478/v10039-011-0023-1]

[9]  Eşrefoğlu M, Gül M, Ateş B, Yilmaz I. Ultrastructural clues for the protective effect of ascorbic acid and N-acetylcysteine against oxidative damage on caerulein-induced pancreatitis. *Pancreatology* 2006; 6: 477-85 [PMID: 16864970]

[10]  Esrefoglu M. Experimental and clinical evidence of antioxidant therapy in acute pancreatitis. *World J Gastroenterol* 2012; 18: 5533-41 [PMID: 23112545 DOI: 10.3748/wjg.v18.i39.5533]

[11]  Valle-Prieto A, Conget PA. Human mesenchymal stem cells efficiently manage oxidative stress. *Stem Cells Dev* 2010; 19: 1885-93 [PMID: 20380515 DOI: 10.1089/scd.2010.0093]

[12]  Torrente D, Avila M, Cabezas R, Morales L, Gonzalez J, Samudio I, Barreto G. Paracrine factors of human mesenchymal stem cells increase wound closure and reduce reactive oxygen species production in a traumatic brain injury in vitro model. *Hum Exp Toxicol* 2013 Oct 31. [Epub ahead of print] [PMID:24178889]

[13]  Arslan F, Lai RC, Smeets MB, Akeroyd L, Choo A, Aguor EN, Timmers L, van Rijen HV, Doevendans PA, Pasterkamp G, Lim SK, de Kleijn DP. Mesenchymal stem cell-derived exosomes increase ATP levels, decrease oxidative stress and activate PI3K/Akt pathway to enhance myocardial viability and prevent adverse remodeling after myocardial ischemia/reperfusion injury. *Stem Cell Res* 2013; 10: 301-12 [PMID: 23399448 DOI: 10.1016/j.scr.2013.01.002].

[14]  Tu XH, Song JX, Xue XJ, Guo XW, Ma YX, Chen ZY, Zou ZD, Wang L. Role of bone marrow-derived mesenchymal stem cells in a rat model of severe acute pancreatitis. *World J Gastroenterol* 2012; 18: 2270-9 [DOI: 10.3748/wjg.v18.i18.2270 PMID: 22611322]

[15]  Bouwens L, Houbracken I, Mfopou JK. The use of stem cells for pancreatic regeneration in diabetes mellitus. *Nat Rev Endocrinol* 2013 9: 598-606 [PMID: 23877422 DOI: 10.1038/nrendo]

[16]  Dor Y, Brown J, Martinez OI, Melton DA. Adult pancreatic beta-cells are formed by self-duplication rather than stem-cell differentiation. *Nature* 2004; 429: 41–6 [PMID: 15129273]

[17]  Smukler SR, Arntfield ME, Razavi R, Bikopoulos G, Karpowicz P, Seaberg R, Dai F, Lee S, Ahrens R, Fraser PE, Wheeler MB, van der Kooy D. The adult mouse and human pancreas contain rare multipotent stem cells that express insulin. *Cell Stem Cell* 2011; 8: 281–293 [PMID: 21362568 DOI: 10.1016/j.stem.2011.01.015].

[18]  Xu X, D'Hoker J, Stangé G, Bonné S, De Leu N, Xiao X, Van de Casteele M, Mellitzer G, Ling Z, Pipeleers D, Bouwens L, Scharfmann R, Gradwohl G, Heimberg H. Beta

cells can be generated from endogenous progenitors in injured adult mouse pancreas. Cell 2008; 132: 197–207 [PMID: 18243096 doi: 10.1016/j.cell.2007.12.015]

[19]   Zhou Q, Law AC, Rajagopal J, Anderson WJ, Gray PA, Melton DA. A multipotent progenitor domain guides pancreatic organogenesis. *Dev Cell* 2007; 13: 103–14 [PMID: 17609113]

[20]   Gong J, Tian F, Ren J, Luo G. Experimental evidence supporting the lack of primary stem cells in adult pancreatic tissue. *Pancreatology* 2010; 10: 620-30 [PMID: 21051917 DOI: 10.1159/000321586]

[21]   Wang Y, Lanzoni G, Carpino G, Cui CB, Dominguez-Bendala J, Wauthier E, Cardinale V, Oikawa T, Pileggi A, Gerber D, Furth ME, Alvaro D, Gaudio E, Inverardi L, Reid LM. Biliary tree stem cells, precursors to pancreatic committed progenitors: evidence for possible life-long pancreatic organogenesis. Stem Cells 2013; 31: 1966–19 [PMID: 23847135 DOI: 10.1002/stem.1460].

[22]   Bonner-Weir S, Toschi E, Inada A, Reitz P, Fonseca SY, Aye T, Sharma A. The pancreatic ductal epithelium serves as a potential pool of progenitor cells. Pediatr Diabet 2004; 5: 16–22 [PMID: 15601370]

[23]   Inada A, Nienaber C, Katsuta H, Fujitani Y, Levine J, Morita R, Sharma A, Bonner-Weir S. Carbonic anhydrase II-positive pancreatic cells are progenitors for both endocrine and exocrine pancreas after birth. *Proc Natl Acad Sci U S A* 2008; 105: 19915–9 [PMID: 19052237 DOI: 10.1073/pnas.0805803105].

[24]   Strobel O, Rosow DE, Rakhlin EY, Lauwers GY, Trainor AG, Alsina J, Fernández-Del Castillo C, Warshaw AL, Thayer SP. Pancreatic duct glands are distinct ductal compartments that react to chronic injury and mediate Shh-induced metaplasia. *Gastroenterology* 2010;138: 1166–77 [PMID: 20026066 DOIi: 10.1053/j.gastro.2009.12.005]

[25]   Stanger BZ, Tanaka AJ, Melton DA. Organ size is limited by the number of embryonic progenitor cells in the pancreas but not the liver. Nature 2007; 445: 886–91 [PMID: 17259975]

[26]   Rovira M, Scott SG, Liss AS, Jensen J, Thayer SP, Leach SD. Isolation and characterization of centroacinar/ terminal ductal progenitor cells in adult mouse pancreas. Proc Natl Acad Sci U S A 2010; 107: 75–80 [DOI: 10.1073/pnas.0912589107 PMID: 20018761]

[27]   Pasca di Magliano M, Forsmark C, Freedman S, Hebrok M, Pasricha PJ, Saluja A, Stanger BZ, Holt J, Serrano J, James SP, Rustgi AK. Advances in Acute and Chronic Pancreatitis: From Development to Inflammation and Repair. Gastroenterology 2013; 144: e1–e4 [DOI:: 10.1053/j.gastro.2012.11.018 PMID: 23159450]

[28]   Rountree CB, Barsky L, Ge S, Zhu J, Senadheera S, Crooks GM. A CD133-expressing murine liver oval cell population with bilineage potential. Stem Cells 2007; 25: 2419–29 [PMID: 17585168]

[29] Hald J, Sprinkel AE, Ray M, Serup P, Wright C, Madsen OD. Generation and characterization of Ptf1a antiserum and localization of Ptf1a in relation to Nkx6.1 and Pdx1 during the earliest stages of mouse pancreas development. *J Histochem Cytochem* 2008; 56: 587–595 [DOI: 10.1369/jhc.2008.950675 PMID: 18347078].

[30] Lynn FC, Smith SB, Wilson ME, Yang KY, Nekrep N, German MS. Sox9 coordinates a transcriptional network in pancreatic progenitor cells. *Proc Natl Acad Sci U S A* 2007, 104:10500–10505 [PMID: 17563382]

[31] Maestro MA, Boj SF, Luco RF, Pierreux CE, Cabedo J, Servitja JM, German MS, Rousseau GG, Lemaigre FP, Ferrer J. Hnf6 and Tcf2 (MODY5) are linked in a gene network operating in a precursor cell domain of the embryonic pancreas. *Human Mol Genet* 2003, 12: 3307–14 [PMID: 14570708]

[32] Jensen J. Gene regulatory factors in pancreatic development. *Dev Dyn* 2004, 229: 176–200 [PMID: 14699589]

[33] Villasenor A, Chong DC, Henkemeyer M, Cleaver O. Epithelial dynamics of pancreatic branching morphogenesis. *Development* 2010; 137: 4295–305 [DOI: 10.1242/dev.052993. PMID: 21098570]

[34] Solar M, Cardalda C, Houbracken I, Martín M, Maestro MA, De Medts N, Xu X, Grau V, Heimberg H, Bouwens L, Ferrer J. Pancreatic exocrine duct cells give rise to insulin-producing β cells during embryogenesis but not after birth. *Dev Cell* 2009, 17: 849–60 [DOI: 10.1016/j.devcel.2009.11.003 PMID: 20059954]

[35] Seymour PA, Freude KK, Dubois CL, Shih HP, Patel NA, Sander M. A dosage-dependent requirement for Sox9 in pancreatic endocrine cell formation. *Dev Biol* 2008; 323:19–30 [DOI: 10.1016/j.ydbio.2008.07.034 PMID: 18723011]

[36] Anderson KR, Singer RA, Balderes DA, Hernandez- Lagunas L, Johnson CW, Artinger KB, Sussel L. The L6 domain tetraspanin Tm4sf4 regulates endocrine pancreas differentiation and directed cell migration. *Development* 2011; 138:3213–24 [DOI: 10.1242/dev.058693 PMID: 21750032]

[37] Cole L, Anderson M, Antin PB, Limesand SW. One process for pancreatic beta-cell coalescence into islets involves an epithelial-mesenchymal transition. *J Endocrinol* 2009; 203: 19–31 [DOI: 10.1677/JOE-09-0072 PMID: 19608613]

[38] Rukstalis JM, Habener JF. Snail2, a mediator of epithelial-mesenchymal transitions, expressed in progenitor cells of the developing endocrine pancreas. *Gene Exp Patterns* 2007; 7: 471–9 [PMID: 17185046].

[39] Afelik S, Jensen J. Notch signaling in the pancreas: patterning and cell fate specification. *Wiley Interdiscip Rev Dev Biol* 2013; 2: 531–44 [DOI: 10.1002/wdev.99 PMID: 24014421]

[40]  Taguchi M, Yamaguchi T, Otsuki M. Induction of PDX-1-positive cells in the main duct during regeneration after acute necrotizing pancreatitis in rats. J Pathol 2002; 197: 638–46 [PMID: 12210084]

[41]  Bhushan A, Itoh N, Kato S, Thiery JP, Czernichow P, Bellusci S, Scharfmann R. Fgf10 is essential for maintaining the proliferative capacity of epithelial progenitor cells during early pancreatic organogenesis. *Development* 2001; 128: 5109–17 [PMID: 11748146]

[42]  Scharfmann R. Control of early development of the pancreas in rodents and humans: implications of signals from the mesenchyme. *Diabetologia* 2000; 43: 1083–92 [PMID: 11043853]

[43]  Apelqvist A, Li H, Sommer L, Beatus P, Anderson DJ, Honjo T, Hrabe de Angelis M, Lendahl U, Edlund H. Notch signalling controls pancreatic cell differentiation. *Nature* 1999; 400: 877–881 [PMID: 10476967]

[44]  Zulewski H, Abraham EJ, Gerlach MJ, Daniel PB, Moritz W, Müller B, Vallejo M, Thomas MK, Habener JF. Multipotential nestin-positive stem cells isolated from adult pancreatic islets differentiate ex vivo into pancreatic endocrine, exocrine, and hepatic phenotypes. *Diabetes* 2001; 50: 521–33 [PMID: 11246871]

[45]  Sangiorgi E, Capecchi MR. Bmi1 lineage tracing identifies a self-renewing pancreatic acinar cell subpopulation capable of maintaining pancreatic organ homeostasis. *Proc Natl Acad Sci U S A* 2009; 106: 7101–6 [DOI: 10.1073/pnas.0902508106 PMID: 19372370].

[46]  Sharma A, Zangen DH, Reitz P, Taneja M, Lissauer ME, Miller CP, Weir GC, Habener JF, Bonner-Weir S. The homeodomain protein IDX-1 increases after an early burst of proliferation during pancreatic regeneration. *Diabetes* 1999; 48: 507–13 [PMID: 10078550]

[47]  Sander M, German MS. The beta cell transcription factors and development of the pancreas. J Mol Med (Berl) 1997; 75: 327–40 [PMID: 9181474]

[48]  Jonsson J, Carlsson L, Edlund T, Edlund H. Insulin-promoter-factor 1 is required for pancreas development in mice. *Nature* 1994; 371: 606–9 [PMID: 7935793]

[49]  Gradwohl G, Dierich A, LeMeur M, Guillemot F. neurogenin3 is required for the development of the four endocrine cell lineages of the pancreas. *Proc Natl Acad Sci U S A* 2000; 97: 1607–11 [PMID: 10677506]

[50]  Esrefoglu M. Role of stem cells in repair of liver injury: experimental and clinical benefit of transferred stem cells on liver failure. *World J Gastroenterol* 2013; 19: 6757-73 [PMID:24187451 DOI: 10.3748/wjg.v19.i40.6757]

[51]  Vieyra DS, Jackson KA, Goodell MA. Plasticity and tissue regenerative potential of bone marrow-derived cells. *Stem Cell Rev* 2005; 1: 65–9 [PMID: 17132877]

[52] Meirelles Lda S, Nardi NB. Murine marrow-derived mesenchymal stem cell: isolation, in vitro expansion, and characterization. *Br J Haematol* 2003; 123: 702–11 [PMID: 14616976]

[53] Lagasse E, Connors H, Al-Dhalimy M, Reitsma M, Dohse M, Osborne L, Wang X, Finegold M, Weissman IL, Grompe M. Purified hematopoietic stem cells can differentiate into hepatocytes in vivo. *Nat Med* 2000; 6: 1229–34 [PMID: 11062533]

[54] Hagiwara M, Shen B, Chao L, Chao J. Kallikrein-modified mesenchymal stem cell implantation provides enhanced protection against acute ischemic kidney injury by inhibiting apoptosis and inflammation. *Hum Gene Ther* 2008; 19: 807–19 [DOI: 10.1089/hgt.2008.016 PMID: 18554097]

[55] Jung KH, Song SU, Yi T, Jeon MS, Hong SW, Zheng HM, Lee HS, Choi MJ, Lee DH, Hong SS. Human bone marrow-derived clonal mesenchymal stem cells inhibit inflammation and reduce acute pancreatitis in rats. *Gastroenterology* 2011; 140: 998–1008 [DOI: 10.1053/j.gastro.2010.11.047 PMID: 21130088]

[56] García-Olmo D, García-Arranz M, Herreros D, Pascual I, Peiro C, Rodríguez-Montes JA. A phase I clinical trial of the treatment of Crohn's fistula by adipose mesenchymal stem cell transplantation. *Dis Colon Rectum* 2005; 48: 1416–23 [PMID: 15933795]

[57] English K, Barry FP, Mahon BP. Murine mesenchymal stem cells suppress dendritic cell migration, maturation and antigen presentation. *Immunol Lett* 2008; 115: 50–8 [PMID: 18022251]

[58] Orlic D, Kajstura J, Chimenti S, Jakoniuk I, Anderson SM, Li B, Pickel J, McKay R, Nadal-Ginard B, Bodine DM, Leri A, Anversa P. Bone marrow cells regenerate infracted myocardium. *Nature* 2001; 410: 701–5 [PMID: 11287958]

[59] Deng YB, Yuan QT, Liu XG, Liu XL, Liu Y, Liu ZG, Zhang C. Functional recovery after rhesus monkey spinal cord injury by transplantation of bone marrow mesenchymal-stem cell-derived neurons. Chin Med J (Engl) 2005; 118: 1533–41 [PMID: 16232330]

[60] Humphreys BD, Bonventre JV. Mesenchymal stem cells in acute kidney injury. *Annu Rev Med* 2008; 59: 311-25 [PMID: 17914926]

[61] Williams AR, Hare JM. Mesenchymal stem cells: biology, pathophysiology, translational findings, and therapeutic implications for cardiac disease. *Circ Res* 2011; 109: 923-40 [DOI: 10.1161/CIRCRESAHA.111.243147 PMID: 21960725]

[62] Jung KH, Shin HP, Lee S, Lim YJ, Hwang SH, Han H, Park HK, Chung JH, Yim SV. Effect of human umbilical cord blood-derived mesenchymal stem cells in a cirrhotic rat model. *Liver Int* 2009; 29: 898-909 [DOI: 10.1111/j.1478-3231.2009.02031.x. PMID: 19422480]

[63] Moodley Y, Atienza D, Manuelpillai U, Samuel CS, Tchongue J, Ilancheran S, Boyd R, Trounson A. Human umbilical cord mesenchymal stem cells reduce fibrosis of

bleomycin-induced lung injury. *Am J Pathol* 2009; 175: 303-13 [DOI: 10.2353/ajpath. 2009.080629 PMID: 19497992]

[64] Yi T, Song SU. Immunomodulatory properties of mesenchymal stem cells and their therapeutic applications. *Arch Pharm Res* 2012; 35: 213-21 [doi: 10.1007/ s12272-012-0202-z. PMID: 22370776]

[65] Cui HF, Bai ZL. Protective effects of transplanted and mobilized bone marrow stem cells on mice with severe acute pancreatitis. *World J Gastroenterol* 2003; 9: 2274-7 [PMID: 14562392]

[66] Chen Z, Lu F, Fang H, Huang H. Effect of mesenchymal stem cells on renal injury in rats with severe acute pancreatitis. *Exp Biol Med (Maywood)* 2013; 238: 687-95 [DOI: 10.1177/1535370213490629 PMID: 23918880

[67] Sun XC, Wu JS, Wu JM, Huang ZM, Yu Z. [Effects of intraperitoneal injection of marrow mesenchymal stem cells on intestinal barrier in acute pancreatitis]. *Zhonghua Yi Xue Za Zhi* 2013; 93: 951-5 [PMID: 23863684]

[68] Wang L, Tu XH, Zhao P, Song JX, Zou ZD. Protective effect of transplanted bone marrow-derived mesenchymal stemcells on pancreatitis-associated lung injury in rats. *Mol Med Rep* 2012; 6: 287-92 DOI: 10.3892/mmr.2012.922 PMID: 22613963]

[69] Marrache F, Pendyala S, Bhagat G, Betz KS, Song Z, Wang TC. Role of bone marrow-derived cells in experimental chronic pancreatitis. *Gut* 2008; 57: 1113-20 [DOI: 10.1136/gut.2007.143271 PMID: 18367560]

[70] Tran TT, Kahn CR. Transplantation of adipose tissue and stem cells: role in metabolism and disease. Nat Rev Endocrinol 2010; 6: 195–213 [DOI: 10.1038/nrendo.2010.20. PMID: 20195269]

[71] Baek SJ, Kang SK, Ra JC. In vitro migration capacity of human adipose tissue-derived mesenchymal stem cells reflects their expression of receptors for chemokines and growth factors. *Exp Mol Med* 2011; 43: 596–603 [DOI: 10.3858/emm.2011.43.10.069 PMID: 21847008]

[72] Wen Z, Liao Q, Hu Y, Liu S, You L, Zhao Y. Human adipose-derived stromal/stem cells: a novel approach to inhibiting acute pancreatitis. *Med Hypotheses* 2013; 80: 598–600 [DOI: 10.1016/j.mehy.2013.01.034 PMID: 23419667]

[73] Yang B, Bai B, Liu CX, Wang SQ, Jiang X, Zhu CL, Zhao QC. Effect of umbilical cord mesenchymal stem cells on treatment of severe acute pancreatitis in rats. *Cytotherapy* 2013; 15: 154-62 [DOI: 10.1016/j.jcyt.2012.11.007 PMID: 23321327]

[74] Zhou CH, Li ML, Qin AL, Lv SX, Wen-Tang, Zhu XY, Li LY, Dong Y, Hu CY, Hu DM, Wang SF. Reduction of fibrosis in dibutyltin dichloride-induced chronic pancreatitis using rat umbilical mesenchymal stem cells from Wharton's jelly. Pancreas 2013; 42: 1291-302 [DOI: 10.1097/MPA.0b013e318296924e PMID: 24152954]

# 3

# Acute and Chronic Pancreatitis — Complications

Rone Antônio Alves de Abreu and
Manlio Basilio Speranzini

## 1. Introduction

Over the course of pancreatitis, the first two to four days of symptoms are the most important because this is the period during which 15% to 25% of patients evolve to its severe form. According to clinical and experimental data, this period is characterized by an initial state of hypovolemia.

It is known that the morbidity of severe acute pancreatitis appears in two stages. The first two weeks are characterized by a systemic inflammatory response syndrome (SIRS), which results from release of inflammatory mediators.

Organ failure is common and often occurs even in the absence of infection. The early mortality rate is 42 to 60%.

The second stage begins around two weeks after the start of symptoms and is characterized by sepsis-related complications that result from the infection of pancreatic necrosis. Thus, there is an association with systemic complications, like pulmonary insufficiency, kidney failure and cardiovascular insufficiency, known as multiple organ failure syndrome (MOFS).

The inflammatory mediators are primarily released from the area of the viscera and they rise to the systemic compartment mainly through the lymphatic circulation and the circulation of the portal and suprahepatic veins. The lungs are the first organ to be reached by blood and lymph that are rich in activated polymorphonuclear cells, cytokines and other active biological compounds. Failure of the gastrointestinal barrier that enables translocation of bacteria and endotoxins is considered to be one of the major factors responsible for the development of local infection and multiple organ failure that is seen in severe acute pancreatitis, which is responsible for the majority of the deaths.

Independent of the etiology of the acute pancreatitis, once the inflammatory events of the acinar cells have started, this will lead to progression to SIRS. Among the commonest complications, those of the lungs occur most frequently and are potentially the most serious. The spectrum of these complications goes from hypoxemia to acute respiratory distress syndrome (ARDS). [1]

## 2. Hypoxemia without radiological alterations

Tachypnea, moderate respiratory alkalosis and hypoxemia are observed in around two thirds of the patients with acute pancreatitis, over the first 48 hours. This hypoxemia does not match the severity of alterations indicated by examinations. Radiological alterations are only present in 11% of the cases.

However, a study by Lankish *et al.* (1996) [2] showed that around 30% of the patients present PaO2 values lower than 60 mmHg and 63% lower than 70 mmHg.

Respiratory failure develops in around:

- 10% of the cases of mild acute pancreatitis;
- 47% of the cases of sterile pancreatic necrosis;
- 74% of the cases of infected necrosis.

The main cause of hypoxemia is disorders of ventilation/perfusion, which may give rise to an intrapulmonary shunt in around 30% of the cardiac output. The incidence of respiratory failure is unrelated to etiological factors, patients' ages, amylase values, calcium levels or use of fluid therapy. In several studies, a correlation has been found between the degree of hypoxemia and mortality, reaching rates of 14% when PO2 is lower than 60 mmHg.

Some authors have considered that not recognizing hypoxemia and hypovolemia immediately is the most important factor in occurrences of multiple organ failure triggered during the first week. [1]

## 3. Hypoxemia with radiological alterations

In one third of the patients with acute pancreatitis, respiratory complications are detected radiologically. Pulmonary infiltrates or atelectasis are found in 15%, pleural effusion in 4% to 17% and pulmonary edema in 8% to 50%. The morbidity and mortality rates are significantly higher than those in cases of hypoxemia without radiological alterations.

**Pleural effusion** is today considered to be a sign of poor prognosis, with associated mortality of 20% to 30%. It is usually of small proportions and occasionally hemorrhagic, and is characterized by high amylase levels (up to 30 times higher than in serum) and high protein and lactate dehydrogenase levels. Most cases of pleural effusion occur on the left side (68%), while

22% are bilateral and 10% are on the right side. The two main causes are transdiaphragmatic lymphatic blockage and pancreatic-pleural fistulas due to rupture of the pancreatic canal or a pseudocyst. (Fig. 1)

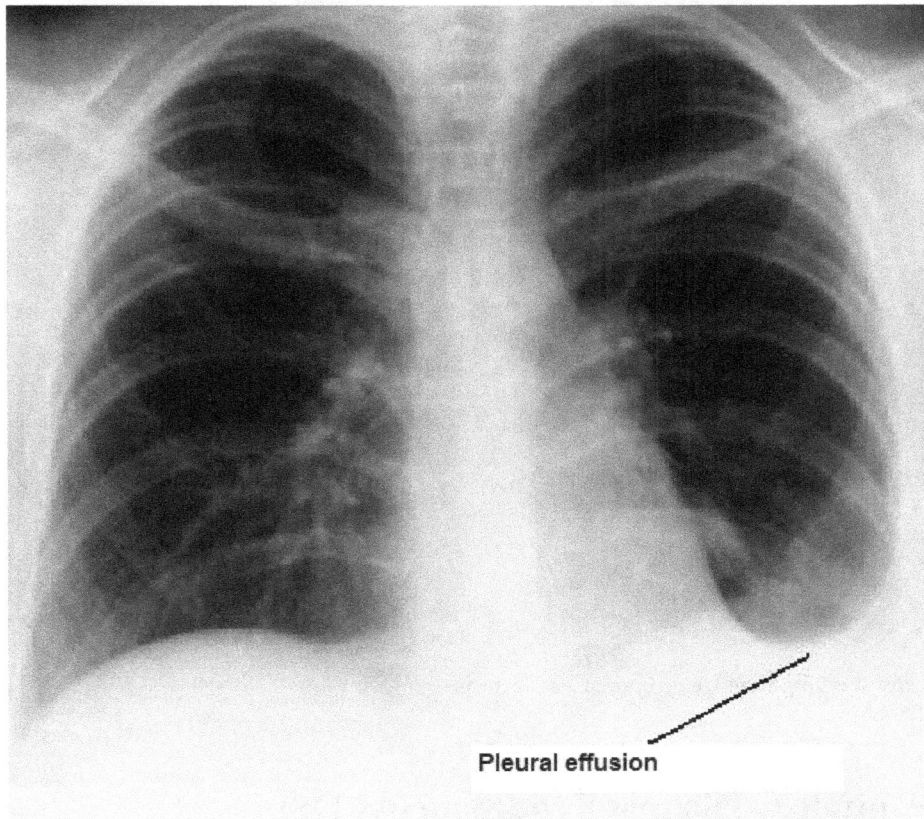

Pleural effusion

**Figure 1.** Chest x-ray showing left-side pleural effusion

The treatment for pleural effusion is often initially conservative. However, large pleural effusions frequently become symptomatic are require thoracocentesis and endotracheal intubation. When the abdominal pathological condition has been resolved, the pleural effusions are often also resolved. Chronic pleural effusions often necessitate an abdominal approach: drainage of the pseudocyst or abscess and, possibly, resection of the path of the fistula, so as to completely resolve the condition.

**Atelectasis** occurs due to diminution of the quantity of surfactant and is a frequent complication. Because the primary lesion is at the alveolar-interstitial level, this decreases the pulmonary compliance and increases the ventilatory effort, thus leading more quickly to diaphragm fatigue. As previously mentioned, pro-inflammatory cytokines have a preponderant role in the systemic complications of acute pancreatitis. Some experimental studies have shown that TNF-$\alpha$ and IL-1 have a negative inotropic synergic effect on the contractility of the diaphragm, i.e. showing that cytokines also contribute towards atelectasis through diminishing ventilation. [1, 3] (Fig. 2)

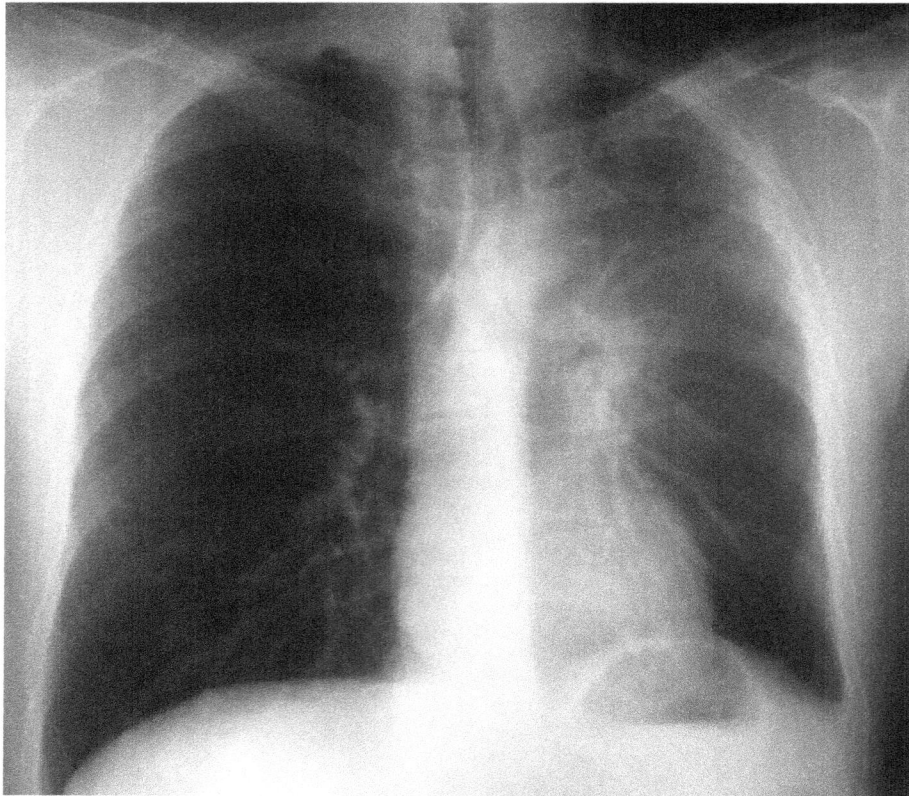

**Figure 2.** Chest x-ray showing left-side pulmonary atelectasis

## 4. Acute Respiratory Distress Syndrome (ARDS)

ARDS is the most severe pulmonary complication. It occurs in 15% to 20% of the patients with acute pancreatitis and its mortality rate is 56%. It is responsible for 50% to 90% of all deaths due to pancreatitis. Despite being more frequent in cases of severe acute pancreatitis, it may occur in cases of mild forms, in around 10% of these cases.

ARDS usually manifests between the second and seventh day after the start of acute pancreatitis, but it may have faster evolution. Clinically, it presents with severe dyspnea and extreme hypoxemia that is refractory to supplementation with high concentrations of oxygen. Multilobular pulmonary infiltrates are also observed.

The physiopathology of ARDS remains unclear, but the action of the pancreatic enzymes and inflammatory mediators released by the pancreatic lesion seems to have a key role. ARDS has been described as increased pulmonary vascularization with protein transudation to the alveolar space and decreased pulmonary compliance, manifested clinically by refractory hypoxemia and radiologically by diffuse pulmonary infiltrates. Experimental studies have suggested that acute pancreatitis and its respiratory complications should be treated by combating the pro-inflammatory response, thereby necessitating better comprehension of the physiopathology and the drugs that potentially inhibit this response. [1]

# 5. Kidney failure

Kidney failure is present in around 15% of the cases of mild acute pancreatitis and in 35% to 43% of the cases of severe pancreatitis.

The evolution to kidney failure is influenced by the severity of the episode of acute pancreatitis. The presence of kidney failure notably worsens the prognosis for cases of acute pancreatitis, given that the mortality rate is much higher than in cases without kidney failure. Higher urea levels are one of the items in Ranson's criteria, thus corroborating the relationship between renal alterations and the severity of the episode. The kidney failure that accompanies acute pancreatitis is of pre-renal origin in most cases. It is worth emphasizing that episodes of acute pancreatitis should not be ruled out as a cause of kidney failure even in the absence of hyperamylasemia. There should be strong diagnostic suspicion, given that normal amylase levels are found in around 19% to 32% of the patients with acute pancreatitis. [1]

# 6. Pseudocysts

Pancreatic pseudocysts can be defined as organized accumulations that are rich in pancreatic enzymes, which arise as a consequence of and remain after an episode of acute pancreatitis or after exacerbation of chronic pancreatitis. Their content is variable but is predominantly fluid. They may or may not present necrotic material and debris, and they are rich in amylase and lipase. Biochemical studies on their content have demonstrated that the carcinoembryonic antigen (CEA) levels are low but that the CA 19.9 levels may be high. These pseudocysts have low viscosity and cytological evaluations show that inflammatory cells predominate.

These are the commonest cystic lesions associated with pancreatic diseases. They are a relatively common complication in adult patients with a diagnosis of pancreatitis, occurring in 16%-50% of the cases of acute pancreatitis and in 20%-40% of the cases of chronic pancreatitis.

Pseudocysts are initially connected to the pancreatic duct system, either directly or indirectly via the pancreatic parenchyma. Two thirds of the patients with pseudocysts have demonstrable connections between the pseudocyst and the pancreatic duct, when the duct is ruptured on the posterior face. In one third of the cases, there is a very significant inflammatory reaction that seals the connection such that it is not demonstrable. [4]

## 6.1. Etiology

Alcoholic pancreatitis seems to be the biggest cause of pseudocysts in countries in which alcohol consumption is high, and this accounts for 59% to 78% of all the cases. Biliary pancreatitis is most commonly in second place among the causes. Patients with chronic pancreatitis who develop acute exacerbations seem to have greater incidence of pseudocysts than do patients with acute pancreatitis. Patients with biliary acute pancreatitis present it with a lower incidence. [4]

## 6.2. Classification

Pancreatic cystic lesions were classified by D'Egidio and Schein, in 1992, as follows:

- Type I: post-necrotic, arising after episodes of acute pancreatitis, without identifiable abnormalities in the pancreatic ducts; rarely, they are in communication with a pancreatic canal;

- Type II: occurring in cases of chronic pancreatitis that become acute; recognized through alterations in the pancreatic ducts, with which the pseudocysts are often in communication;

- Type III: retention pseudocysts from calcifying chronic pancreatitis, proven by characteristic ductal alterations or the presence of intracanalicular calculi (calcifications).

In 2002, Nealon and Walser proposed another classification system that was more detailed, composed of seven different types that were based on the ductal anatomy and its relationships with the pseudocyst. [5]

## 6.3. Differential diagnosis between pseudocysts and cystic tumors

The main differential diagnosis for pancreatic pseudocysts is made in relation to cystic neoplasia of the pancreas. The main categories are summarized in Box 1, along with their essential characteristics. (Table 1)

|  | SCA | MCN | IMPN | SCPN | Pseudocyst |
|---|---|---|---|---|---|
| **Age** | Middle age | Middle age | Elderly | Young | Variable |
| **Gender** | Female | Female | Male | Female | Male |
| **Presentation** | Mass/pain | Mass/pain | Pancreatitis | Mass/pain | Pain |
| **Location** | Entire pancreas | Tail and body | Head | Entire pancreas | Entire pancreas |
| **Malignant potential** | Very low | Moderate to high | Variable | Low | None |

**SCA**-serous cystadenoma; **MCN**-mucinous cystic neoplasm; **IMPN**-intraductal mucinous papillary neoplasm; **SCPN** – solid-cystic pseudopapillary neoplasm

**Table 1.** Differential diagnosis of cystic lesions of the pancreas

The examinations most used for making the differential diagnosis and for making therapeutic decisions are multichannel computed tomography (CT) scans, magnetic resonance imaging (MRI) with pancreatic resonance, endoscopic retrograde cholangiopancreatography (ERCP) and endoscopic ultrasound (US). (Fig. 3)

The sensitivity varies. If on the one hand, ERCP should be weighted carefully because of its complications, on the other hand it provides a dynamic and anatomical view of the pancreatic duct.

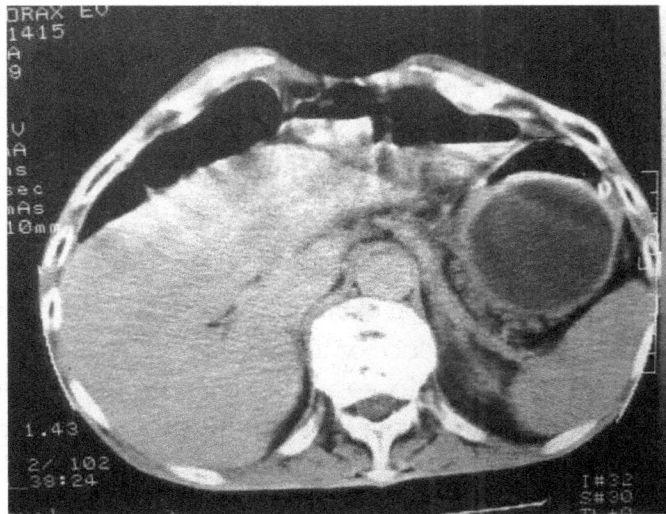

**Figure 3.** Abdominal CT scan showing pancreatic pseudocyst

Pancreatic resonance does not present the complications of ERCP, but it does not provide the same standard of imaging and information about the pancreatic duct. CT is more widely used, but it does not define the anatomy of the pancreatic duct so well. Endoscopic US has the advantage of also supplying punctured material from inside the accumulation for biochemical and other analyses, but it is not yet universally available. Recent studies have proven the relevance of such information for making the differential diagnosis of pseudocysts, as shown (Table 2). [6]

|  | SCA | MCN | MCA | Pseudocyst |
|---|---|---|---|---|
| **CEA** | low | high | high | low |
| **CA 125** | variable | variable | high | low |
| **CA 19-5** | variable | variable-high | variable-high | variable |
| **Amylase** | low-high | low-high | low-high | high |
| **Lipase** | low | low | low | high |

**SCA**-serous cystadenoma; **MCN**-mucinous cystic neoplasm; **MCA**-mucinous cystadenoma

**Table 2.** Differential diagnosis of cystic lesions of the pancreas

## 6.4. Box 2

Before dealing with any peripancreatic accumulation, the differential diagnosis between pseudocysts and cystic neoplasms of the pancreas needs to be established. In this process, a variety of factors need to be comprehended, reviewed and investigated, such as the history of the disease and previous imaging examinations (when available). In some cases, biochemical and cytological analyses should be performed on the peripancreatic fluid.

If a peripancreatic fluid accumulation becomes established due to an episode of acute pancreatitis and then persists for several weeks, the diagnosis of pseudocyst is confirmed. This direct relationship between episodes of pancreatitis and appearance of pseudocysts may be particularly more difficult to establish in cases of chronic pancreatitis. On the other hand, cystic neoplasms may give rise to a moderately inflammatory process in the pancreas that, in turn, may mimic chronic pancreatitis. This situation is particularly more frequent in cases of intraductal mucinous papillary tumors. [7]

It is important to review all the radiological examinations on the patient that are available. An abdominal CT scan may define the presence or absence of cystic lesions over time. When this possibility does not exist, MRI and endoscopic US examinations may aid in making the differential diagnosis. Both of these may reveal septal divisions, solid components inside the cyst or communication between the cyst and the main pancreatic duct. [8]

It is worth emphasizing that communication between the main pancreatic duct and the cyst may occur both in cases of chronic pancreatitis with an association pseudocyst and in cases of mucinous papillary neoplasia of the main duct. In the first case, other signs are generally seen to be associated with the chronic pancreatitis, such as calcifications and multiple ductal stenosis. In the second case, the cystic lesion is associated with dilatation of the main pancreatic duct. If the diagnosis nonetheless still remains undefined, aspiration should be performed on the cyst, for histological analysis and biochemical tests. [9]

## 6.5. Clinical picture

The clinical presentation of pancreatic pseudocysts may vary from asymptomatic to major abdominal repercussions caused by the possible complications. The acute complications include bleeding (generally from pseudoaneurysms of the splenic or hepatic artery), infection and rupture. The chronic complications include obstruction of the pylorus, biliary obstruction and thrombosis of the splenic or portal vein with development of gastric varices.

## 6.6. Treatment

For acute fluid accumulations, no intervention is necessary, since most of these tend to resolve spontaneously. If pseudocysts develop, the current knowledge suggests that, depending on their characteristics and location, they can be treated expectantly unless they present related symptoms or complications: abdominal pain, early satiety, weight loss and persistent fever [9]

## 6.7. Surgical treatment

The classical surgical options are cystogastrostomy, cystoduodenostomy and Roux-en-Y cystojejunostomy, depending on the location of the cyst. Laparoscopic approaches have progressively become more used over the last decade. Even so, and despite the growth of less invasive techniques such as endoscopic, percutaneous and ultrasound-guided drainage, controversy still exists in the literature regarding the best form of therapeutic approach for pancreatic pseudocysts. [11]

## 6.8. Percutaneous drainage

A recent cohort study showed that percutaneous drainage is associated with high mortality, prolonged hospital stay and greater incidence of complication than seen with surgical drainage. Although percutaneous drainage seems to be convenient for both physicians and patients, it should only be performed in patients with acute pseudocysts that are radiologically associated with normal ductal anatomy, or in cases in which the associated comorbidities make surgery a high-risk procedure. The main predictors for failure of this method are sudden ductal obstruction (cutoff), communication between the cyst and the pancreatic duct and an association with chronic pancreatitis. [11, 12]

## 6.9. Endoscopic drainage

ERCP is better than magnetic resonance cholangiopancreatography (MRCP) for characterizing the pancreatic duct. In cases of chronic pancreatic pseudocyst, endoscopic treatment is currently used as an initial option, except in patients with chronic pain, biliary obstruction or pseudocysts involving the pancreatic tail. Two different types of approach are used: (1) transmural endoscopic drainage (transgastric or transduodenal); and (2) transpapillary drainage.

The transpapillary approach requires that the pseudocyst is in communication with the main pancreatic duct and that there is no significant septum formation that would impede complete drainage. Any ductal stenosis that might be identified can be dilated using a balloon, and then an endoprosthesis is placed inside the pancreatic duct.

For transmural drainage to be performed safely, certain inclusion criteria need to be observed: six weeks of clinical treatment without regression; size greater than or equal to 4 cm; distance between the gastroduodenal wall and the pseudocyst wall less than or equal to 1 cm; absence of associated neoplastic processes; and evident bulging of the gastroduodenal wall. [13]

## 6.10. Technique

- Endoscopic retrograde pancreatography is performed in order to study the duct and classify the cyst;

- The area of the gastroduodenal segment with the greatest bulging, as seen on tomography and endoscopy, is identified;

- The area selected is punctured using an endoscopic sclerosis needle (10 x 4 mm), in order to confirm its proximity to the cyst;

- A fistula is constructed from the gastrointestinal tract (duodenum or stomach) to the pseudocyst, by means of a semi-open polypectomy loop connected to an electrocauterization device, using only the coagulation function, in monopolar mode, at an intensity of 30 watts;

- The cyst is immediately cannulated using a cholangiography catheter and nonionic iodinated contrast is injected to document and certify the cyst, with placement of one or two pigtail biliary stents of caliber 10 Fr, which should be short (maximum of 6 cm) Once the fluid has drained through the stent, the procedure can be terminated. (Figs. 4-8).

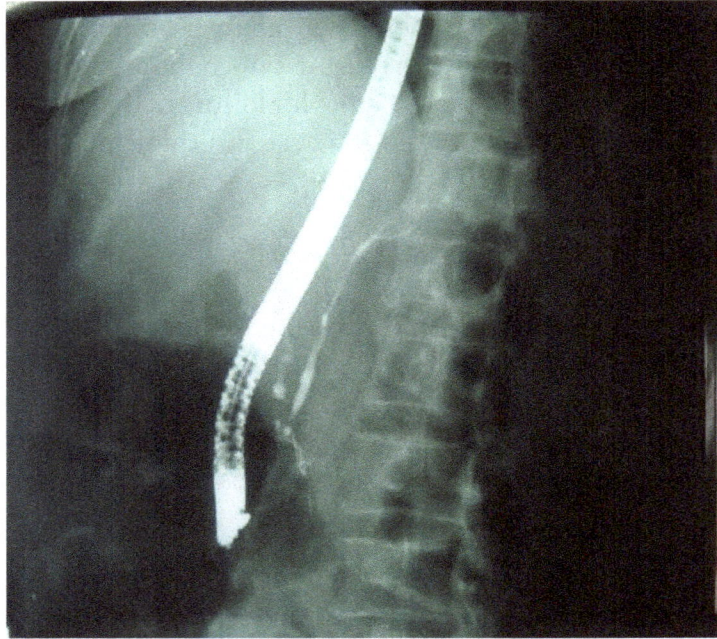

**Figure 4.** Pancreatography showing absence of communication between the Wirsung duct and the pseudocyst

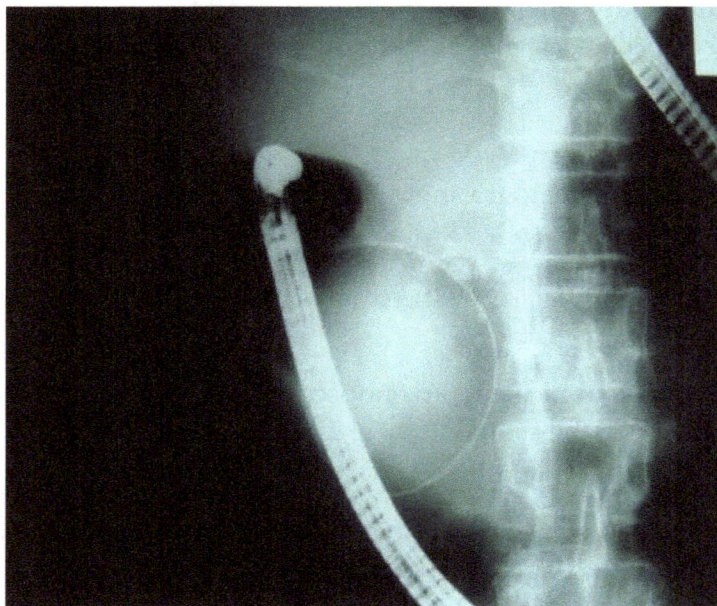

**Figure 5.** ERCP showing guidewire inside the pancreatic pseudocyst

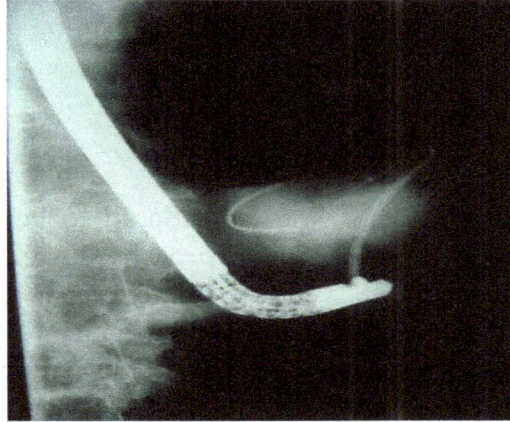

**Figure 6.** ERCP showing location of the endoprosthesis through the anterior wall of the stomach

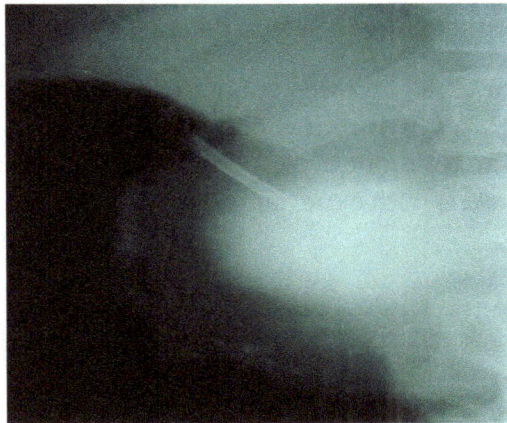

**Figure 7.** Final appearance showing stent providing communication between the pseudocyst and the gastrointestinal tract

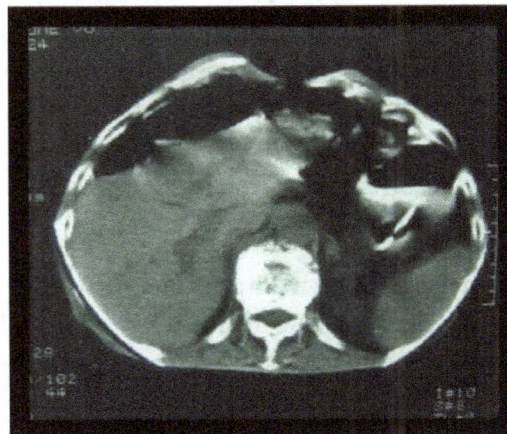

**Figure 8.** Abdominal CT on the 14th day after drainage, showing stent (arrow) providing communication between the pseudocyst and the stomach

We have had the opportunity to treat and follow up 14 patients initially, with five years of follow-up, and we concluded that transmural endoscopic drainage could be used as the first choice, provided that the inclusion criteria were rigorously respected. [13]

### 6.11. Infected pseudocyst

For a long time, infected pseudocysts were considered to be a contraindication against construction of a cystenterostomy. Endoscopic approaches have come to simplify this procedure and expand its indications. Today, cystenterostomy is considered to be the first choice in these cases. The limit for not performing the procedure, when infection coexists, is the patient's clinical state and the presence of sepsis and associated hemodynamic instability. In these cases, it is more prudent to use a conservative approach with external drainage. However, it is emphasized in the literature that the endoscopic approach is particularly attractive under these circumstances, since it achieves the therapeutic objectives with less surgical trauma and without creation of an external fistula that is difficult to manage. In addition to infected pseudocysts, other complex situations such as infected pancreatic necrosis have been successfully managed by means of endoscopy in selected cases.

The debate between the various techniques is far from being exhausted. Comprehension of the physiopathology and natural history has helped in choosing the best form of treatment. The important point is that the therapeutic principles can be attained through careful assessment and actions by professionals with experienced of the various types of treatment available. [14, 15]

# 7. Vascular complications

Although pseudoaneurysms and obstruction or thrombosis of the splenic vein, with consequent segmental, selective or left-side portal hypertension, are rare, they follow a course with high morbidity and mortality, especially if not identified and treated effectively. Recent studies have shown that vascular complications of chronic pancreatitis occur more frequently than had been supposed in the past. It is therefore necessary for physicians to be alert in relation to the clinical situations from which these complications may arise, and for them to know the options available for making the diagnosis and implementing effective treatment. These complications have high morbidity and mortality, such that the mortality rate may reach levels close to or even exceeding 50%.

Among the causes of digestive hemorrhage in situations of chronic pancreatic disease, not only the commonest causes like peptic ulcer disease and acute lesions of the gastroduodenal mucosa should be considered, but also the vascular complications of chronic pancreatitis. [16]

### 7.1. Arterial complications

When the vascular involvement is arterial, it can evolve in two distinct manners: free hemorrhage in the abdominal cavity or formation of a vascular cystic mass called a pseudoaneurysm.

The splenic artery is the one most commonly involved, followed by the gastro-duodenal, pancreatico-duodenal and hepatic arteries. [16, 17]

## 7.1.1. Pseudoaneurysm of the splenic artery

Pseudoaneurysm of the splenic artery generally results from the action of proteolytic enzymes that are released during the pancreatic inflammatory process. These enzymes cause arterial erosion that may result in free hemorrhage into the gastrointestinal tract or directly into the peritoneal cavity (thereby leading to hemoperitoneum), or may result in formation of pseudoaneurysm. (Diagram 1.)

Pathogenesis of obstruction of thrombosis of the splenic vein

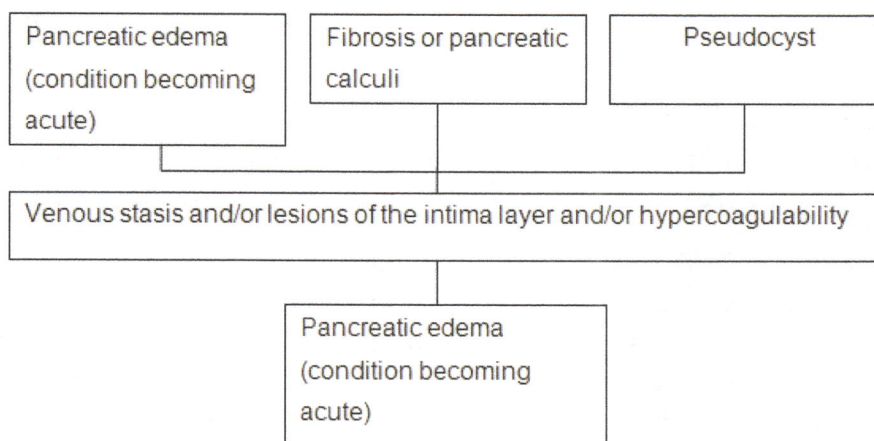

| Pancreatic edema (condition becoming acute) | Fibrosis or pancreatic calculi | Pseudocyst |
|---|---|---|

Venous stasis and/or lesions of the intima layer and/or hypercoagulability

Pancreatic edema (condition becoming acute)

**Diagram 1**

Pseudoaneurysms originate when weakening of the arterial wall leads to aneurysmatic vascular dilation, generally of an artery adjacent to a pancreatic pseudocyst. The latter then tends to involve the aneurysmatic sac. Pseudocysts occur in 10% to 40% of the patients with chronic pancreatitis and up to 10% of these patients present associated pseudoaneurysms. Bleeding occurs in up to 75% of the cases and is often severe. The mortality rate ranges from 18% to 29% among the patients undergoing treatment and may reach 90%-100% among untreated individuals.

### 7.1.1.1. Clinical picture

Clinically, the bleeding that results from pseudoaneurysms can manifest in different forms, from intermittent gastrointestinal bleeding to massive hemorrhage with collapse of the circulation and death. Rupture of the pseudoaneurysm into the pancreatic duct, with subsequent gastrointestinal bleeding, known as *hemosuccus pancreaticus* or Wirsungorrhage, should be considered as a complication in patients with chronic pancreatitis and digestive hemorrhage, and it is potentially fatal. This complication generally presents as intermittent digestive hemorrhage in association with abdominal pain, hyperamylasemia and/or hyperlipasemia resulting from acute distension of the pancreatic duct due to the hemorrhage. Through the Wirsung duct, the blood crosses the ampulla of Vater and flows into the gastrointestinal tract, which may result in melena, hematemesis or hematochezia. In cases in which the pseudoaneurysm is not in communication with the pancreatic duct, the bleeding originating from its rupture may continue to be held inside the pseudocyst and is manifested in the form of abdominal pain, a rapid increase in pseudocyst volume (identified on physical examination or through image evaluation methods) and a decrease in hematocrit. [19]

### 7.1.1.2. Diagnosis

Some authors have suggested that abdominal ultrasound should be the first examination to be performed. Ultrasound used in association with Doppler is very useful, since it allows the pulsatile arterial flow to be viewed inside cystic masses, thus strengthening the diagnosis of pseudoaneurysm.

Dynamic CT with venous contrast in a bolus seems to be the best noninvasive method for diagnosing arterial complications in patients with chronic pancreatitis, especially in relation to identifying pseudoaneurysms, with sensitivity of around 80% to 100%.

In comparison with CT, MRI presents the advantage of not requiring ionizing radiation. Moreover, it can be performed with intravenous administration of gadolinium, which is a substance equivalent to the iodinated contrast medium of CT, but free from its adverse effects. Thus, this method can be used safely in individuals with a previous history of hypersensitivity to contrast and also in those with kidney disorders. Vascular anatomical studies conducted using MRI (angioresonance) have provided images similar to those obtained through conventional angiography. Thus, during the arterial phase, after intravenous administration of gadolinium in bolus form, it is possible to analyze the vascular anatomy in detail and identify cases of pseudoaneurysm formation.

ERCP has less usefulness in cases of complications vasculares pancreatitis chronic (CVPC) in particular, except that on rare occasions it is able to demonstrate active bleeding originating from the ampulla of Vater.

Out of all the methods available, angiography is still the most trustworthy of them and it continues to be the gold standard for diagnosing the arterial complications of chronic pancreatitis. It makes it possible to diagnose pseudoaneurysms, even if they are small, which is an advantageous characteristic given that up to 20% of these are not large enough to be detected through other imaging methods. Furthermore, if it is performed during the active phase of hemorrhaging, it allows the exact site of bleeding to be located, identified from the extravasation of contrast from a given vessel. It should always be performed before the surgical procedure, of the patient's hemodynamic state allows this, thus ensuring safety and success in the operation. The main reason for this is that identifying the bleeding vessel during surgery may be difficult due to the inflammation, necrosis and friability of adjacent tissues (caused by the pancreatitis), which may result in incorrect ligature of a vessel or even total inability to control the bleeding. Angiography also offers the advantage that, in selected patients, it also constitutes a therapeutic method, as will be seen below. [18-19].(Fig. 9-10)

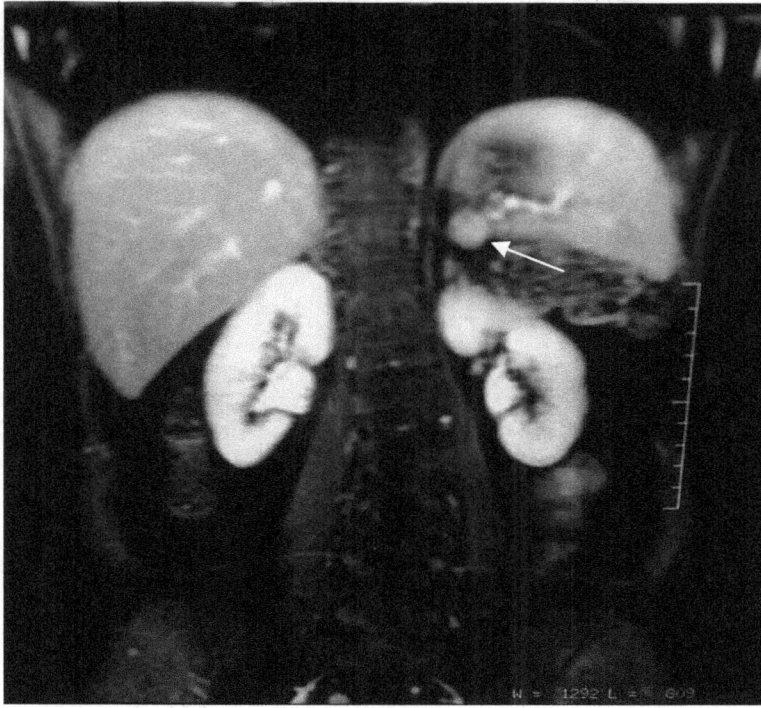

**Figure 9.** RM, arrow showing pseudoaneurysm of splenic artery

## 7.1.1.3. Treatment

After diagnostic confirmation and angiographic identification of the origin of the bleeding, treatment should be instituted as soon as possible. The ideal strategy for pseudoaneurysms is still a matter of debate, but the choices are surgical treatment, therapeutic angiography or a combination of these two. Nonetheless, the choice has to be guided by two main factors: the patient's hemodynamic condition and identification of the exact site from which the bleeding originates.

In patients who are unstable from a hemodynamic point of view, the preferred treatment is surgical, which should be performed immediately. However, there is no consensus among the various authors regarding the ideal surgical procedure to perform. Most authors have recommended surgical resection of the pseudoaneurysm in association with resection of the pancreatic area affected. On the other hand, others have suggested performing proximal and distal ligature of the vessel that has been identified as the source of the bleeding, in association with internal drainage of the pseudocyst, without the need for pancreatic resection.

Locating the exact point of origin of the bleeding is essential for determining the best therapeutic option, given that it has been observed that pseudoaneurysms located in the body or tail of the pancreas are more easily dealt with surgically than are those located in the head of

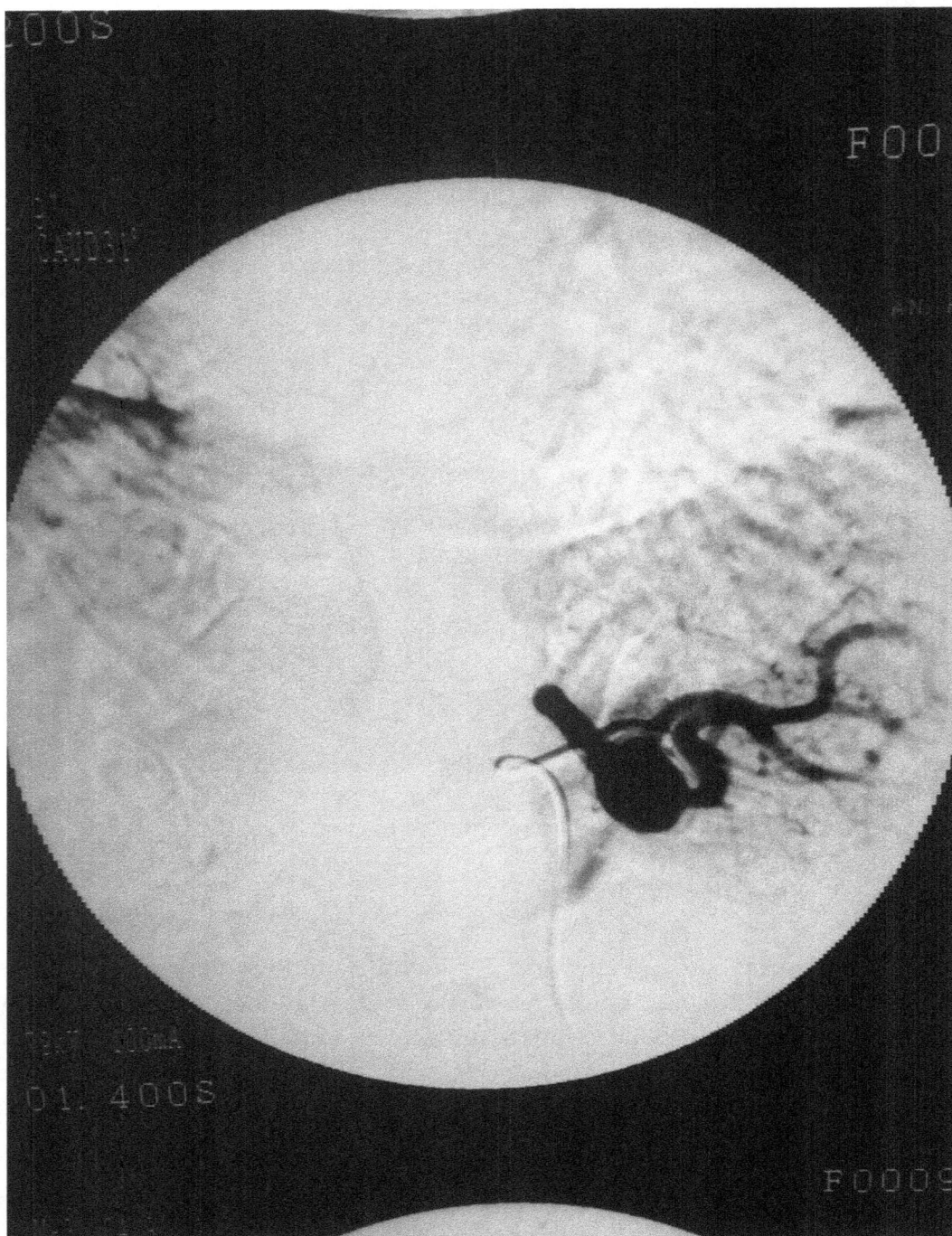

**Figure 10.** Arteriography showing pseudocyst of splenic artery

the organ. The latter generally require the Whipple procedure (duodeno-pancreatectomy), a procedure that leads to much higher surgical mortality. From reviewing the literature, Marshal et al reported that the overall mortality was 16% when pancreatic resection was performed as therapy for pseudoaneurysms located in the body or tail of the pancreas, but when the same procedure was performed to treat pseudoaneurysms located in the head of the pancreas, the mortality rate was much higher, estimated as 43% (Fig. 11)

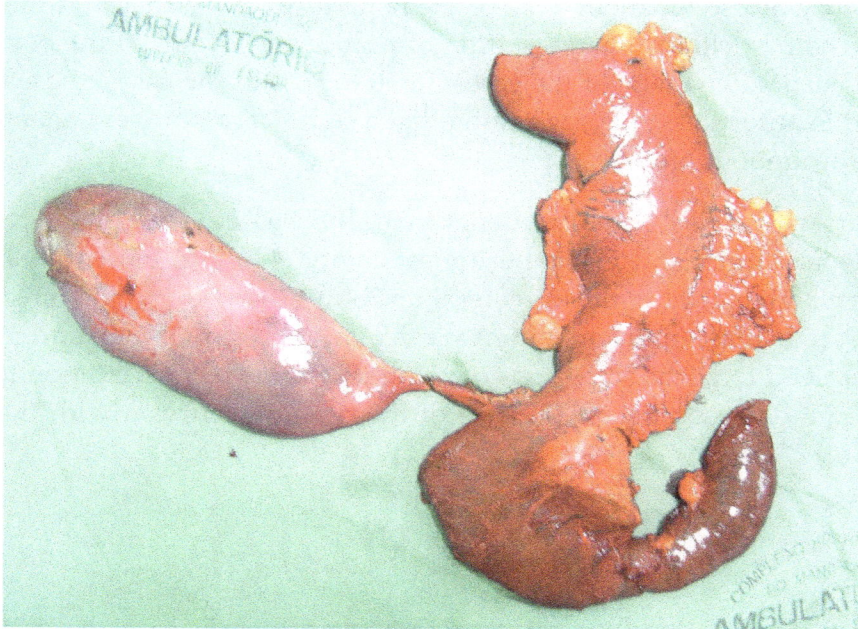

**Figure 11.** Whipple procedure (gastroduodenopancreatectomy)

Although surgical manipulation is frequently necessary for treating the arterial complications of chronic pancreatitis, its use as emergency therapy is becoming progressively lower, as experience with transcutaneous angiographic embolization is being acquired. This method can be used as definitive therapy, or even as temporary therapy. The latter allows bleeding to be controlled so that a surgical procedure can subsequently be performed more safely.

Temporary angiographic embolization consists of selective embolization using gel foam or by means of occlusion using a balloon in the celiac trunk. In both of these procedures, the aim is to reduce the bleeding and bring it under control, to the point at which the patient can be sent for surgery more safely. In some cases, the angiographic procedure may cause not only reduction of the bleeding but also its complete control, thus reducing the need for subsequent surgical treatment. In these cases, angiographic embolization may constitute the definitive therapy. [18, 19]

### 7.1.2. Pseudoaneurysms of the hepatic artery

Pseudoaneurysms of the hepatic artery occur only rarely, but when present, they often rupture (in 56% of the cases). The mortality rate varies, but may reach 40%. The variants that most influence the prognosis for these patients are the individual clinical conditions, the bleeding characteristics of the lesion and the surgical procedure used.

Patients with pseudoaneurysms of the hepatic artery are frequently asymptomatic or present vague pain in the upper quadrant or epigastrium. Symptoms generally appear when complications arise: these are mainly due to extrinsic compression of the biliary tract or rupturing of the pseudoaneurysm. [17]

The natural history of pseudoaneurysms of the hepatic artery is unclear, unlike those of the splenic artery. The first clinical manifestation of pseudoaneurysms of the hepatic artery is a rupture, which occurs in 64-80% of the cases. In 30 to 50% of the cases, these aneurysms are only discovered in autopsies, thus suggesting that a significant number of aneurysms remain asymptomatic throughout life.

Rupturing occurs with almost equal frequency in the biliary tree (41%) (in the common hepatic duct or right hepatic duct) and in the peritoneal cavity (44%). In the latter situation, this is associated with a high mortality rate (greater than 35%). Among the remaining cases, 10% are manifested within the gastrointestinal tract, particularly the duodenum, and 5% in the portal vein, which may lead to portal hypertension. Unlike what is seen in relation to aortic aneurysms, there are no data correlating the size of the pseudoaneurysm with the likelihood of rupture (Diagram 2.).

Arterial complications of chronic pancreatitis

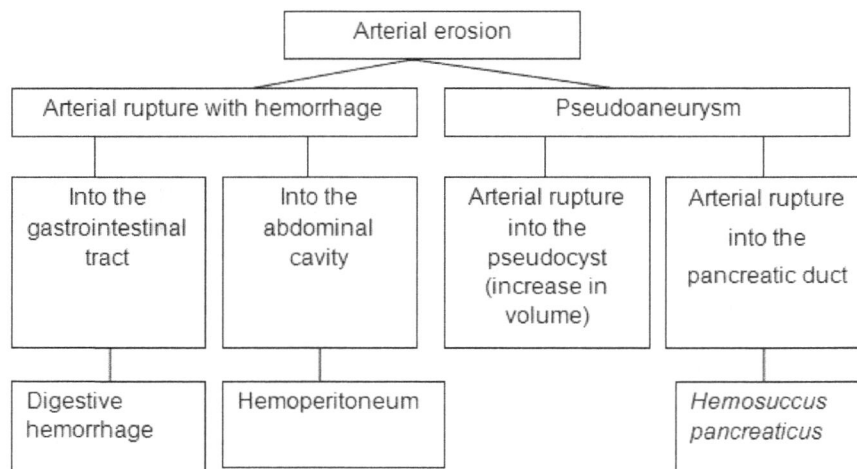

```
                              ┌─────────────────────┐
                              │   Arterial erosion   │
                              └─────────────────────┘
              ┌──────────────────────────┐   ┌──────────────────────────┐
              │ Arterial rupture with     │   │     Pseudoaneurysm        │
              │ hemorrhage                │   │                           │
              └──────────────────────────┘   └──────────────────────────┘
     ┌──────────────┐  ┌──────────────┐  ┌──────────────┐  ┌──────────────┐
     │ Into the      │  │ Into the      │  │ Arterial      │  │ Arterial      │
     │ gastrointestinal│  │ abdominal    │  │ rupture       │  │ rupture       │
     │ tract         │  │ cavity        │  │ into the      │  │ into the      │
     │               │  │               │  │ pseudocyst    │  │ pancreatic duct│
     │               │  │               │  │ (increase in  │  │               │
     │               │  │               │  │ volume)       │  │               │
     └──────────────┘  └──────────────┘  └──────────────┘  └──────────────┘
     ┌──────────────┐  ┌──────────────┐                    ┌──────────────┐
     │ Digestive     │  │ Hemoperitoneum│                    │ Hemosuccus    │
     │ hemorrhage    │  │               │                    │ pancreaticus  │
     └──────────────┘  └──────────────┘                    └──────────────┘
```

**Diagram 2**

Obstructive jaundice may result from hemorrhaging within the biliary tree and secondary obstruction due to coagulum or from extrinsic compression of the duct by a pseudoaneurysm that has not yet ruptured, and this is found in 51% of the patients. The pain presented may be a consequence of coagulum inside the biliary tree or of compression of this, and it is typical of biliary colic.

It is generally difficult to make this diagnosis before the operation and it depends on whether there is a high degree of suspicion. The diagnosis may particularly be suspected in cases of upper digestive hemorrhage in which endoscopy fails to reveal its origin. Regarding diagnostic means, the propaedeutics are the same as cited above for aneurysms of the splenic artery.

Currently, the preferred treatment is embolization by means of angiography. In patients who are hemodynamically unstable, the management indicated is emergency surgery. Some

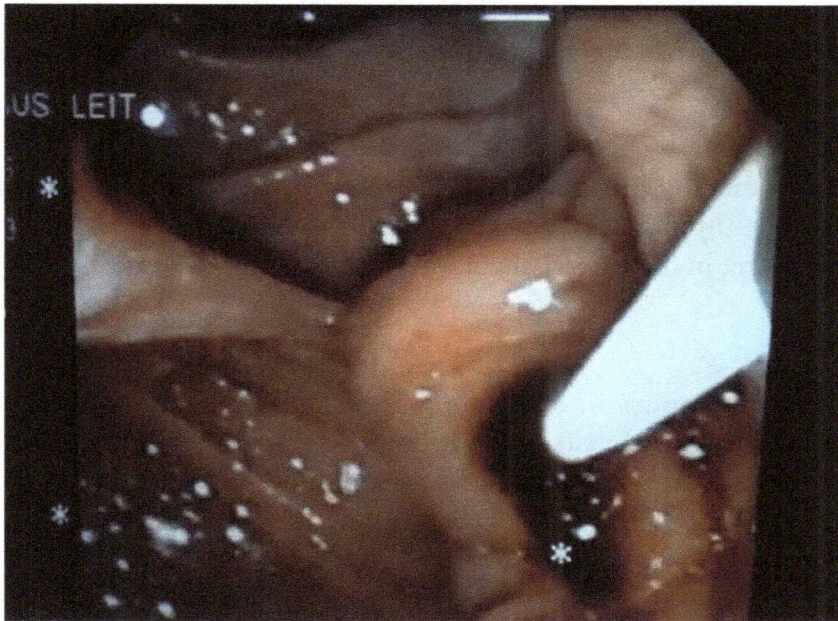

**Figure 12.** ERCP showing hemobilia

exceptional cases without immediate risk of rupture and without progressive increase in size or hemodynamic instability can be managed using conservative therapy, through serial imaging examinations and appropriate treatment of the associated infections. [18, 19-20]

## 7.2. Venous complications

### 7.2.1. Extrahepatic portal hypertension

The main cause of hypertension of the portal vein system is cirrhosis, while pancreatitis is an uncommon etiology. It may be limited to the superior mesenteric vein (which is a branch of the splenic vein) or it may involve the entire splenic-mesenteric-portal system. The portal hypertension caused by pancreatitis usually results from extrinsic venous compression due to a pseudocyst or pseudotumor, which are the most frequent complications of chronic pancreatitis. It can be classified into two forms: occlusive and non-occlusive. [21]

Its pathogenesis involves various factors. It is believed that the inflammatory process causes the initial damage, with degeneration of the vascular wall, venous spasms, stasis and thrombosis. The anatomical location and contiguity processes have the effect that the splenic vein is more vulnerable to this process, because of its location close to the posterosuperior border of the pancreas. It has been observed that simple dilation of the pancreas is sufficient to produce an obstruction of the splenic vein.

Venous drainage of the spleen usually takes place not only through the splenic vein but also through the short gastric veins and from these to the right and left gastric veins. Thus, if the splenic vein is obstructed, dilation of the venous system of the submucosa of the stomach may occur, with formation of gastric varices, separately or in association with esophageal varices.

Although it has been observed that gastric varices alone are highly suggestive of obstruction of the splenic vein, with consequent left segmental hypertension, an association with esophageal varices is not uncommon. [22, 23]

Another drainage route for the spleen is through the gastroepiploic veins, which drain to the superior mesenteric vein and then to the portal vein. In the presence of left segmental hypertension, the left gastroepiploic vein may also drain through tributaries of the inferior mesenteric vein, thus resulting in formation of colonic varices. [22]

### 7.2.1.1. Clinical picture

The presence of gastric varices in association with splenomegaly, with preserved hepatic function, should suggest a diagnosis of left segmental hypertension with consequent O/TVS (obstruction / thrombosis of the splenic vein), although not all patients present this complete trio. Clinically, the evolution may be either asymptomatic or symptomatic. [22]

### 7.2.1.2. Diagnosis

By performing upper digestive endoscopy, gastric and/or gastroesophageal varices and their characteristics, including signs or current or recent bleeding, can be viewed. The diagnosis can be complemented with abdominal US with color Doppler, MRI (angioresonance), angiography and, more recently, endoscopic US. [23]

### 7.2.1.3. Treatment

Among symptomatic patients, splenectomy is the most effective surgical procedure for permanently controlling the gastrointestinal bleeding in patients with O/TVS and left segmental hypertension. Among asymptomatic patients, even if they present varices in the gastric fundus but without evidence of bleeding, there is controversy regarding the case management. It has been proposed that these patients should be treated expectantly, considering that only a small percentage will possibly present bleeding and that these patients would only require a surgical procedure at that time. For patients for whom surgery is impossible, endoscopic treatment comprising sclerotherapy can be attempted. [24]

## 8. Cavity effusion

Cavity effusion in cases of chronic pancreatitis can be explained by two theories: they may arise through the outflow of pancreatic juices anteriorly to the peritoneum (pancreatic ascites) or posteriorly through the diaphragm to the pleura (pleural effusion), through rupturing of the main pancreatic duct or one of its branches. Pleural effusion may also be caused by the passage of blood and lymph that are rich in pancreatic enzymes, close to the pleura, thus causing reactional pleurisy with small-scale effusion. [25]

Both of these are rare complications, but they are significant in cases of chronic pancreatitis and have a mortality rate of 20% if they are not adequately treated.

Both the volume of ascites and the abdominal pain vary in intensity. Most patients present painless voluminous ascites and almost always believe that they have alcoholic cirrhosis with ascites. Recent histories of acute pancreatitis are rarely present.

Pleural effusion is more common on the left side and it consists of an exudate rich in amylase and lipase. When the patients are symptomatic, they most commonly present thoracic pain, dyspnea and weight loss. [25, 26]

The diagnosis depends on there being great clinical suspicion and can be confirmed through imaging examinations and analysis of pleural and ascitic fluid in which high amylase and protein content is demonstrated.

In up to 25% of the patients, simultaneous presence of pancreatic ascites and pancreatic pleural effusion can be seen.

Imaging examinations with CT and MRI are useful because, in calcifications of the pancreatic parenchyma, they show dilatation and stenosis of the Wirsung duct and the presence of pseudocysts and fistulas. ERCP is indicated in all cases of internal pancreatic fistulas with ascites and pleural effusion, to search for ductal pathological conditions and to locate the paths of fistulas. [27, 28]

Non-surgical treatment is indicated for patients with pancreatic ascites and pleural effusion of pancreatic origin. The rationale of the treatment consists of diminishing the exocrine pancreatic secretion, thereby stimulating closure of the pancreatic duct at the rupture site. The treatment includes suspension of the oral diet, use if a diet administered via an enteral probe and use of paracentesis or thoracocentesis, as appropriate. For patients who are not treated using clinical means, surgical treatment is indicated after delineating the anatomy of the pancreatic duct, by means of ERCP. Most patients with pancreatic ascites or pleural effusion present extravasation from an incompletely formed or ruptured pseudocyst, whereas a minority present direct extravasation through the duct. Use of endoscopic treatment with sphincterotomy or insertion of a prosthesis into the pancreatic duct to aid in evaluating a small number of patients has been reported, and occlusion of the ductal extravasation can be attempted. [28]

The surgical treatment is based on the findings from pancreatography. Rupture of the pancreatic duct or extravasation from a pseudocyst into the body or tail of the pancreas can be treated by means of distal pancreatectomy or Roux-en-Y pancreatojejunostomy at the extravasation site. Extravasation from the pancreatic duct in the more proximal parts of the gland are treated by means of Roux-en-Y pancreatojejunostomy at the rupture site. [29]

## 9. Obstruction of the bile ducts and gastrointestinal tract

Obstruction of the bile ducts and gastrointestinal tract occurs more in chronic pancreatitis cases because of the repeated upsurges. Over time, these cause replacement of the pancreatic parenchyma by fibrous tissue that, in turn, causes extrinsic compression of the pancreatic duct, end of the bile duct and the second portion of the duodenum and may also cause mechanical obstruction of these structures. [30]

## 9.1. Biliary obstruction

The incidence of biliary obstruction in patients with chronic pancreatitis ranges from 4% to 30%. In 80% to 85% of all individuals, the distal bile duct is completely surrounded by the pancreas, and in the remaining 15% to 20%, it is closely related to the posterior wall of the head of the pancreas. The extent of the bile duct stenosis caused by pancreatic fibrosis depends on the length of the intra-pancreatic portion of the bile duct, which ranges from 1.5 to 6.0 cm. The compression of the bile duct may be of definitive nature, when produced by pancreatic fibrosis in advanced cases, or of transitory nature, as occurs in the majority of the initial forms of the disease. It is caused by edema during acute inflammatory upsurges. The obstruction occurs in such a way that it does not cause total obstruction of the biliary flow, unlike in malignant processes. [30, 31]

### 9.1.1. Clinical manifestations of biliary obstruction

Biliary obstruction is characterized by episodes of exacerbation and remission. In some patients, it may be totally asymptomatic and an incidental finding. Jaundice occurs in 30% to 50% of the patients and may be transitory, recurrent or persistent. Fever, hot and cold flushes and abdominal pain may also occur. Other symptoms include weight loss, weakness, nausea and vomiting.

### 9.1.2. Laboratory tests

Elevation of alkaline phosphatase levels is the most reliable early sign of biliary obstruction, even in the absence of hyperbilirubinemia. Persistently high levels (twice the normal values) are indicative of bile duct obstruction in patients with chronic pancreatitis. Nonetheless, elevated alkaline phosphatase levels are unrelated to the severity of the condition. Transitory increases in alkaline phosphatase and plasma bilirubin levels, which occur frequently during upsurges with acute transformation of chronic pancreatitis, result from pancreatic edema and are only rarely associated with bile duct stenosis. Because of low sensitivity, bilirubin should only serve for providing diagnostic suspicion when there is persistent hyperbilirubinemia.

### 9.1.3. Radiological examinations

US and CT are the methods for investigating obstruction of the biliary tree. CT enables greater diagnostic precision, since it more clearly identifies the nature of the lesion. It also allows evaluations of the pancreatic anatomy and alterations, such as the presence of calcifications, which are indicative of chronic pancreatitis. CT is the main examination for the initial investigation of patients with obstructive jaundice. (Fig. 13)

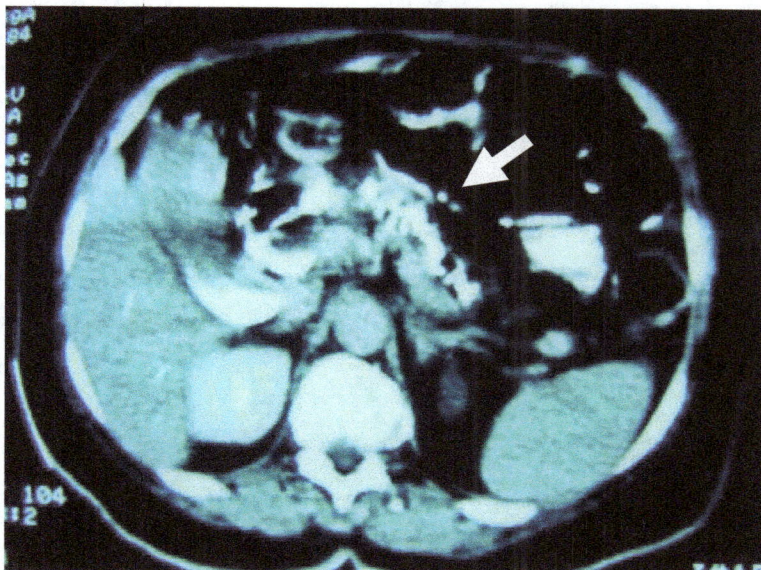

**Figure 13.** Abdominal CT showing pancreatic calcifications

The definitive proof of biliary obstruction comes from cholangiography via ERCP or transhepatic puncture. Another means of obtaining confirmatory images is through using MRI, which enables evaluation of the bile duct without administration of contrast.

The differential diagnosis between cholestasis caused by chronic pancreatitis and by pancreatic adenocarcinoma may be difficult, particularly among patients with preexisting chronic pancreatitis. The parameters that are most useful for this differentiation are age (lower among patients with chronic pancreatitis) and bilirubin levels (higher among patients with adenocarcinoma). The cholangiographic appearance of the progressive compression of the bile duct in chronic pancreatitis cases may be useful for distinguishing it from adenocarcinoma. [25]

*9.1.4. Treatment*

The decision on the management to be used in treating biliary obstruction in patients with chronic pancreatitis should be based on the form of clinical presentation and on an assessment of the risks involved in expectant management. The clinical and laboratory data that favor interventionist management include the presence of jaundice and elevated bilirubin and alkaline phosphatase levels for a period of more than one month, presence of associated cholangitis and/or choledocolithiasis, biliary cirrhosis diagnosed by means of liver biopsy and suspected presence of cancer. Another indication for biliary drainage in patients with chronic pancreatitis is a finding of compression of the bile duct in patients with an indication for surgical treatment of their chronic pancreatitis in order to control pain. (Fig.14)

## 9.2. Duodenal obstruction

Duodenal obstruction in patients with chronic pancreatitis occurs much less frequently than biliary obstruction. The precise mechanism for the duodenal obstruction caused by chronic

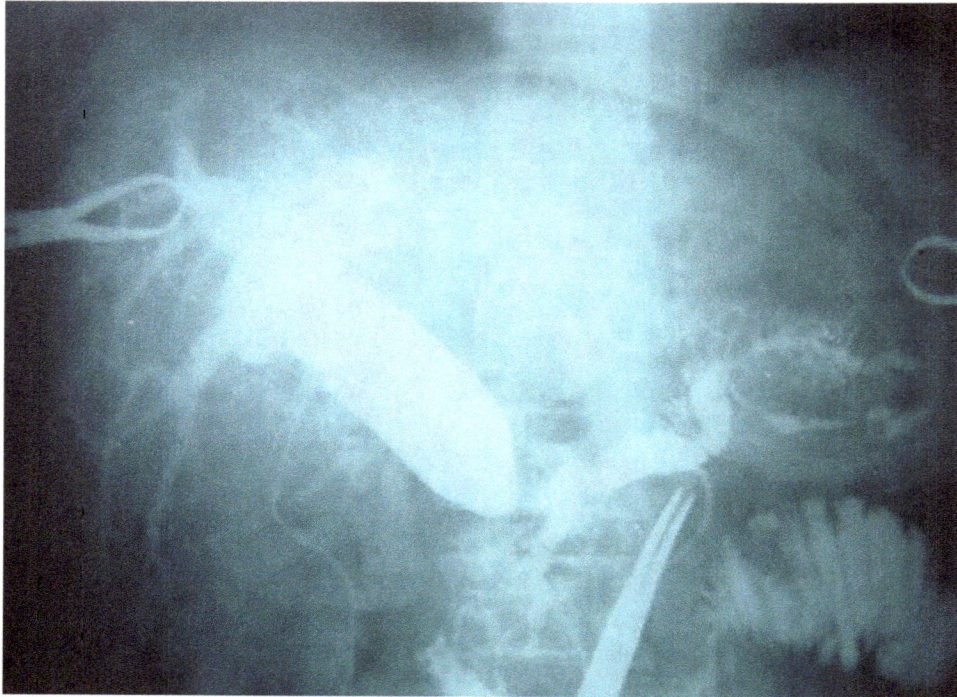

**Figure 14.** During the operation: dilation of the Wirsung duct and bile ducts

pancreatitis is unknown. It can present in two forms: transitory obstruction (more frequent) caused by the edema that is characteristic of periods when the disease becomes acute; and, more rarely, obstruction that is more prolonged or even permanent, caused by fibrosis located in the cephalic portion of the pancreas. The factors responsible for transformation of the edema in the fibrosis that causes the obstructive process are not fully known, but several studies have shown that pancreatic-duodenal ischemia (which is known to occur in experimental and clinical chronic pancreatitis) has a role. [25]

### 9.2.1. Clinical manifestations

The main symptoms of duodenal obstruction are persistent nausea and vomiting of increasing intensity, without accompanying pain. This diagnosis should be suspected when the symptoms persist for more than two weeks after the start of the clinical treatment. Vomiting generally occurs soon after meals and brings back the recently ingested food. It may be bilious if the obstruction is distal to the duodenal papilla.

### 9.2.2. Radiological and endoscopic diagnosis

Duodenal obstruction caused by chronic pancreatitis can be demonstrated through upper digestive endoscopy or contrasted radiological examination of the stomach and duodenum. The appearance is nonspecific, but the contrasted examination generally shows long uniform compression in the second portion of the duodenum, while the endoscopic examination demonstrates a fixed extrinsic concentric obstruction in the post-bulbar portion [26-28]. (fig 15)

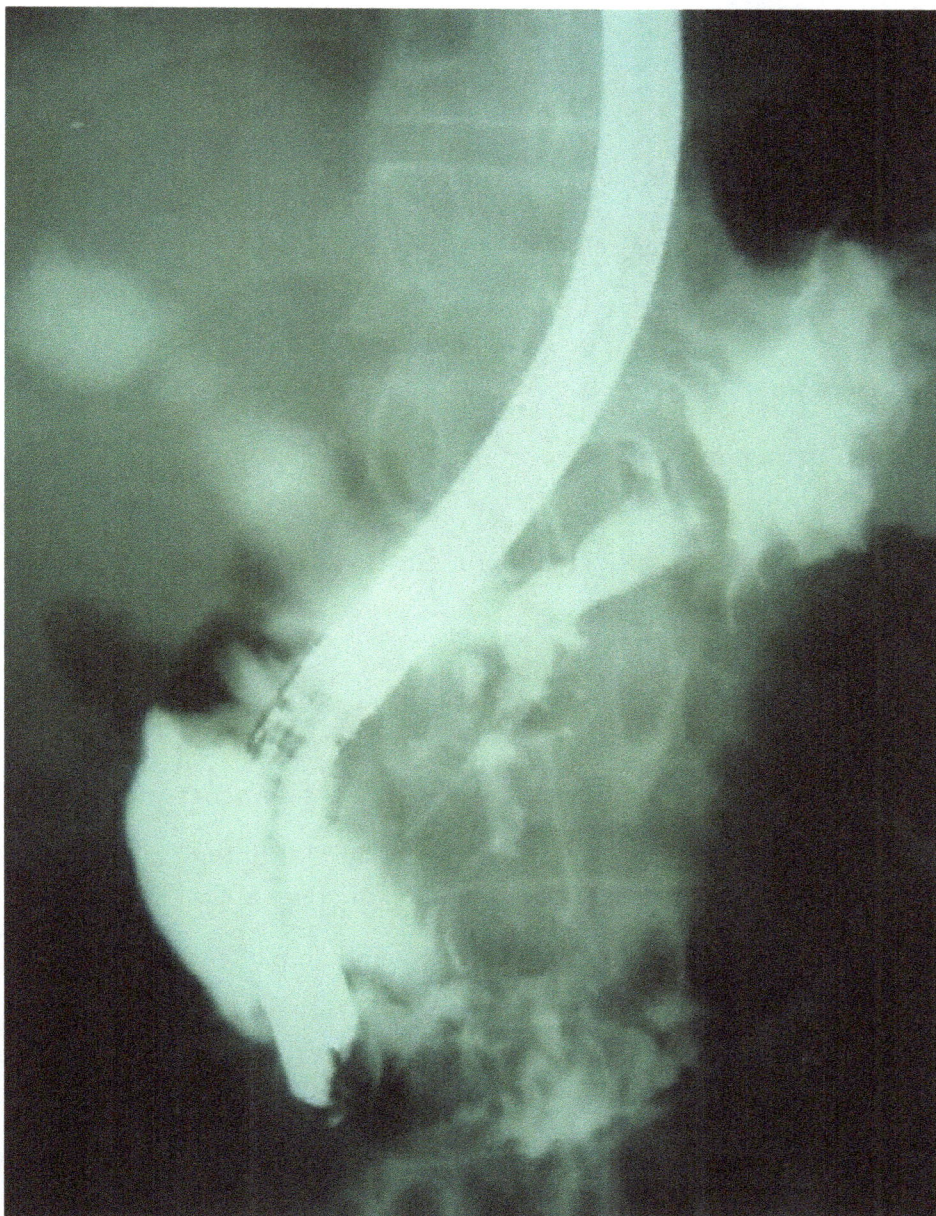

**Figure 15.** ERCP showing dilation of Wirsung duct and bile duct

## 9.2.3. Treatment

In most cases, the duodenal obstruction caused by pancreatic edema during crises of acute transformation of chronic pancreatitis responds favorably to clinical treatment consisting of fasting and parenteral nutrition. Persistence of the obstructive condition for more than four weeks of conservative treatment is very rare, but constitutes an indication for a surgical bypass. Patients with previous episodes of intermittent obstruction of the upper digestive tract probably have obstructions caused by fibrosis of the pancreas and are also candidates for surgical treatment. [29-32]

## Author details

Rone Antônio Alves de Abreu[1,2,3*] and Manlio Basilio Speranzini[4,5]

*Address all correspondence to: roneabreu@uol.com.br

1 Faculty of Medicine ITPAC-Araguaína – Tocantins, Brazil

2 Federal University of São Paulo – UNIFESP, Brazil

3 General Surgery of Hospital Reference Araguaína – Tocantins, Brazil

4 Department of Gastroenterology, Faculty of Medicine, University of São Paulo (retired), Brazil

5 Hospital Complex of Mandaqui-São Paulo, Brazil

## References

[1] Malaquias, Ana Rita Santos Patrício. "Complicações da pancreatite aguda." (2008).

[2] Lankish PG, Burchard-Reckert S, Peterson M, et al. Etiology and age have a limited influence on the course of acute pancreatitis. Pancreas. 1996.13;344-349.

[3] Bollen, TL, et al. The Atlanta Classification of acute pancreatitis revisited. Br Journal Surgery. 2008;95 6-21.

[4] Eulálio, JMR. Pseudocisto Pancreatico. I Consenso Brasileiro de Pancreatite Crônica. 2010;1 71-80.

[5] Habashi Samir, Draganov Peter V. Pancreatit Pseudocyst. World J Gastroenterology. 2009; 15 38-47

[6] Abreu, RAA, et al. Drenagem endoscópica transmural de pseudocisto pancreatico: resultados a longo prazo. Arq Gastroenterol. 2007;44(1)29-34.

[7] Nealon, WH.Walser, E. Main pancreatic ductal anatomy can direct choice of modality for treating pancreatic pseudocyst (surgery versus percutaneous drainage). Ann Surgery. 2002;235 752-758.

[8] Nealon WH, Walser E. Duct drainage alone is sufficient in the operative management of pancreatic pseudocyst in patients with chronic pancreatitis. Ann Surgery. 2003;237 614-662.

[9] Morton JM et al. A national comparison of surgical versus percutaneous drainage of pancreatic pseudocyst. J Gastrointestinal Surgery.2001;9 15-25.

[10] Mendes, AF; Galvão MC; Alves JG. Pancreatite crônica e suas complicações vasculares. I Consenso Brasileiro de Pancreatite Crônica. 2010;1 81-89.

[11] Santvoor, HC. Et al. Describing peripancreatic collections in severe acute pancreatitis using morphologic terms: an international interobserverver agreement study. Pancreatology.2008;8 593-599.

[12] Atabek, U. Amin, D. Camishion, RC. Pancreatic cystograstrostomy by combined upper endoscopy and percutaneous transgatric instrumentation. Journal Laparoendoscopy Surgery. 1993;3 501-504.

[13] Obermeyer, RJ et al. Laparoscopic pancreatic cystogastrostomy. Laparosc Endos Percutan Technol.2003;13 250-253.

[14] Coelho, D. et al. Management of infected and sterile pancreatic necrosis by programmed endoscopic necrosectomy. Dig Dis. 2008;26 364-369.

[15] Dumonceau Jean-Marc, Gomez Carlos Macias. Endoscopic management of complications of chronic pancreatitis. World J Gastroenterology. 2013;19(3) 7308-7315

[16] Tsu-Jun-Te *et al.* Management and outcomes of blending pseudoanurysm associated with chronic pancreatitis. BMC gastroenterology. 2006;6(2) 3-7.

[17] Yu Yeon Hwa et al. Hepatic artery pseudoaneurysm caused by acute idiopathic pancreatitis. World J Gastroenterology. 2012;18 2291-2294.

[18] Raymundo Selma Regina O. Pseudo aneurisma de artéria hepática: Relata de Caso. Cirurgia Vascular e Angiologia.2004;16 136-144.

[19] Oseguera Guillermo Alberto Ballinas et al. Manejo del pseudoaneurisma de la arteria esplénica. Informe de dos casos. Cirugía y Cirujanos.2011;79(3) 268-273.

[20] Malatesi et al. Pseudoaneurisma dell'arteria splenica: insolito caso de emorragia gastrointestinale in paziente com pancreatite cronica. G Chir.2010; 32 394-396.

[21] Lu ke *et al.* Risk factors and outcomes of intra-abdominal hypertension in patients with severe acute pancreatitis. World Journal of Surgery. 2012;36 171–178.

[22] Izbicki Jakob R. et al. Extra hepatic portal hypertension in Chronic Pancreatitis. Annals of surgery. 2012;236(1) 82–89.

[23] Mifkovic A, et al. Intra-abdominal hypertension and acute pancreatitis. Bratisl Lek Listy. 2013;114(3) 166-171.

[24] Shaikh Zohaib Farooque. Pancreatic ascites in the setting of portal hypertension. BMJ case report. 2011;10 1136-2011.

[25] Cavalcanti, D; Cordeiro, N; Basile, R. Derrames cavitários na Pancreatite Crônica. I Consenso Brasileiro de Pancreatite Crônica.2010;1 91-92.

[26] Cheung Cherry X, et al. Chylous Ascites Post Open Cholecystectomy After Severe Pancreatitis. JOP. J Pancreas.2012;13 278-281.

[27] Matin J. M. Gomez Chylous ascites secondary to acute pancreatitis: a case report and review of literature. Nutr Hosp. 2012;27 314-318.

[28] Smith Emily K *et al*. Acute chylous ascites mimicking acute appendicitis in a patient with pancreatitis. World J Gastroenterology. 2009;15(7) 4849-4852,

[29] Khan Fahmi Yousef, Matar Issa. Chylous ascites secondary to hyperlipidemic pancreatitis with normal serum amylase and lipase. World Journal of Gastroenterology. 2007;13 480-482.

[30] Garcia Jose A´ ngel Flores et al, Estómago de retención por estenosis duodenal secundaria a pancreatitis crónica. Cirurgia Espanhola.2013;91 43.

[31] Varghese JC, Masterson A, Lee MJ. Value of MR pancreatography in the evaluation wih chronic pancreatitis. Clinic Radiol. 2002;57 939-957.

[32] Vitellas KM, et al. MR cholangiopancreatography of bile and pancreatic duct abnormalities with emphasis on the single-shot fast spin-echo technique. Radiographics. 2000;20 939-957.

# 4

# Etiology of Pancreatitis and Risk Factors

Eugenia Lauret, María Rodríguez-Peláez and
Luis Rodrigo Sáez

## 1. Introduction

### 1.1. Etiology of pancreatitis and risk factors

Acute pancreatitis (AP) is one of the most common gastrointestinal diseases requiring hospitalization worldwide, with a rising incidence ranging from 13 to 45 per 100,000 persons/ year. The burden of this disease on patients and society is expected to increase even more. Chronic pancreatitis (CP) is a progressive fibro-inflammatory disorder which eventually culminates in permanent impairment of the exocrine and/or endocrine pancreatic function. Although the incidence and prevalence of CP is lower than the reported for AP, this disease significantly reduces patients' quality of life. The annual incidence of CP in industrialized countries has been estimated at 5-12 per 100,000, with a prevalence of about 50 per 100,000 persons [1].

Many conditions are known to potentially cause pancreatitis with varying degrees of certainty, and although some variations have been described between countries, most of cases are attributed to biliary stones or sludge, followed by alcohol abuse. Advances in imaging, molecular biology and genetics have broadened the list of possible etiologies, and the number of presumed idiopathic cases (10-15%) will decrease as our understanding of the disease improves [1,2].

The etiology of pancreatitis should be determined on admission or in the early course of the disease, as this allows the clinician to choose the most appropriate management strategies and therapy in acute phase, and prevent recurrence. A detailed personal history (including data such as previous acute pancreatitis or gallstone disease, alcohol abuse, drug intake, metabolic syndromes, trauma or recent invasive procedures, concomitant autoimmune diseases) and family history of pancreatic disorders can provide guidance for a first etiological approach.

Physical examination, biochemical tests (liver enzymes, calcium, triglycerides) and the appropriate performance of imaging studies will help to make a differential diagnosis among biliary, alcoholic and other causes of pancreatitis.

In this chapter, the aim will be to conduct a comprehensive and updated review of the possible causes of pancreatitis (Table 1) and associated risk factors.

## 2. Risk factors of pancreatitis

### 2.1. Age and sex

Although the incidence of AP do not differ according to sex, CP is more common among men. The risk of AP increases with age, whereas CP mainly affects middle-age individuals. Besides, age and sex distribution is different by etiology. Usually, alcohol-related pancreatitis is more common in middle-aged men. By contrast, pancreatitis in women is more frequent related to gallstones, instrumental procedures, autoimmune diseases or to be idiopathic. Geographic variations observed in age and sex distribution can be partly explained by differences in etiology [1,3].

### 2.2. Race

The risk of pancreatitis is 2 to 3-fold higher among the black population than the whites. Little is known about the possible reasons of this racial disparity and further studies are needed to determine whether these observed differences may be related to dietary, genetic or other factors [1,4].

### 2.3. Lifestyle factors

#### 2.3.1. Diet

The role of dietary factors in the etiology of pancreatitis is unclear. The consumption of high glycemic foods has been associated with an increased risk of non-gallstone-related acute pancreatitis. By contrast, it has been suggested that vegetables and fruit consumption are associated with reduced risk for pancreatic diseases [5,6].

It also should be noted that celiac disease increases the risk of pancreatitis by approximately 3-fold. Diffuse inflammation of the duodenum and papillary stenosis may be the mechanisms involved [7].

Dietary pattern is an area for future research, with other new issues to analyze as the role of the microbiota in pancreatic diseases [8].

#### 2.3.2. Obesity

It has been found that abdominal adiposity increases the risk and severity of AP. The overweight has similar effect for gallstone and non-gallstone-related inflammation [5,9].

*2.3.3. Diabetes*

Some studies found that type 2 diabetes mellitus increases the risk of AP by 1.5 to 3-fold, particularly in younger diabetic patients [10]. This risk may be attributed to diabetes itself, but also to other associated factors with this metabolic disorder (gallstones, hypertriglyceridemia) or the use of antidiabetic drugs such as dipeptidyl peptidase 4 inhibitors (sitagliptin) or glucagon-like peptide 1 agonist (exenatide) [11].

# 3. Etiology of pancreatitis

## 3.1. Obstructive disorders

Mechanical ampullary obstruction can be induced mainly by gallstone, but also for a wide variety of other disorders [1,2].

*3.1.1. Gallstones*

Gallstones (including microlithiasis) are the most common etiology of AP, accounting for at least 35-45% of cases. However, only 3 to 7% of patients with gallstones develop pancreatitis. The risk increases with the age, female gender and small gallstones. The rising incidence of obesity is likely to contribute to AP by promoting gallstone formation.

Proposed mechanisms in the pathogenesis of this disorder include reflux of bile into the pancreatic duct due to transient ampullary obstruction and/or secondary to edema resulting from the passage of stones. Both events may lead to increase pressure in the pancreatic duct, resulting in injury of the gland with release of pancreatic enzymes causing autodigestion and triggering AP [12].

Biliary sludge is a viscous suspension in gallbladder bile that may contain small (< 5mm) stones (i.e., microlithiasis). Its formation has been associated with mechanical or functional conditions that promote bile stasis, such as distal bile duct obstruction, prolonged fasting, total parenteral nutrition or use of ceftriaxone [13]. It is commonly found up to 20-40% of patients initially diagnosed with idiopathic pancreatitis, and in the absence of any other etiology this could be considered as probable cause of the disease.

Gallstones are not recognized as etiology of CP. However, prolonged ductal obstruction may lead to development of CP.

*3.1.2. Pancreatic/ampullary obstruction*

Pancreatic and periampullary tumors can cause pancreatitis. The intraductal papillary mucinous neoplasm is the most commonly involved, due to obstruction of main and/or side branches of pancreatic duct by the tumor itself and/or by mucus secretion [14]. Pancreatic adenocarcinoma can also present as pancreatitis, and the acute attacks may precede the diagnosis of overt malignancy in the gland by several months [15]. It has been estimated that approximately 5-14% of patients with benign or malignant pancreatobiliary tumors are initially diagnosed as idiopathic AP [16]. Unexplained recurrent pancreatitis from the middle age should raise the suspicion of underlying tumor, especially in patients with worrisome associated symptoms (weight loss, new-onset diabetes).

---

### OBSTRUCTIVE

• Gallstones, microlithiasis, "biliary sludge"

• Benign and malignant strictures, ampullary or pancreatic tumors, mucin (*intraductal papillary mucinous neoplasms*)

• Anatomic variants: *Pancreas divisum, annular pancreas, choledochal cyst, choledochocele, duodenal duplication, duodenal diverticula*

• Sphincter of Oddi dysfunction

• Parasites (*Ascaris, Anisakis*)

---

### TOXICS

• Alcohol, Tobacco

• Organophosphorous insecticides

• Venoms (*Scorpion, spider*)

• Estricnine

• Heroin, cocaine

• Drugs: *Pentamidine, Thiazide, Furosemide, Azathioprine, 6-Mercaptopurine, Sulindac, Salicylates, L-asparaginase, Valproic acid, Calcium, Estrogen, Tamoxifen, Sulfonamide, Tetracycline.*

---

**METABOLIC.** Hypertriglyceridemia, Hypercalcemia

---

### HEREDITARY / GENETIC

• Hereditary pancreatitis

• Cystic fibrosis

---

### TRAUMA/IATROGENIC

• Post-endoscopic retrograde cholangiopancreatography

• Transparietohepatic cholangiography

• Pancreas biopsy / Fine-needle aspiration

• Transcatheter arterial embolization for hepatocellular carcinoma

• Posoperative

---

### INFECTIONS

• Viruses: *Mumps, Coxsackievirus, Cytomegalovirus, Varicella-zoster, Herpes simplex, EpsteinBarr, Human immunodeficiency virus, Hepatitis A, B and C*

• Bacteria: *Mycoplasma, Mycobacterium tuberculosis, Leptospira, Legionella, Salmonella Typhi*

• Fungi: *Aspergillus*

• Parasites: *Toxoplasma, Cryptosporidium, Clonorchis sinensis*

---

**VASCULAR DISEASE**

- Hypotension/Ischemia
- Vasculitis
- Atheromatosis, emboli to pancreatic vessels
- Hypothermia
- Haemolysis

**AUTOIMMUNE**

**MISCELLANEOUS.** Celiac disease, Crohn´s disease, Severe Burns, Tropical pancreatitis, Posterior Penetrating Duodenal Ulcer

**IDIOPHATIC**

**Table 1.** Etiological factors associated with acute pancreatitis.

### 3.1.3. Anatomic/Functional abnormalities

Other conditions that have been associated with obstructive pancreatitis include anatomic variants and physiologic anomalies of the pancreatic drainage that occur in 10-15 % of the population, including pancreas divisum and sphincter of Oddi dysfunction (SOD).

### 3.1.4. Pancreas divisum

It is the most common congenital malformation of the pancreas. It is due to the fusion failure between the dorsal and ventral pancreas, resulting in separate pancreatic ductal systems. It is found in approximately 7% of autopsy series. The implication of this anatomic variant as a potential cause of AP remains controversial. The proposed pathogenic mechanism is the relative obstruction to pancreatic juice flow through the minor papilla, leading to increased intraductal pressure. However, since the rate of AP in patients with pancreas divisum is similar to the general population, it has been suggested that the involvement of other factors is required to the development of the disease. In this regard, the prevalence of this malformation in patients with mutations in the cystic fibrosis transmembrane conductance regulator *(CFTR)* was found to be higher than in patients with idiopathic or alcohol-related AP, or control subjects [13,17].

### 3.1.5. Sphinter of Oddi dysfunction

SOD is also a controversial cause of AP (Table 2). The involved mechanism is associated with spasm or stenosis of the sphincter muscle controlling the bile and pancreatic flow into the duodenum. Pancreatic-type SOD ranges from patients with pancreatic-type pain, raised serum amylase or lipase and pancreatic duct dilatation (Type I), to those with pancreatic-type pain and no other abnormalities (Type III). The importance of this condition as cause of recurrent AP is not clearly established, although it has been considered to cause up to one third of all cases of idiopathic pancreatitis [16].

| Biliary type | Pancreatic type |
|---|---|
| **Type I**<br>• Biliary-type pain<br>• And all of the following:<br>- Abnormal aminotransferases or alkaline phosphatase (>2 times normal on at least 2 ocassions)<br>- Dilated bile duct (>8 mm) | **Type I**<br>• Pancreatic-type pain<br>• And all of the following:<br>- Amylase/lipase (>1.5 times normal)<br>- Pancreatic duct >6 mm in head or >5mm in body<br>- Delayed drainage of contrast after ERCP (>9 minutes) |
| **Type II**<br>• Biliary-type pain<br>• And one of the following:<br>- Abnormal aminotransferases or alkaline phosphatase (>2 times normal on at least 2 ocassions)<br>- Dilated bile duct (>8 mm) | **Type II**<br>• Pancreatic-type pain<br>• And one or two of the following:<br>- Amylase/lipase (>1.5 times normal)<br>- Pancreatic duct >6 mm in head or >5mm in body<br>- Delayed drainage of contrast after ERCP (>9 minutes) |
| **Type III**<br>Biliary-type pain only | **Type III**<br>Pancreatic-type pain only |

**Table 2.** Sphincter of Oddi dysfunction. Revised Classification Milwaukee. The Rome III Consensus Statement.

## 3.2. Toxics

### 3.2.1. Alcohol

The prevalence of AP is approximately 4-fold higher among subjects who are alcohol consumers compared to nondrinkers. However, the absolute risk of developing alcohol-related pancreatitis is lower than that for chronic alcohol liver diseases and ranges from 5% to 10% for large consumers [18,19]. Alcohol intake is the single most common cause of CP, and the second after gallstones for AP being responsible for about 30-35% of cases of acute attacks.

The risk of acute alcohol-induced pancreatitis increases in a dose-dependent manner, with a threshold for CP of approximately 4-5 drinks/day. Chronic alcoholic patients eventually develop CP after 10 to 20 years of continuous alcohol abuse. The contribution of the beverage type to this risk requires further studies [19,20].

Although the exact mechanism of pancreatic injury remains unclear, alcohol may act directly on the acinar cells as a toxic by promoting the synthesis of enzymes, activation of pancreatic proteases, changes in cellular lipid metabolism, induction of oxidative stress, activation of stellate cells and/or by increasing the sensitivity of the gland to other genetic and environmental factors.

Two pathogenic theories have been described. In one, alcohol-related injury is the result of perturbations in exocrine function leading to an increase of the lithogenicity of pancreatic juice and the formation of protein plugs and stones. Atrophy and fibrosis develop as a result of the obstructive process. The other theory proposed a stepwise progression to fibrosis after recurrent attacks of AP. Inflammation and necrosis from the initial episodes of AP lead to areas of scarring, ductal obstruction, stasis and subsequent stone formation. However, given the low rate of pancreatitis among heavy drinkers, it has been suggested that other genetic and environmental cofactors would be required for the development of alcoholic pancreatitis [19,21].

### 3.2.2. Smoking

Tobacco and alcohol are cofactors that increase the risk of pancreatitis. Furthermore, both habits often coexist and are enhanced in a dose-dependent manner. However, large studies have suggested that smoking alone is an independent risk factor for both AP and CP [22,23].

It has been reported that smoking increases by approximately 2-fold the risk of non-gallstone-related AP, but not for gallstone-related pancreatitis. This risk was higher in patients who consumed alcohol, current smokers and those with more than 20 packs-years of smoking, particularly if they met the three characteristics (relative risk, 4.12) [24].

Regarding CP, smoking alone has been attributed 25% of the risk for this disease. It has been calculated a risk more than 2-fold among subjects who smoked less than one pack/day, and more than 3-fold for those with higher consumption [25].

At this time, there is very little information about the pathogenesis of smoking-induced pancreatitis compared with those of other causes. Data from animal models suggest several potential mechanisms such as altered gene expression in the exocrine pancreas and activation of pancreatic enzymes with acinar cell damage. Nicotine has also been shown to modulate the oxidative stress and lipid peroxidation and these processes might be involved in the pathophysiology of acute and chronic pancreatitis. As is becoming evident with respect to alcohol, there may be other environmental and/or genetic factors that may promote pancreatic injury with smoking [26].

### 3.2.3. Drugs

AP due to drugs is a rare event (2%). Over one hundred of different medications have been related in the development of the disease by several mechanims. These include immunologic reactions (azathioprine, 6-mercaptopurine, aminosalicylates, sulfonamides), a direct toxic effect (diuretics, sulfonamides), accumulation of toxic metabolites (valproic acid, didanosine, pentamidine, tetracycline), ischemia (diuretics, azathioprine), intravascular thrombosis (estrogen), and increased viscosity of pancreatic juice (diuretics and steroids). No medications are known to cause CP.

Drug-induced pancreatitis has been classified (I-IV) (Table 3) according to the number of registered cases, latency period and reaction with rechallenge: Class Ia drugs (at least 1 case report with positive rechallenge, excluding all other causes, such as alcohol, hypertriglyceridemia, gallstones, and other drugs), Class Ib drugs (at least 1 case report with positive rechallenge; however, other causes, such as alcohol, hypertriglyceridemia, gallstones, and other drugs were not ruled out), Class II drugs (at least 4 cases in the literature and consistent latency in ≥75% of cases), Class III drugs (at least 2 cases in the literature with no consistent latency among cases and no rechallenge) and Class IV drugs (Not fitting into the earlier-described classes, single case report published in medical literature, without rechallenge). Classes I and II have the greatest potential for causing AP. The time interval between beginning of the drug and the development of the disease is highly variable, depending on the substance involved and its pathogenic mechanism. Therefore, a high index of suspicion and a detailed drug history are essential for making the diagnosis [27,28].

### 3.2.4. Others toxics

Organophosphate pesticides, arachnids and reptiles venoms have been described to cause AP by cholinergic stimulation [2]. Cocaine consumption may cause pancreatitis by vasoconstrictor and ischemic effects [29].

**Class IA**

| | | | |
|---|---|---|---|
| α-methyldopa | Cytosine | Mesalamine | Simvastatin |
| Azodisalicylate | Arabinoside | Metronidazole | Stibogluconate |
| Bezafibrate | Dapsone | Pentamidine | Sulfamethoxazole |
| Cannabis | Enalapril | Pravastatin | Sulindac |
| Carbimazole | Furosemide | Procainamide | Tetracycline |
| Codeine | Isoniazid | Pyritonol | Valproic acid |

**Class IB**

| | | | |
|---|---|---|---|
| All-trans-retinoic acid | Lamivudine | Meglumine | Premarin |
| Amiodarone | Losartan | Methimazole | Sulfamethazole |
| Azathioprine | Lynesterol/ | Nelfinavir | Trimethoprim- |
| Clomiphene | Metho-xyethinylestradiol | Norethindronate/ | sulfamethazole |
| Dexamethasone | 6- Mercaptopurine | mestranol | |
| Ifosfamida | | Omeprazole | |

**Class II**

| | | | |
|---|---|---|---|
| Acetaminophen | Didanosine | L-asparaginase | Propofol |
| Chlorthiazide | Erythromycin | Pegasparagase | Tamoxifen |
| Clozapine | Estrogen | | |

**Class III**

| | | | |
|---|---|---|---|
| Aledronate | Cimetidine | Interferon/ribavirin | Metformin |
| Atorvastatin | Clarithromycin | Irbesartan | Minocycline |
| Carbamazepine | Cyclosporin | Isotretinoin | Mirtazapine |
| Captopril | Gold | Ketorolac | Naproxen |
| Ceftriaxone | Hydrochlorothiazide | Lisinopril | Paclitaxel |
| Chlorothalidone | Indomethacin | Metalozone | Prednisone |
| | | | Prednisolone |

**Class IV**

| | | | |
|---|---|---|---|
| Adrenocorticotrophic hormone | Cisplatin | Diclofenac | Fluvastatin |
| Ampicillin | Colchicine | Difenoxylate | Gemfibrozil |

| | | | |
|---|---|---|---|
| Bendroflumethiazide | Cyclophosphamide | Doxorubicin | Interleukin-2 |
| Benzapril | Cyproheptidine | Ethacrinic acid | Ketoprofen |
| Betamethazone | Danazol | Famciclovir | Lovastatin |
| Capecytabine | Diazoxide | Finasteride | Mefanamic acid |
| | | 5-fluorouracil | Nitrofurantoin |

*Data modified from Badalov N et al [28].*

**Table 3.** Summary of the medications associated with pancreatitis based on Drug Class.

## 3.3. Metabolic disorders

### 3.3.1. Hypertriglyceridemia

This type of hyperlipidemia induces AP in about 1-4% of cases, and this is an uncommon etiology of CP. The disease typically develops in patients with a history of familiar hyperlipidemia and/or an associated secondary factor as uncontrolled diabetes, alcohol consumption, hypothyroidism, nephrotic syndrome, drug intake or pregnancy. The risk is particularly increased in patients with AP not due to alcoholic or obstructive causes and with high serum triglyceride concentrations above 1000 mg/dL. Mild-to-moderate hyperlipidemia is often secondary to alcoholic AP, and should not be confused with marked hypertriglyceridemia causing AP [2].

The mechanism of hypertriglyceridemia induced pancreatitis is unclear though some authors suggest stimulation of amylase release, cell damage from free fatty acids and chylomicrons in acinar cells, and sluggish flow in the capillaries resulting in ischemic injury [13].

### 3.3.2. Hypercalcemia

This is a rare cause of AP and almost always happens as result of concomitant hyperparathyroidism. Pancreatitis has been reported to be related to endogenous hypercalcemia by disseminated carcinoma and after iatrogenic effect, for example with total parenteral nutrition or vitamin D poisoning. Proposed mechanisms include deposition of calcium in pancreatic duct and calcium activation of trypsinogen within the pancreatic parenchyma. Because the incidence of pancreatitis is low in patients with chronic hypercalcemia, additional factors are probable necessary to induce acute episodes [13,30].

## 3.4. Hereditary/genetic pancreatitis

In pancreatitis, alterations in several genes have so far been described [31].

Hereditary pancreatitis is an autosomal dominant disorder with high penetrance rates up to 80%. This disorder is associated with mutations in the trypsinogen gen *PRSS1* that promotes the premature conversion of trypsinogen to active trypsin, resulting in pancreatic autodigestion. This genetic syndrome is characterized by a strong family history of pancreatic disease, and most patients develop recurrent pancreatitis from childhood, with progressive evolution to CP and a significant increase in risk of pancreatic cancer.

Severe homozygote mutations in *CFTR* gene cause cystic fibrosis. Patients who are compound heterozygotes for mild mutations have 40 to 80-fold increased risk of developing CP compared with the general population, without presenting other manifestations of cystic fibrosis and with a normal sweat chloride test.

Mutations in the serine protease inhibitor kazal type 1 gene (*SPINK1*) and chymotrypsin C (CTRC) are associated with acute and chronic pancreatitis. Patients who have severe mutations typically develop CP in childhood. Other mutations predispose to the development, but do not necessarily cause pancreatitis.

## 3.5. Trauma and medical procedures

### 3.5.1. Blunt or penetrating trauma

Both types of injuries may cause pancreatitis in about 0.2% and 1% cases respectively, ranging from a mild contusion to a severe damage [2]. These conditions can lead to acute duct rupture and pancreatic ascites. The low rates of AP after trauma result from the retroperitoneal location of the gland. The injury healing may result in a narrowing of the main pancreatic duct, causing obstructive pancreatitis in the gland downstream from the stricture.

Rarely a posterior duodenal ulcer can penetrate into the pancreas and thereby induce AP. This complication may present as gastrointestinal bleeding.

### 3.5.2. Post-ERCP

The result of instrumentation of the gland as in endoscopic retrograde cholangiopancreatography (ERCP) can result in post-ERCP pancreatitis. This injury occurs in 3-5% of unselected patients and although the episodes are usually mild, up to 11% of cases the disease is severe. The risk of post-ERCP pancreatitis may be increased up to 25% in those with suspected SOD or in those with a prior history of post-ERCP pancreatitis. Other risk factors for the development of this complication include young age, female sex, repeated attempts of papilla cannulation and poor emptying of pancreatic duct after contrast injection. Proposed underlying mechanisms that may be involved in the pathogenesis of post-ERCP pancreatitis are mechanic damage from manipulation, and/or chemical, hydrostatic or thermal injury around the papillary orifice or over pancreatic duct [32,33].

### 3.5.3. Postoperative pancreatitis

This complication can occur after abdominal or thoracic surgery. It has been described in about 0.4-7.6% after cardiopulmonary bypass and 6% after liver transplantation. Significant risks for postoperative pancreatitis include renal insufficiency, hypotension, and infections. Intraoperative or postoperative medications may also cause pancreatitis [34,35].

Other procedures have also been described as cause of iatrogenic pancreatitis (transparietohepatic cholangiography, pancreatic biopsy/fine-needle aspiration). Pancreatitis after transarterial embolization for the treatment of hepatocellular carcinoma results from a retrograde injection of the chemotherapeutic or embolic agents into pancreatic arteries, giving rise to ischemic pancreatitis [36].

## 3.6. Infectious diseaSES

Many infectious agents are associated with AP (Table 1), but no microorganism has ever been identified within the pancreas. Mumps and Coxsackie B virus are the most common causes of infectious pancreatitis. Other viruses (Cytomegalovirus, Herpes simplex, Varicella-zoster, Hepatitis B), bacteria (*Salmonella typhi, Leptospira, Legionella*), fungi (*Aspergillus*) and parasites (*Toxoplasma, Cryptosporidium*) have all been associated with AP. *Clonorchis sinensis* and *Ascaris* cause pancreatitis by invading and blocking the pancreatic duct [2,37].

AP may be caused by HIV infection or secondary to anti-retroviral treatment. In acquired immunodeficiency syndrome (AIDS), other infectious agents may cause pancreatitis including Cytomegalovirus, *Candida, Cryptosporidium neoformans, Toxoplasma gondii, Pneumocystis carinii* and *Mycobacterium avium* complex [38].

## 3.7. Vascular diseases

Pancreatic ischemia has been reported in the following circumstances: hypotension, hemor-rhagic shock, vasculitis (systemic lupus erythematosus and polyarteritis nodosa), atheroemb-olism, hypothermia, haemolysis and emboli to pancreatic vessels. It has been described episodes of AP in long-distance runners, on an ischemic basis [2].

## 3.8. Autoimmune pancreatitis

Less than 5% of patients evaluated in a tertiary center with pancreatitis on admission, were diagnosed as autoimmune pancreatitis (AIP). This disease may present in a variety of ways and among patients with this disease, only 10% to 25% have features of AP o CP at the time of presentation.

AIP has distinct clinical and histological features. Two subtypes are known, the type 1 (lymphoplasmacytic sclerosing pancreatitis) is a multi-organ disease associated with IgG4, and type 2 (idiopathic duct centric pancreatitis) appears to be a pancreas-specific disorder with characteristic granulocyte-epithelial lesions [39]. Immunologic abnormalities including hypergammaglobulinemia, elevated serum IgG4 levels and the presence of autoantibodies against lactoferrin and carbonic anhydrase are important serological markers of the type 1 AIP.

Because the diagnosis can be elusive, several criteria have proposed to diagnose AIP. The most widely used in the United States are the HISORT criteria (histology, imaging, serology, other organ involvement and response to therapy) [40]. Abnormal imaging can be observed in computed tomography, magnetic resonance imaging or endoscopic ultrasound as multifocal or diffuse pancreatic-ductal narrowing, and abnormal enhancement or enlargement of the pancreas. Histologic confirmation is desirable and can be obtained by endoscopic ultrasound-guided biopsy of the pancreas. Ampullary biopsy with IgG4 immunostaining may be a safer alternative with a specificity approaching 100% but a sensitivity of about 50% [41]. AIP clearly responds to steroid therapy although spontaneous resolution without treatment has also been described; however relapses are relatively common. In some cases, other immunosuppressive agents are necessary.

## 3.9. Miscellaneous conditions

### 3.9.1. Celiac disease

There is an increased risk of developing pancreatitis in patients with celiac disease and between 10% and 20% of newly diagnosed patients may develop pancreatic insufficiency. It has been described that celiac disease is associated with a 3-fold increased risk of development any form of pancreatitis and even higher for CP (HR: 19.8). This increased risk was only found among celiac individuals diagnosed in adulthood, and was generally noted in the first year of diagnosis especially for CP and enzyme supplementation, but remained even 5 years after [7].

Several factors might contribute to the association between celiac disease and pancreatitis [13]. The earliest proposed mechanism was malnutrition, which impairs the secretion of pancreatic enzymes and influences the composition of the bile inducing microlithiasis, thus predisposing to development of pancreatitis. Malnutrition has also been described to be associated with increased levels of pro-inflammatory cytokines as well as pancreatic acinar cell damage, ductal disruption and other structural changes, such as acinar atrophy. Other proposed mechanisms include altered levels of autoregulatory enteric hormones (cholecystokinin) and papillary stenosis resulting from localized duodenal inflammation. Another potential explanation involves immunopathogenetic mechanisms, by T helper cell class 1 (TH1) cytokine up-regulation in celiac disease through polymorphisms in tumor necrosis factor-$\alpha$, a TH1 proinflammatory cytokine, which plays an important role in the pathogenesis of severe pancreatitis. Villous atrophy is associated with pancreatic insufficiency, and restored pancreatic enzyme levels are observed after introduction of a gluten-free diet.

By contrast, the relationship between autoimmune pancreatitis and celiac disease has not been demonstrated, since there is only so far a case report of this association [42].

### 3.9.2. Inflammatory bowel disease

Pancreatitis has been associated with inflammatory bowel disease, either secondary to the use of drugs that may potentially cause this disorder or by other mechanisms as duodenal Crohn´s disease leading to pancreatic flow obstruction, or as a result of the granulomatous disease or the autoimmune process directly involving the pancreas [43].

## 3.10. Idiopathic pancreatitis

This condition is defined as pancreatitis with unknown etiology established after initial laboratory and imaging studies. In some patients the cause may be found after further investigations, but in others no definitive etiology is detected. These patients should be evaluated at centers of excellence focusing on pancreatic diseases. It is recommended to complete a comprehensive study, since biliary sludge/microlithiasis may be detected in up to 75% of patients with recurrent AP initially labeled as unknown origin, and it has been estimated that up to 15% of patients with benign or malignant tumors may present as apparent idiopathic pancreatitis. Additionally, the role of genetic testing in idiopathic pancreatitis has yet to be determined, but the study of genetic abnormalities is being increasingly recognized [16,44].

## 4. Conclusions

Pancreatitis is a common digestive disorder with a broad spectrum of etiologies. Although most cases are secondary to biliary stones/sludge or alcohol abuse, other potential causes should be considered once the two most common etiologies have been excluded. One of the primary goals in the diagnostic process of the pancreatitis should be to reduce the rate of idiopathic pancreatitis, because the identification of the cause of the disease may help to prevent subsequent relapses when the etiological factor is eliminated.

## Author details

Eugenia Lauret*, María Rodríguez-Peláez and Luis Rodrigo Sáez

*Address all correspondence to: meugelb@hotmail.com

Gastroenterology Unit, Central University Hospital of Asturias, Asturias, Spain

## References

[1] Yadav D, Lowenfels AB. The epidemiology of pancreatitis and pancreatic cancer. Gastroenterology 2013;144:1252-1261.

[2] Forsmark CE, Baillie J, AGA Institute Clinical Practice and Economics Committee, AGA Institute Governing Board. AGA Institute technical review on acute pancreatitis. Gastroenterology 2007;132:2022-2044.

[3] Yadav D, O'Connell M, Papachristou GI. Natural history following the first attack of acute pancreatitis. Am J Gastroenterol 2012;107:1096-1103.

[4] Yang AL, Vadhavkar S, Singh G, Omary MB. Epidemiology of alcohol-related liver and pancreatic disease in the United States. Arch Intern Med 2008;168:649-656.

[5] Alsamarrai A, Das SL, Windsor JA, Petrov MS. Factors That Affect Risk for Pancreatic Disease in the General Population: A Systematic Review and Meta-analysis of Prospective Cohort Studies. Clin Gastroenterol Hepatol 2014, Feb 5. [Epub ahead of print].

[6]   Oskarsson V, Sadr-Azodi O, Orsini N, Andrén-Sandberg Å, Wolk A. High dietary glycemic load increases the risk of non-gallstone-related acute pancreatitis: a prospective cohort study. Clin Gastroenterol Hepatol 2014;12:676-682.

[7]   Ludvigssons JF, Montgomery SM, Ekbom A. Risk of pancreatitis in 14,000 individuals with celiac disease. Clin Gastroenterol Hepatol 2007;5:1347-1353.

[8]   Farrell JJ, Zhang L, Zhou H, et al. Variations of oral microbiota are associated with pancreatic diseases including pancreatic cancer. Gut 2012;61:582-588.

[9]   Sadr-Azodi O, Orsini N, Andren-Sandberg A, et al. Abdominal and total adiposity and the risk of acute pancreatitis: a population-based prospective cohort study. Am J Gastroenterol 2013;108:133-139.

[10]  Yang L, He Z, Tang X, Liu J. Type 2 diabetes mellitus and the risk of acute pancreatitis: a meta-analysis. Eur J Gastroenterol Hepatol 2013;25:225-231.

[11]  Singh S, Chang HY, Richards TM, Weiner JP, Clark JM, Segal JB. Glucagonlike peptide 1-based therapies and risk of hospitalization for acute pancreatitis in type 2 diabetes mellitus: a population-based matched case-control study. JAMA Intern Med 2013;173:534-539.

[12]  Wang GJ, Gao CF, Wei D, Wang C, Ding SQ. Acute pancreatitis: etiology and common pathogenesis. World J Gastroenterol 2009;15:1427-1430.

[13]  Khan AS, Latif SU, Eloubeidi MA. Controversies in the etiologies of acute pancreatitis. JOP 2010;11:545-552.

[14]  Venkatesh PG, Navaneethan U, Vege SS. Intraductal papillary mucinous neoplasm and acute pancreatitis. J Clin Gastroenterol 2011;45:755-758.

[15]  Munigala S, Kanwal F, Xian H, Scherrer JF, Agarwal B. Increased risk of pancreatic adenocarcinoma after acute pancreatitis. Clin Gastroenterol Hepatol 2014;12:1143-1150.

[16]  Lee JK, Enns R. Review of idiopathic pancreatitis. World J Gastroenterol 2007;13: 6296-6313.

[17]  Bertin C, Pelletier AL, Vullierme MP, et al. Pancreas divisum is not a cause of pancreatitis by itself but acts as a partner of genetic mutations. Am J Gastroenterol 2012;107:311–317.

[18]  Yadav D, Eigenbrodt ML, Briggs MJ, Williams DK, Wiseman EJ. Pancreatitis: prevalence and risk factors among male veterans in a detoxification program. Pancreas 2007;34:390-394.

[19]  Herreros-Villanueva M, Hijona E, Bañales JM, Cosme A, Bujanda L. Alcohol consumption on pancreatic diseases. World J Gastroenterol 2013;19:638-645.

[20] Irving HM, Samokhvalov AV, Rehm J. Alcohol as a risk factor for pancreatitis. A systematic review and meta-analysis. JOP 2009;10:387-392.

[21] Tapia JA, Salido GM, González A. Ethanol consumption as inductor of pancreatitis. World J Gastrointest Pharmacol Ther 2010;1:3-8.

[22] Tolstrup JS, Kristiansen L, Becker U, Grønbæk M. Smoking and Risk of Acute and Chronic Pancreatitis Among Women and Men. A Population-Based Cohort Study. Arch Intern Med 2009;169:603-609.

[23] Luaces-Regueira M, Iglesias-García J, Lindkvist B, et al. Smoking as a risk factor for complications in chronic pancreatitis. Pancreas 2014;43:275-280.

[24] Sadr-Azodi O, Andrén-Sandberg Å, Orsini N, Wolk A. Cigarette smoking, smoking cessation and acute pancreatitis: a prospective population-based study. Gut 2012;61:262-267.

[25] Andriulli A, Botteri E, Almasio PL, et al. Smoking as a cofactor for causation of chronic pancreatitis: a meta-analysis. Pancreas 2010;39:1205-1210.

[26] Alexandre M, Pandol SJ, Gorelick FS, Thrower EC. The emerging role of smoking in the development of pancreatitis. Pancreatology 2011;11:469-474.

[27] Spanier BW, Tuynman HA, Van der Hulst RW, et al. Acute pancreatitis and concomitant use of pancreatitis-associated drugs. Am J Gastroenterol 2011;106:2183-2188.

[28] Badalov N, Baradarian R, Iswara K, et al. Drug-induced acute pancreatitis: an evidence-based review. Clin Gastroenterol Hepatol 2007;5:648-661.

[29] Vázquez-Rodríguez S, Soto S, Fernández E, Baltar R, Vázquez-Astray E. [Cocaine induced acute pancreatitis]. Gastroenterol Hepatol 2009;32:588-589. Spanish.

[30] Abboud B, Daher R, Boujaoude J. Digestive manifestations of parathyroid disorders. World J Gastroenterol 2011;17: 4063-4066.

[31] Ooi CY, Gonska T, Durie PR, Freedman SD. Genetic testing in pancreatitis. Gastroenterology 2010;138:2202-2206.

[32] ASGE Standards of Practice Committee. Complications of ERCP. Gastrointest Endosc 2012;75:467-473.

[33] Donnellan F, Byrne MF. Prevention of Post-ERCP Pancreatitis. Gastroenterol Res Pract 2012;ID 796751. doi: 10.1155/2012/796751.

[34] Perez A, Ito H, Farivar RS, et al. Risk factors and outcomes of pancreatitis after open heart surgery. Am J Surg 2005;190:401-405.

[35] Papachristou GI, Abu-Elmagd KM, Bond G, et al. Pancreaticobiliary complications after composite visceral transplantation: incidence, risk, and management strategies. Gastrointest Endosc 2011;73:1165-1173.

[36] Alcívar-Vásquez JM, Ontanilla-Clavijo G, Ferrer-Ríos MT, Pascasio-Acevedo JM. Acute necrotizing pancreatitis after transarterial chemoembolization of hepatocellular carcinoma: An unusual complication. Rev Esp Enferm Dig 2014;106:147-149.

[37] Parenti DM, Steinberg W, Kang P. Infectious causes of acute pancreatitis. Pancreas 1996;13:356-371.

[38] Dutta SK, Ting CD, Lai LL. Study of prevalence, severity, and etiological factors associated with acute pancreatitis in patients infected with human immunodeficiency virus. Am J Gastroenterol 1997;92:2044-2048.

[39] Chari ST, Kloeppel G, Zhang L, et al. Histopathologic and clinical subtypes of autoimmune pancreatitis: The Honolulu consensus document. Pancreas 2010;39:549-554.

[40] Chari ST. Diagnosis of autoimmune pancreatitis using its five cardinal features: introducing the Mayo Clinic's HISORt criteria. J Gastroenterol 2007;42 (Suppl 18): 39-41.

[41] Moon SH, Kim MH, Park DH, et al. Ig G4 immunostaining of duodenal papillary biopsy specimens may be useful for supporting a diagnosis of autoimmune pancreatitis. Gastrointest Endosc 2010; 71:960-966.

[42] Masoodi I, Wani H, Alsayari K, et al. Celiac disease and autoimmune pancreatitis: an uncommon association. A case report. Eur J Gastroenterol Hepatol 2011;23:1270-1272.

[43] Navaneethan U, Shen B. Hepatopancreatobiliary manifestations and complications associated with inflammatory bowel disease. Inflamm Bowel Dis 2010;16:1598-1619.

[44] Tenner S, Baillie J, DeWitt J, Vege SS. American College of Gastroenterology guideline: management of acute pancreatitis. Am J Gastroenterol 2013;108:1400-1415.

# 5

# The Role of Advanced Endoscopy in Management of Acute Pancreatitis

Charing Ching Ning Chong,
Anthony Yuen Bun Teoh, Paul Bo San Lai,
James Yun Wong  Lau and Francis Ka Leung Chan

## 1. Introduction

Acute pancreatitis is the inflammation of the pancreas as a result of pre-mature activation of the pancreatic enzymes leading to auto-digestion and inflammation.

The Atlanta's classification is the most commonly used classification of acute pancreatitis. [1] It defines acute pancreatitis as acute inflammation of the pancreas which is further classified into mild, moderate and severe forms. Mild acute pancreatitis refers to an attack with no organ dysfunction, local or systemic complications and usually resolves in the first week. Moderately severe acute pancreatitis is defined by the presence of transient organ failure, local complications or exacerbation of co-morbid disease. Severe acute pancreatitis is associated with persistent organ failure, with or without local complications, for more than 48 hours. Local complications include peripancreatic fluid collections, pancreatic and peripancreatic necrosis (sterile or infected), pseudocyst and walled-off necrosis (sterile or infected).

The majority of patients suffer from mild disease but around 20% may suffer from severe disease with local and systemic complications. [2, 3]The use of advanced endoscopy is dramatically changing the management of these patients. Although morbidity and mortality is usually encountered in the group with severe pancreatitis,, it is wise to treat every patient aggressively until disease severity has been established. The goals of initial management are fluid replacement, electrolyte balance, caloric support, and prevention of local and systemic complications.

Gallstone is the leading cause of pancreatitis and accounts for 30-60% of patients in most series. [4-8] Endoscopic retrograde cholangiopancreatography (ERCP) is most helpful in patients with incarcerate bile duct stones and concomitant cholangitis and pancreatic ductal disruption. Endoscopic ultrasound (EUS) guided therapy is replacing surgery in the management of pancreatic fluid collections.

## 2. Role of early endoscopic retrograde cholangiopancreatography

Acute biliary pancreatitis is believed to result from transient obstruction of the common bile duct (CBD). [6-8] The majority of stones will pass out spontaneously. However, some patients will suffer from persistent obstruction and the duration of CBD obstruction is believed to be a critical factor contributing to the severity of pancreatitis. [6] In patients suffering from acute cholangio-pancreatitis, ERCP may provide drainage and relieve the obstruction caused by the presence of a persistent common bile duct stone.

Two early meta-analyses summarized the outcomes from 4 initial randomized trials. [9, 10] The results were controversial. (Table 1) The results from the United Kingdom and Hong Kong studies showed that early ERCP reduced the odds of having complications in patients with predicted severe disease. [11, 12] However, the effect was not significant in mild disease and the reduction in mortalities was also not significant. On the other hand, the Germany study, which only included patients with acute pancreatitis without obstructive jaundice, showed no significant differences in mortalities and morbidities in both groups. [13] The Polish study was the only study demonstrating the significant reduction in mortalities and morbidities in both mild and severe disease. However, the results of this study should be reviewed with caution and the study was only published in abstract form. [14]

After that, two more randomized studies had shown that ERCP in patients without biliary obstruction and cholangitis offered no benefit. [15, 16] These results were included in two more recent meta-analyses which showed that early ERCP in patients with biliary pancreatitis without acute cholangitis did not result in reduced risk of local pancreatic complications, overall complications and mortalities. [17, 18] The Dutch Acute Pancreatitis Study Group had performed a prospective, multicenter study on 153 patients with predicted severe acute biliary pancreatitis without cholangitis who were randomized to conservative treatment or ERCP within 72 hours after symptom onset. [19] Patients without and with cholestasis and/or dilated common bile duct were analyzed separately. They found that early ERCP was only beneficial to the cholestasis group by lowering the complications rate.

The current AGA guideline on gallstone pancreatitis is that, urgent ERCP should be performed in patients with concomitant cholangitis and this should be done within 24 hours after admission. [20] While in patients with high suspicion of a persistent common bile duct stone, early ERCP should be performed within 72 hours after admission. A numbers of studies have attempted to look at the predictive value of ultrasound, biochemical or clinical factors in patients with low to intermediate probability of ductal stones. [21-25] Where used in isolation, these factors all suffer from low sensitivity. However, when used in combination, the variables can help the clinician predict the probability of the presence a CBD stone.

|  | United Kingdom [11] | Hong Kong [12] | Germany [13] | Poland [14] |
|---|---|---|---|---|
| No. of patients | 121 | 195 | 238 | 280 |
| Timing of ERCP | <72 hours | <24 hours | <72 hours | <24 hours |
| Inclusion | Acute pancreatitis | Acute pancreatitis | Acute pancreatitis without obstructive jaundice | Acute pancreatitis |
| Intervention | ERCP +/- ES | ERCP +/- ES | ERCP +/- ES | ERCP +/- ES |
| Reduction in mortality | 18% vs 4% (P =NA), (Severe group) | 18% vs 3% (P = NA) (Severe group) | NS | 13% vs 2% (P<0.001) |
| Reduction in morbidity | 61% vs 24% (P = NA) (Severe group) | 54% vs 13% (P = NA) (Severe group) | NS | 36% vs 17% (P<0.001) |
| Other significant outcomes | Reduction in hospital stay (Severe group) | / | No difference between mild and severe group | Reduction in both mild and severe groups |

ERCP: Endoscopic Retrograde Cholangiopancreatography; ES: Endoscopic Sphincterotomy;

NA: Not Available; NS: Not Significant

**Table 1.** Outcomes from Initial Randomized Trials

## 3. Who to perform endoscopic ultrasound on?

Endoscopic Ultrasound (EUS) combines endoscopic visualization with 2-dimensional ultrasound and is well suited for biliary imaging given the close proximity of the extrahepatic bile duct to the proximal duodenum. (Figure 1) Both radial and linear array echo-endoscopes are excellent in detecting common bile duct stones, with a reported sensitivity of 89% to 94% and specificity of 94% to 95%. [26, 27] The benefit of EUS would be most pronounced in patients with intermediate probability of CBD stones. The advantages include the avoidance of the risk associated with a diagnostic ERCP and ERCP can be performed in the same session if stones were detected. [28]

Two meta-analyses have showed that both EUS and magnetic resonance cholangiopancreatography (MRCP) demonstrated excellent efficacy in diagnosing choledocholithiasis. [26, 27] The reported pooled sensitivity and specificity were around 90% for EUS and >95% for MRCP. Furthermore, the use of EUS to select patients for therapeutic ERCP has a significantly lower risk of complications as compared to performing diagnostic ERCP for detecting CBD stones.

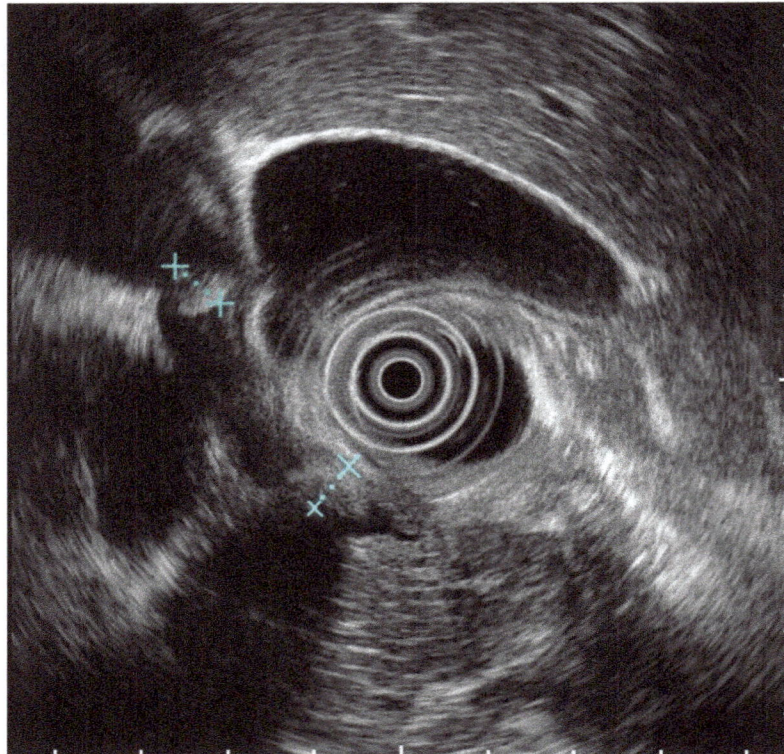

**Figure 1.** Endoscopic Ultrasound Image of Two Stones in Common Bile Duct

## 4. Pancreatic pseudocyst

It is estimated that 15 to 30% of patients will suffer from severe pancreatitis that is characterized by the presence of local complications including pancreatic necrosis, pseudocyst and abscess and organ failure. [20]

Pancreatic pseudocyst is a collection of pancreatic juice enclosed by a wall of fibrous or granulation tissue, occurring at least 4 weeks after the onset of symptoms. (Figure 2) Clinical presentation of pseudocysts varies, ranging form asymptomatic to life threatening condition. Intervention is indicated if patients are symptomatic, suffering from complications, with size greater than > 6 cm, increasing in size or if it does not resolve after 6 weeks.

When compared with surgery and percutaneous methods, endoscopic drainage of pseudocyst is less invasive with decreased risk of morbidities. It can also provide direct access to the cyst.

Endoscopic drainage of pseudocyst can be performed under esophagogastroduodenoscopy (EGD) or EUS guidance. An EGD-guided puncture is essentially a blind procedure, as this requires bulging of cyst into the stomach for localization. Furthermore, there is a risk of bleeding from interposed vessels and also mal-positioning of the stents during the procedure. EUS overcomes these difficulties and has been shown by two randomized studies to be associated with higher rates of success (100% vs 33% & 94% vs 72%) with comparable morbidities. [29, 30]

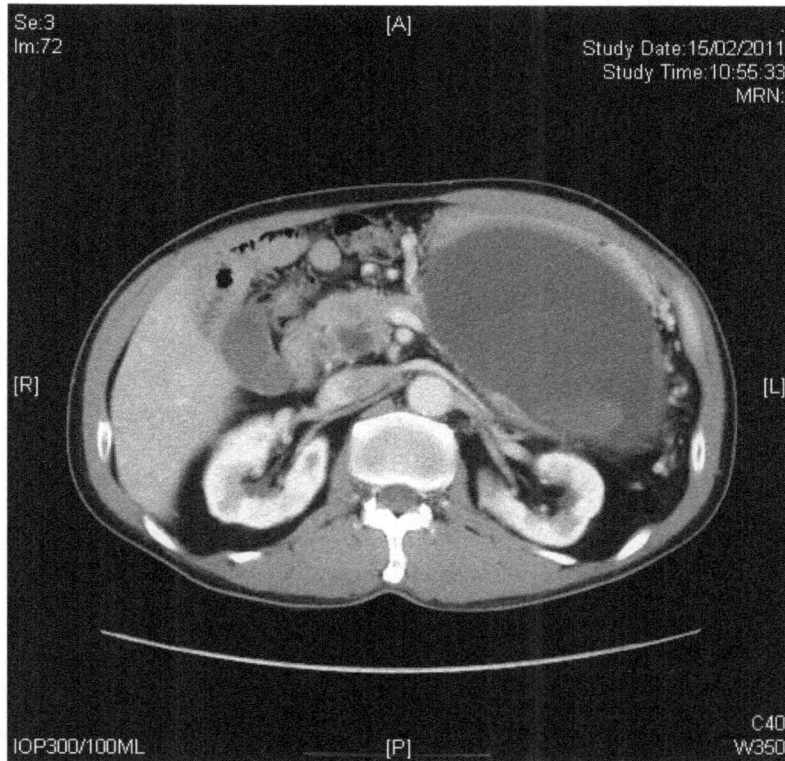

**Figure 2.** CT film demonstrating the presence of an 8cm pseudocyst located at the pancreatic tail region.

The outcomes of EUS-guided pseudocyst drainage were reported in a number of studies. [31-35] A high success rate ranging from 82 to 94% with an acceptable complication rate of 9.1 to 33.3% were reported. These studies demonstrated the feasibility and efficacy of the procedure.

Endoscopic drainage of pseudocyst is usually performed with combined EUS and fluoroscopy guidance. EUS is first used to identify the optimal site of puncture that is free of intervening vascular structures. (Figure 3) The pseudocyst is then punctured with a 19-gauge needle and the track dilated with a needle knife or cystotome. A guide-wire (or double guidewires) is then advanced via the needle under fluoroscopic control. At least two loops should be formed before the needle was withdrawn to prevent dislodgement of guidewire during manipulation. A cysto-gastrostomy is then created and dilated to 6-8mm. Two or more double pigtail stents is then inserted. (Figure 4)

The results of 20 EUS cysto-gastrostomies were compared with 10 surgical cysto-gastrostomies in a retrospective review. The success rate, complication rate and re-intervention rate were similar in both groups. The author concluded that EUS-guided cysto-gastrostomy, should be considered as first-line treatment because of a lower cost and shorter hospital stay, with no difference in clinical outcomes. [36] A recent randomized trial comparing endoscopic and surgical cysto-gastrostomy for pancreatic pseudocyst drainage also produced similar results. [37] Varadarajulu et al showed that endoscopic treatment was associated with shorter hospital stays, better physical and mental health of patients, and lower cost.

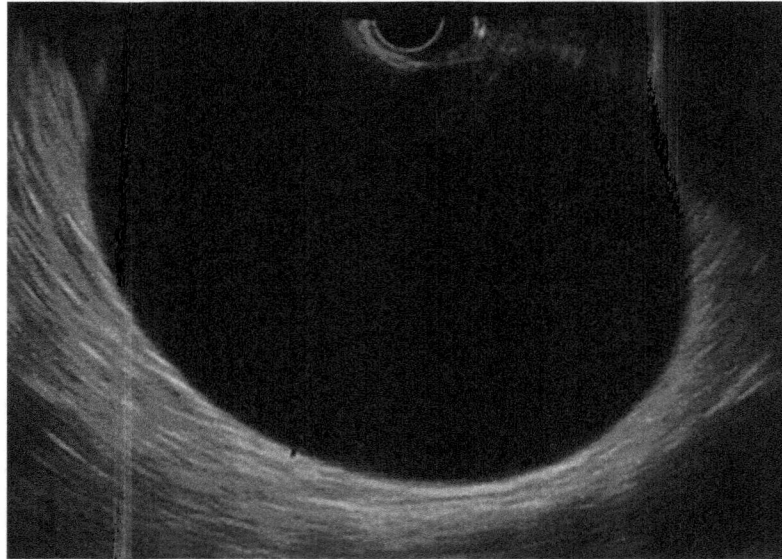

**Figure 3.** Picture of Pancreatic Pseudocyst by Linear Endoscopic Ultrasound (EUS)

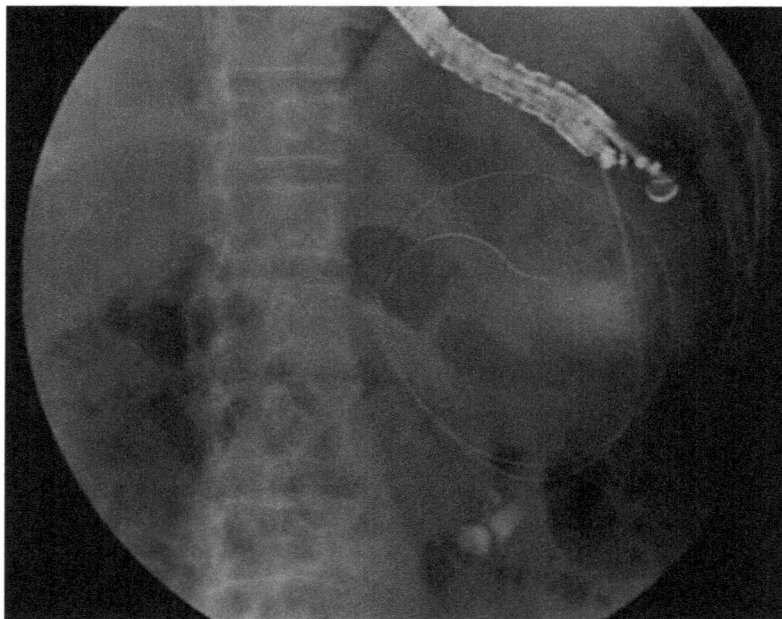

**Figure 4.** Fluoroscopic Picture of EUS-guided Drainage of Pancreatic Pseudocyst Showing the Guidewire Forming Loops within the Pseudocyst.

## 5. Forward-viewing vs oblique-viewing EUS in drainage of pseudocyst

Conventional echoendoscopes are oblique viewing devices and the angle of the instrument channel results in tangential puncturing of the pseudocyst. This may lead to inadequate transmission of force during insertion of the stents. Furthermore, re-cannulation of an angulated track for multiple stent insertion may be difficult after tangential puncturing.

Recently, forward-viewing echoendoscopes have become available. This device allows forward sonographic imaging, with an axis for puncturing and insertion of stents being parallel to the direction of the scanning plane. In contrast to the oblique-viewing device where tangential puncturing results in an angulated track, the forward-viewing endoscope allows for insertion of the needle along the same plane as the direction of scanning.

Voermans et al studied the performance of forward viewing versus oblique viewing EUS in drainage of pseudocyst under a multi-centered setting. [38] Four tertiary centers and 58 patients with pseudocyst greater than 6cm in size were recruited. There were no differences in the procedural time, ease of the procedure, morbidities and success rates.

## 6. Pancreatic necrosis and abscess

Pancreatic necrosis is characterized by diffuse or focal areas of non-viable pancreatic parenchyma, which is typically associated with peri-pancreatic fat necrosis. Radiologically, it is defined as non-enhanced pancreatic parenchyma greater 3 cm or when more than 30% of the area of the pancreas is involved on the computed tomography. (Figure 5)

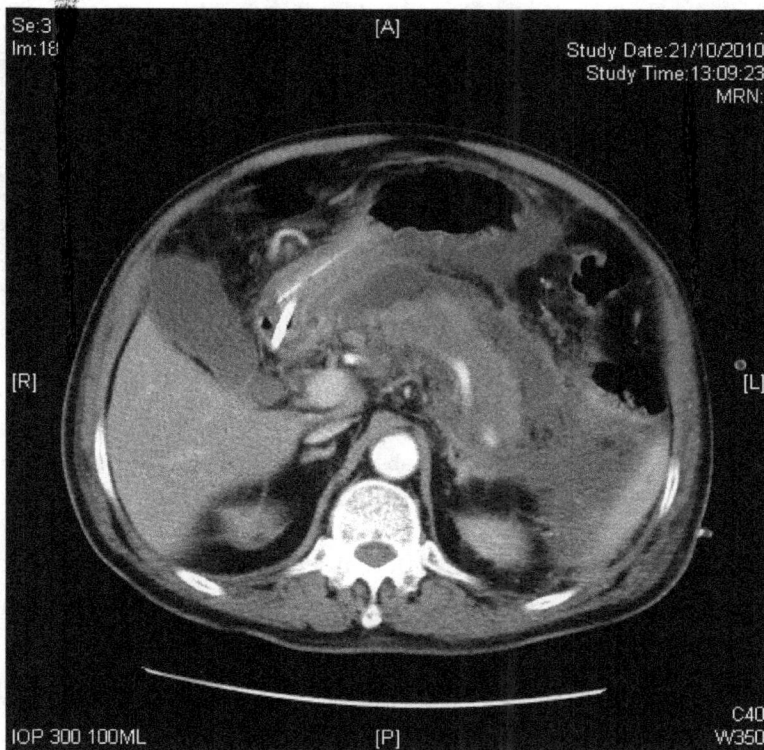

**Figure 5.** This CT film of a patient with pancreatic necrosis characterized by non-enhanced pancreatic parenchyma.

The presence of a sterile necrosis is not an indication for necrosectomy. However, if patients develop worsening symptoms and deteriorating clinical condition, infected necrosis should be suspected. Fine-needle aspiration of the collection should be performed. The sample should be cultured and gram stained to document infection and necrosectomy is indicated in those with documented infection.

Pancreatic abscess is a circumscribed, intra-abdominal collection of pus containing little or no pancreatic necrosis, which arises as a consequence of acute pancreatitis or pancreatic trauma. (Figure 6)

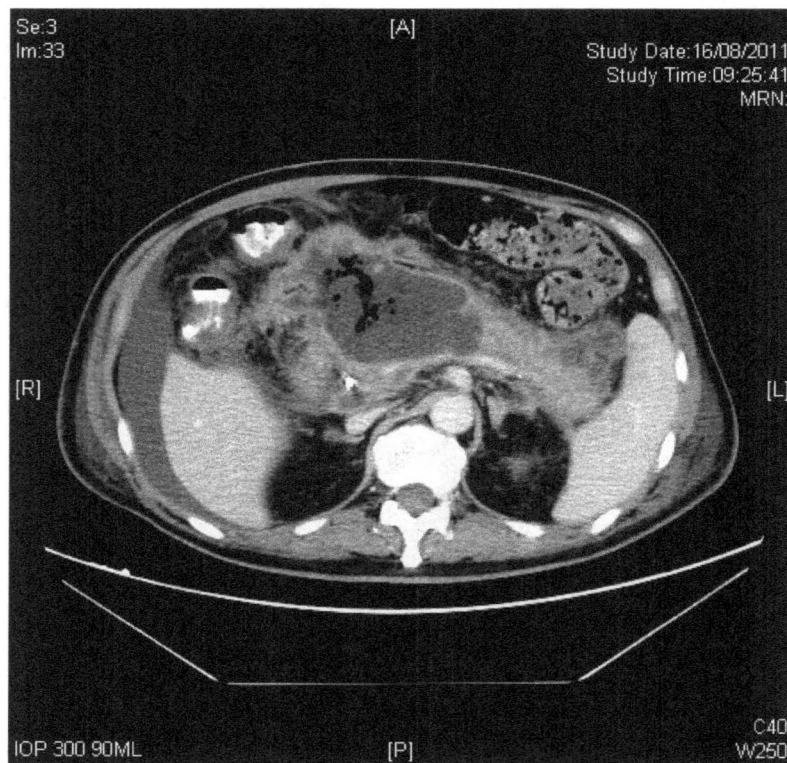

**Figure 6.** CT scan of a patient suffering from pancreatic abscess as evident by the presence of a fluid collection at the neck of the pancreas and associated air locules.

For the treatment of pancreatic necrosis, open necrosectomy was once considered as the standard definitive treatment. (Figure 7) However, it was associated with many problems such as intraoperative collateral tissue damage, bleeding, worsening organ failure due to surgical trauma, multiple operations, stormy postoperative course, lengthy stay in the intensive care unit, incisional hernias, new-onset diabetes, and for the use of pancreatic enzymes, with a high morbidity up to 95%. [39-42] The mortality of open necrosectomy is high, almost 40-75%, particularly if performed early. [40, 43]

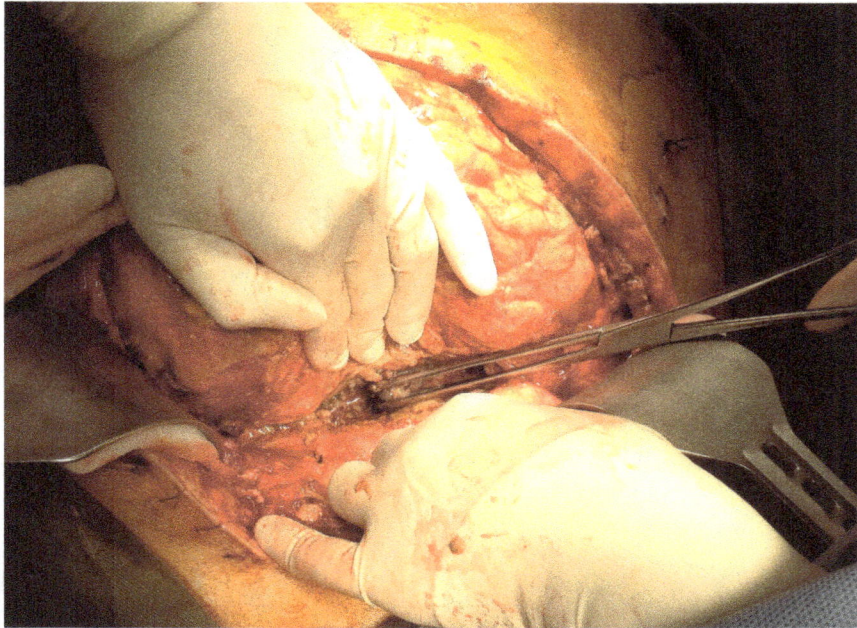

**Figure 7.** Operative picture of open necrosectomy showing the necrotic materials being removed by the forceps.

# 7. Endoscopic necrosectomy

Recently, pancreatic necrosectomy has been performed by the endoscopic approach. [44, 45] This was achieved by either the percutaneous retroperitoneal approach or the transgastric approach. Endoscopic approach has been in favor, as it leads to reduced inflammatory response and decreased complications. [46]

# 8. Percutaneous retroperitoneal approach

Percutaneous retroperitoneal pancreatic necrosectomy allows the use of high volume post-operative lavage that can be performed under local anesthesia. [47, 48] Percutaneous drainage was first achieved with ultrasound-guided pigtail insertion. The track was then dilated to allow for insertion of a 30Fr drain and this would be used later for introduction of a 9.8mm endoscope. On insertion of the endoscope, the necrotic pancreas was seen within the cavity with surrounding pus and turbid material. (Figure 8) The procedure could be done under fluoroscopic guidance. (Figure 9)

The cavity was irrigated generously with saline to flush out the material. Endoscopic necrosectomy was then performed to remove the necrotic pancreas. This could be performed with a number of accessories including forceps, snares or grasping forceps. (Figure 10) The loop snare allowed removal of larger pieces of necrotic material. The process should be repeated until all the necrotic materials were removed.

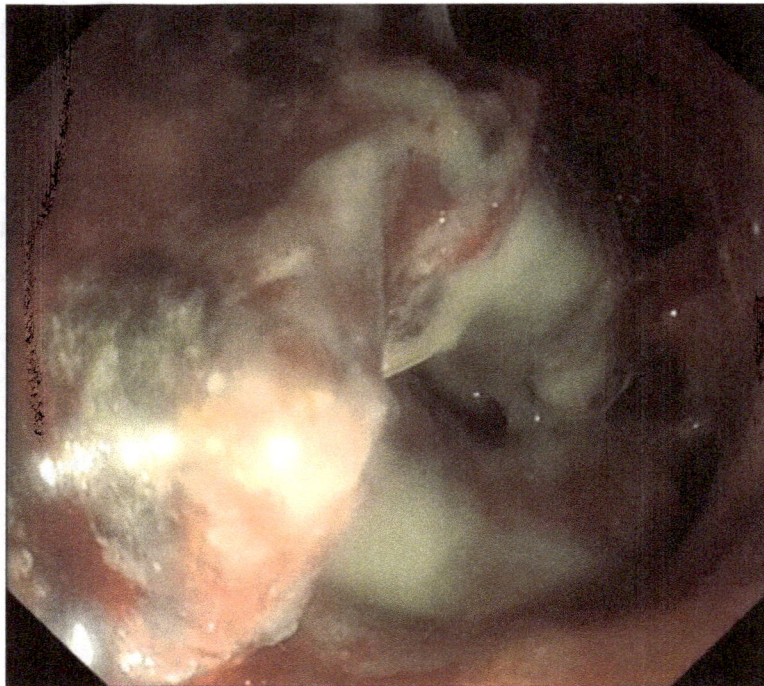

**Figure 8.** Endoscopic Picture of Pancreatic Necrosis

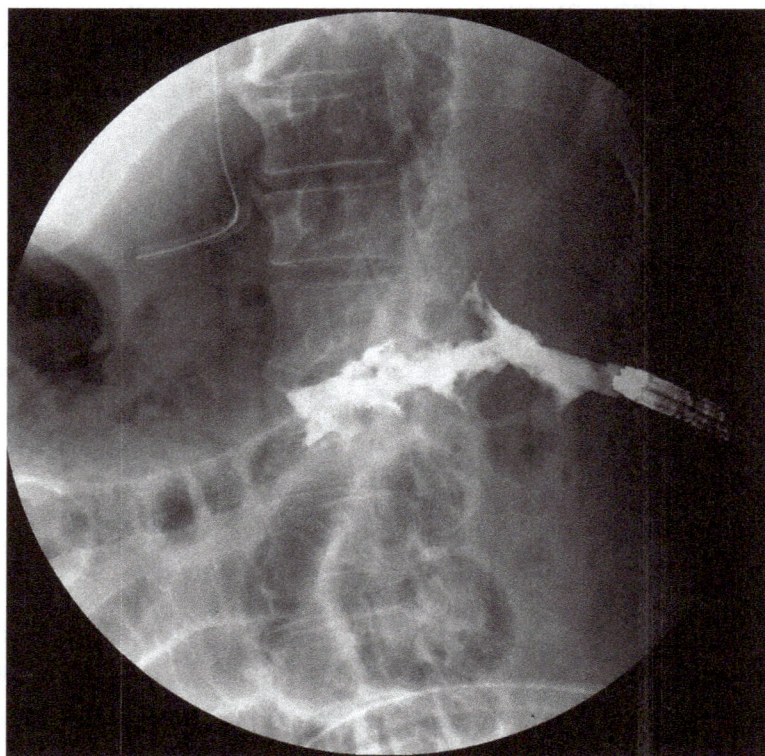

**Figure 9.** Fluoroscopic Image of Percutaneous Retroperitoneal Pancreatic Necrosectomy

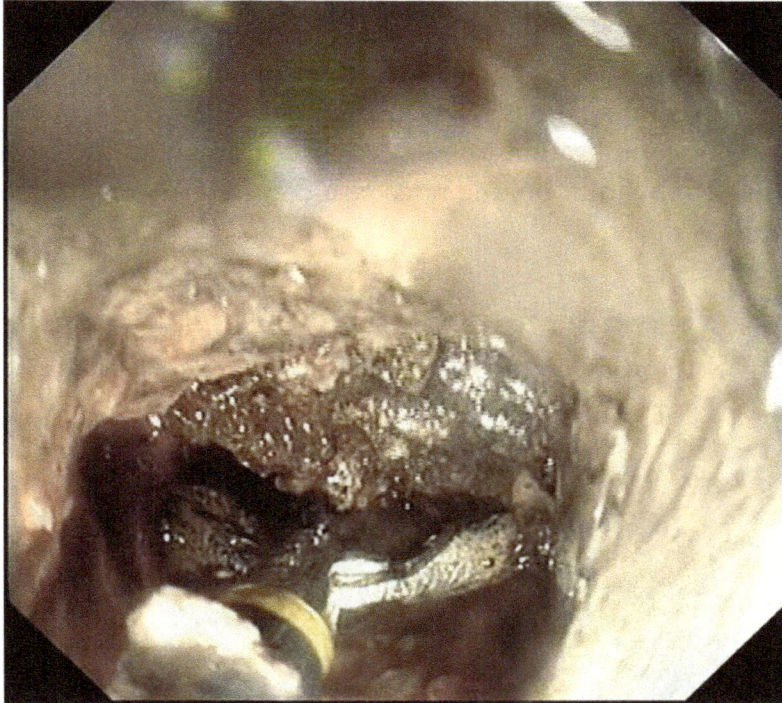

**Figure 10.** Removal of Necrotic Materials with Grasping Forceps via Percutaneous Approach

## 9. Endoscopic transgastric approach

The results and techniques of EUS transgastric drainage in walled off pancreatic necrosis were well reported. [49-52] The procedure begins with the insertion of stents under EUS guidance, followed by the dilation of the track to allow transmural introduction of the endoscope into the walled of pancreatic necrosis for necrosectomy. Repeated endoscopic debridement could be performed via the same route and it is indicated when there is lack of window for percutaneous drainage. Figure 10 showed the necrotic materials that were removed.

The transgastric approach can avoid the complications associated with the percutaneous approach including bleeding, visceral perforation and the risk of pancreatico-cutaneous fistula. Furthermore, the approach provides a more direct approach to the necrotic cavity. However, with this approach, one cannot monitor the output of the drainage material and also, the presence of a fistula may lead to possible contamination of the abscess cavity by gastrointestinal contents.

The outcomes of endoscopic necrosectomy were recently reviewed. [53] Between 1990 and 2009, 10 case series including 260 patients with 1100 endoscopic necrosectomies were performed. The overall mortality was 5% and the mean procedure-related morbidity was 27%. Bleeding was most common complication followed by exacerbation of sepsis and free perforation. Complete resolution of the pancreatic necrosis was achieved by endoscopic means alone in 76% of the patients.

In a Dutch multi-centred randomized study, 88 patients with infected necrotizing pancreatitis were randomized to endoscopic step-up approach or open necrosectomy. [54] In the endoscopic step-up approach, both the percutaneous left retroperitoneal and the transgastric routes were used. The step-up approach had shown a number of benefits, including significantly decreased rates of major complications, new-onset multi-organ failure and also the need for intensive care admission. In addition, the rates of incisional hernias and new-onset diabetes were also significantly reduced.

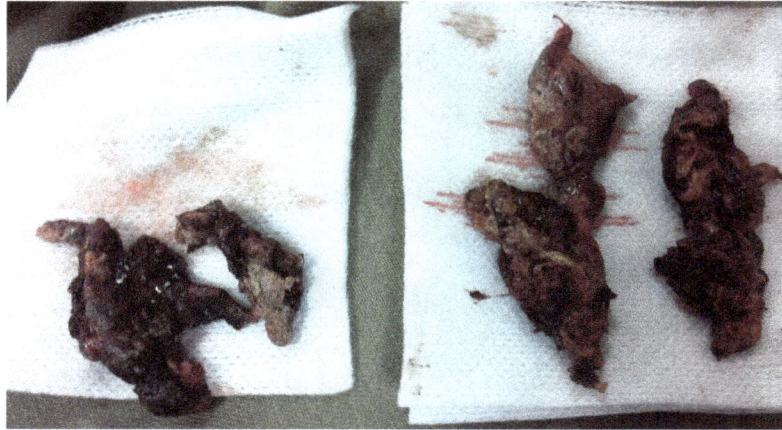

**Figure 11.** Pictures of Necrotic Materials Removed by Endoscopic Transgastric Approach

## 10. Retroperitoneal or transgastric approach for endoscopic necrosectomy

Currently, there is no study comparing which approach is superior. Both approaches are complementary with their respective benefits and risks. Their application will depend on the anatomical location of the collection and should be tailored according to the patient. Bleeding is the most common complication encountered. [54] It could happen during the dilatation of transmural tract debridement of necrotic materials. Care should be taken on necrosectomy as any trauma to blood vessels could result in catastrophic bleeding, especially if branches of the splenic artery or vein were injured. The use of EUS can enhance the identification of vascular structure and reduce the risk of bleeding.

## 11. Is irrigation necessary?

A number of studies have reported on the use of repeat endoscopic irrigation as a part of the treatment in endoscopic necrosectomy to improve outcomes. [49, 51, 55-61] (Table 2) It was performed via an external nasocystic or percutaneous drainage. Dissolution of necroses could be achieved through liquefying the necrotic material through constant flushing and drainage of debris. On the other hand, Jurgensen et al found that neither endoscopic nor external flushing was needed for successful endoscopic treatment for symptomatic necroses once they were grossly cleared mechanically by endoscopy and the discomfort from the use of nasocystic or percutaneous drainage could be avoided. [62] Stenting alone demonstrated good short-and long-term results. It can lead to avoidance of repeated and lengthy procedures, immediate mobilization, better tolerance by patients and potential reduction of hospital stay.

| Reference (year) | N | Mortality / Surgery | Mean no. of Endoscopies for endoscopic necrosectomy and lavage (range) | Use of Irrigation |
|---|---|---|---|---|
| Seewald (2005) [49] | 10 | 0/4 | 23.6 (4-64) | Endoscopic 13/13 Nasocystic 12/13 |
| Charnley (2006) [55] | 13 | 2/4 | 4 (1-6) | Endoscopic 13/13 Nasocystic 5/13 |
| Papchristou (2007) [51] | 22 | 1/NS | 3 (1-12) | Nasocystic 22/22 |
| Voermans (2007) [59] | 25 | 0/2 | 1.7 (1-4) | Nasocystic 20/25 |
| Escourror (2008) [56] | 13 | 0/0 | 1.8 (1-3) | Endoscopic 13/13 Nasocystic 13/13 |
| Hocke (2008) [58] | 19 | 2/2 | NS | Endoscopic 19/19 |
| Coelho (2008) [60] | 36 | 2/6 | 4 (2-8) | Endoscopic 36/36 |
| Gardner (2009) [57] | 17 | 0/1 | 2.2 (NS) | Nasocystic 14/17 |
| Seifert (2009) [61] | 93 | 7/11 | NS | NS |
| Jurgensen (2012) [62] | 35 | 2/0 | 2.9 (1-11) | None |

NS: Not Specified

**Table 2.** Summary of Studies (with more than 10 patients) on Endoscopic Irrigation With Regard of Outcomes

## 12. Is immediate necrosectomy necessary for infected pancreatic necrosis?

While various guidelines have advocated surgical necrosectomy for patients with infected pancreatic necrosis, [63, 64] the issue of conservative versus surgical treatment for infected pancreatic necrosis has been intensely debated. [65] Current evidence suggests that conservative treatment might be successful for infected pancreatic necrosis in a proportion of patients. [66-71] In the recent decades, a number of case series and comparative trials, as well as a meta-analysis, have shown that primary conservative treatment could be successful for infected pancreatic necrosis. [66-68, 72-76] (Table 3) However, patient selection bias and/or publication bias in these case series, which have shown a successful outcome following conservative treatment for infected pancreatic necrosis, could be taken into account when interpreting these results. Mouli et al, in a systemic review and meta-analysis, analyzed 8 studies that have reported conservative treatment as the initial and primary treatment for all consecutive patients with infected necrosis to minimize these biases. [76] They found that conservative management was successful for 64% of patients (95% confidence interval, 51%–78%) and mortality was 12% (95% confidence interval, 6%–18%). Among 324 patients included, 26% of patients required necrosectomy or additional surgery for complications (95% confidence interval, 15%–37%).

Conservative treatment for infected pancreatic necrosis should include intensive care with full organ support, use of effective antimicrobials, and aggressive nutritional support. Percutaneous drainage, despite it is a form of intervention and not truly conservative, has also been considered a part of conservative treatment because it does not involve surgery or formal necrosectomy in some of the reported studies. [77-80]

| Reference (year) | No. of patients with infected pancreatic necrosis on conservative treatment | Patients undergoing percutaneous drainage (%) | Successful conservative treatment (%) | Need for surgery (%) | Median/ mean hospital stay (days) | Mortality (%) |
|---|---|---|---|---|---|---|
| ◉Freeny (1998) [77] | 34 | 100 (34/34) | 47.1 (16/34) | 52.9 (18/34) | 45 | 11.8 (4/34) |
| Runzi (2005) [68] | 28 | 18.75 (3/16) # | 50 (14/28) | 42.9 (12/28) | 54 ± 10 * | 14.3 (4/28) |
| Song (2006) [72] | 19 | NR | 78.9 (15/19) | 21.1 (4/19) | 70 | 5.3 (1/19) |
| ◉Navalho (2006) [78] | 30 | 100 (30/30) | 63.3 (19/30) | 33.3 (10/30) | 24 | 16.6 (5/30) |
| Lee (2007) [67] | 31 | 67.7 (21/31) | 71 (22/31) | 12.9 (4/31) | 37.7 ± 28.5 * | 3.2 (1/31) |
| ◉Bruennler (2008) [79] | 80 | 100 (80/80) | 47.5 (38/80) | 20 (16/80) | 51 | 33.8 (27/80) |
| ◉Mortele (2009) [80] | 13 | 100 (13/13) | 46.2 (6/13) | 53.8 (7/13) | 33 | 7.7 (1/13) |
| Garg (2010) [66] | 77 | 45.45 (35.77) | 54.4 (42/77) | 23.4 (18/77) | 26.5 | 28.6 (22/77) |
| Van Santvoort (2010) [54] | 43 | 95.3 (41/43) | 34.9 (15/43) | 60.4 (26/43) | 50 | 18.6 (8/43) |
| Zerem (2011) [73] | 86 | 80.2 (69/86) | 84.9 (73/86) | 12.8 (11/86) | 13 | 9.3 (8/86) |
| Gluck (2012) [74] | 20 | 100 (20/20) | 70 (14/20) | 15 (3/20) | 54 | 15 (3/20) |
| Alsfasser (2012) [75] | 20 | 50 (10/20) | 65 (13/20) | 30 (6/20) | NR | 5 (1/20) |

◉ Studies reported the results of only those patients who underwent percutaneous drainage for the management of infected pancreatic necrosis

# Eliminated 12 patients required surgical treatment

* Data expressed in mean ± standard deviation NR: Not Reported

**Table 3.** Outcomes of Patients with Infected Pancreatic Necrosis Receiving Primary Conservative Management

The principle for the indication necrosectomy is shifting from infection-based to organ failure- or complication-based. While conservative-first approach is a reasonable approach for the management of infected pancreatic necrosis, it is important to recognize those patients might require necrosectomy later as a step-up therapy at an appropriate time. [76] Indications for necrosectomy include nonresponse to conservative treatment and development of local complications such as bleeding and colonic perforation. Extend and infection of pancreatic necrosis correlated with the development of organ failure and mortality in acute pancreatitis. [81,82] Large amount of thick necrotic debris at difficult-to-drain locations and resistant organisms could be the reasons for failure of conservative therapy. Two studies sought to identify the predictive factors for the need for early surgery. Zerem et al showed that Ranson, Glasgow, and APACHE II scores, CTSI, and C-reactive protein could predict the need for surgery in their patients, but the 95% confidence interval showed that none of the factors were found to be a significant predictor. [73] Garg et al showed that high APACHE II score and serum creatinine level were predictive of mortality. [66] Unfortunately, no predictive factor that could guide a clinician to move towards early surgical intervention was identified in the currently available studies.

## 13. Conclusion

In conclusion, the use of advanced endoscopy is dramatically changing the management of patients with acute pancreatitis. With continued advancement of technology, there is a diminishing need for open surgical intervention. Management of these patients is best under a multidisciplinary team consisting of gastroenterologists, radiologists and surgeons.

## Author details

Charing Ching Ning Chong[1*], Anthony Yuen Bun Teoh[1], Paul Bo San Lai[1],
James Yun Wong Lau[1,2] and Francis Ka Leung Chan[2]

*Address all correspondence to: chongcn@surgery.cuhk.edu.hk

1 Department of Surgery, Prince of Wales Hospital, the Chinese University of Hong Kong, SAR

2 Institute of Digestive Disease, Prince of Wales Hospital, the Chinese University of Hong Kong, SAR

## References

[1] Banks PA, Bollen TL, Dervenis C, Gooszen HG, Johnson CD, Sarr MG, et al. Classification of acute pancreatitis--2012: revision of the Atlanta classification and definitions by international consensus. Gut. 2013;62(1):102-11.

[2]   van Santvoort HC, Bakker OJ, Bollen TL, Besselink MG, Ahmed Ali U, Schrijver AM, et al. A conservative and minimally invasive approach to necrotizing pancreatitis improves outcome. Gastroenterology. 2011;141(4):1254-63.

[3]   Lankisch PG. Natural course of acute pancreatitis: what we know today and what we ought to know for tomorrow. Pancreas. 2009;38(5):494-8.

[4]   Andersson R, Andersson B, Haraldsen P, Drewsen G, Eckerwall G. Incidence, management and recurrence rate of acute pancreatitis. Scandinavian journal of gastroenterology. 2004;39(9):891-4.

[5]   Malecka-Panas E, Juszynski A, Wilamski E. The natural course of acute gallstone pancreatitis. Materia medica Polona Polish journal of medicine and pharmacy. 1996;28(1):8-12.

[6]   Acosta JM, Rubio Galli OM, Rossi R, Chinellato AV, Pellegrini CA. Effect of duration of ampullary gallstone obstruction on severity of lesions of acute pancreatitis. Journal of the American College of Surgeons. 1997;184(5):499-505.

[7]   Runzi M, Saluja A, Lerch MM, Dawra R, Nishino H, Steer ML. Early ductal decompression prevents the progression of biliary pancreatitis: an experimental study in the opossum. Gastroenterology. 1993;105(1):157-64.

[8]   Senninger N, Moody FG, Coelho JC, Van Buren DH. The role of biliary obstruction in the pathogenesis of acute pancreatitis in the opossum. Surgery. 1986;99(6):688-93.

[9]   Sharma VK, Howden CW. Metaanalysis of randomized controlled trials of endoscopic retrograde cholangiography and endoscopic sphincterotomy for the treatment of acute biliary pancreatitis. The American journal of gastroenterology. 1999;94(11): 3211-4.

[10]  Ayub K, Imada R, Slavin J. Endoscopic retrograde cholangiopancreatography in gallstone-associated acute pancreatitis. The Cochrane database of systematic reviews. 2004(4):CD003630.

[11]  Neoptolemos JP, Carr-Locke DL, London NJ, Bailey IA, James D, Fossard DP. Controlled trial of urgent endoscopic retrograde cholangiopancreatography and endoscopic sphincterotomy versus conservative treatment for acute pancreatitis due to gallstones. Lancet. 1988;2(8618):979-83.

[12]  Fan ST, Lai EC, Mok FP, Lo CM, Zheng SS, Wong J. Early treatment of acute biliary pancreatitis by endoscopic papillotomy. The New England journal of medicine. 1993;328(4):228-32.

[13]  Folsch UR, Nitsche R, Ludtke R, Hilgers RA, Creutzfeldt W. Early ERCP and papillotomy compared with conservative treatment for acute biliary pancreatitis. The German Study Group on Acute Biliary Pancreatitis. The New England journal of medicine. 1997;336(4):237-42.

[14] Nowak A, Nowakowska-Dulawa E, Marek TA, Rybicka J. Final results of the prospective, randomized, controlled study on endoscopic sphincterotomy versus conventional management in acute biliary pancreatitis (abstract). Gastroenterology 1995;108:A380.

[15] Acosta JM, Katkhouda N, Debian KA, Groshen SG, Tsao-Wei DD, Berne TV. Early ductal decompression versus conservative management for gallstone pancreatitis with ampullary obstruction: a prospective randomized clinical trial. Annals of surgery. 2006;243(1):33-40.

[16] Oria A, Cimmino D, Ocampo C, Silva W, Kohan G, Zandalazini H, et al. Early endoscopic intervention versus early conservative management in patients with acute gallstone pancreatitis and biliopancreatic obstruction: a randomized clinical trial. Annals of surgery. 2007;245(1):10-7.

[17] Petrov MS, Uchugina AF, Kukosh MV. Does endoscopic retrograde cholangiopancreatography reduce the risk of local pancreatic complications in acute pancreatitis? A systematic review and metaanalysis. Surgical endoscopy. 2008;22(11):2338-43.

[18] Petrov MS, van Santvoort HC, Besselink MG, van der Heijden GJ, van Erpecum KJ, Gooszen HG. Early endoscopic retrograde cholangiopancreatography versus conservative management in acute biliary pancreatitis without cholangitis: a meta-analysis of randomized trials. Annals of surgery. 2008;247(2):250-7.

[19] van Santvoort HC, Besselink MG, de Vries AC, Boermeester MA, Fischer K, Bollen TL, et al. Early endoscopic retrograde cholangiopancreatography in predicted severe acute biliary pancreatitis: a prospective multicenter study. Annals of surgery. 2009;250(1):68-75.

[20] American Gastroenterological Association Institute on "Management of Acute Pancreatits" Clinical P, Economics C, Board AGAIG. AGA Institute medical position statement on acute pancreatitis. Gastroenterology. 2007;132(5):2019-21.

[21] Barkun AN, Barkun JS, Fried GM, Ghitulescu G, Steinmetz O, Pham C, et al. Useful predictors of bile duct stones in patients undergoing laparoscopic cholecystectomy. McGill Gallstone Treatment Group. Annals of surgery. 1994;220(1):32-9.

[22] Alponat A, Kum CK, Rajnakova A, Koh BC, Goh PM. Predictive factors for synchronous common bile duct stones in patients with cholelithiasis. Surgical endoscopy. 1997;11(9):928-32.

[23] van Santvoort HC, Bakker OJ, Besselink MG, Bollen TL, Fischer K, Nieuwenhuijs VB, et al. Prediction of common bile duct stones in the earliest stages of acute biliary pancreatitis. Endoscopy. 2011;43(1):8-13.

[24] Jovanovic P, Salkic NN, Zerem E, Ljuca F. Biochemical and ultrasound parameters may help predict the need for therapeutic endoscopic retrograde cholangiopancrea-

tography (ERCP) in patients with a firm clinical and biochemical suspicion for chole-docholithiasis. European journal of internal medicine. 2011;22(6):e110-4.

[25]  Sotoudehmanesh R, Kolahdoozan S, Asgari AA, Dooghaei-Moghaddam M, Ainechi S. Role of endoscopic ultrasonography in prevention of unnecessary endoscopic ret-rograde cholangiopancreatography: a prospective study of 150 patients. Journal of ultrasound in medicine : official journal of the American Institute of Ultrasound in Medicine. 2007;26(4):455-60.

[26]  Romagnuolo J, Bardou M, Rahme E, Joseph L, Reinhold C, Barkun AN. Magnetic res-onance cholangiopancreatography: a meta-analysis of test performance in suspected biliary disease. Annals of internal medicine. 2003;139(7):547-57.

[27]  Garrow D, Miller S, Sinha D, Conway J, Hoffman BJ, Hawes RH, et al. Endoscopic ultrasound: a meta-analysis of test performance in suspected biliary obstruction. Clinical gastroenterology and hepatology : the official clinical practice journal of the American Gastroenterological Association. 2007;5(5):616-23.

[28]  Liu CL, Fan ST, Lo CM, Tso WK, Wong Y, Poon RT, et al. Comparison of early endo-scopic ultrasonography and endoscopic retrograde cholangiopancreatography in the management of acute biliary pancreatitis: a prospective randomized study. Clinical gastroenterology and hepatology : the official clinical practice journal of the Ameri-can Gastroenterological Association. 2005;3(12):1238-44.

[29]  Varadarajulu S, Christein JD, Tamhane A, Drelichman ER, Wilcox CM. Prospective randomized trial comparing EUS and EGD for transmural drainage of pancreatic pseudocysts (with videos). Gastrointestinal endoscopy. 2008;68(6):1102-11.

[30]  Park DH, Lee SS, Moon SH, Choi SY, Jung SW, Seo DW, et al. Endoscopic ultra-sound-guided versus conventional transmural drainage for pancreatic pseudocysts: a prospective randomized trial. Endoscopy. 2009;41(10):842-8.

[31]  Vosoghi M, Sial S, Garrett B, Feng J, Lee T, Stabile BE, et al. EUS-guided pancreatic pseudocyst drainage: review and experience at Harbor-UCLA Medical Center. MedGenMed : Medscape general medicine. 2002;4(3):2.

[32]  Yasuda I, Iwata K, Mukai T, Iwashita T, Moriwaki H. EUS-guided pancreatic pseu-docyst drainage. Digestive endoscopy : official journal of the Japan Gastroenterologi-cal Endoscopy Society. 2009;21 Suppl 1:S82-6.

[33]  Ahlawat SK, Charabaty-Pishvaian A, Jackson PG, Haddad NG. Single-step EUS-guided pancreatic pseudocyst drainage using a large channel linear array echoendo-scope and cystotome: results in 11 patients. JOP : Journal of the pancreas. 2006;7(6): 616-24.

[34]  Ang TL, Teo EK, Fock KM. EUS-guided drainage of infected pancreatic pseudocyst: use of a 10F Soehendra dilator to facilitate a double-wire technique for initial trans-gastric access (with videos). Gastrointestinal endoscopy. 2008;68(1):192-4.

[35] Khashab MA, Lennon AM, Singh VK, Kalloo AN, Giday SA. Endoscopic ultrasound (EUS)-guided pseudocyst drainage as a one-step procedure using a novel multiple-wire insertion technique (with video). Surgical endoscopy. 2012;26(11):3320-3.

[36] Varadarajulu S, Lopes TL, Wilcox CM, Drelichman ER, Kilgore ML, Christein JD. EUS versus surgical cyst-gastrostomy for management of pancreatic pseudocysts. Gastrointestinal endoscopy. 2008;68(4):649-55.

[37] Varadarajulu S, Bang JY, Sutton BS, Trevino JM, Christein JD, Wilcox CM. Equal efficacy of endoscopic and surgical cystogastrostomy for pancreatic pseudocyst drainage in a randomized trial. Gastroenterology. 2013;145(3):583-90 e1.

[38] Voermans RP, Ponchon T, Schumacher B, Fumex F, Bergman JJ, Larghi A, et al. Forward-viewing versus oblique-viewing echoendoscopes in transluminal drainage of pancreatic fluid collections: a multicenter, randomized, controlled trial. Gastrointestinal endoscopy. 2011;74(6):1285-93.

[39] Buchler MW, Gloor B, Muller CA, Friess H, Seiler CA, Uhl W. Acute necrotizing pancreatitis: treatment strategy according to the status of infection. Annals of surgery. 2000;232(5):619-26.

[40] Connor S, Alexakis N, Raraty MG, Ghaneh P, Evans J, Hughes M, et al. Early and late complications after pancreatic necrosectomy. Surgery. 2005;137(5):499-505.

[41] Traverso LW, Kozarek RA. Pancreatic necrosectomy: definitions and technique. Journal of gastrointestinal surgery : official journal of the Society for Surgery of the Alimentary Tract. 2005;9(3):436-9.

[42] Cirocchi R, Trastulli S, Desiderio J, Boselli C, Parisi A, Noya G, et al. Minimally invasive necrosectomy versus conventional surgery in the treatment of infected pancreatic necrosis: a systematic review and a meta-analysis of comparative studies. Surgical laparoscopy, endoscopy & percutaneous techniques. 2013;23(1):8-20.

[43] Besselink MG, Verwer TJ, Schoenmaeckers EJ, Buskens E, Ridwan BU, Visser MR, et al. Timing of surgical intervention in necrotizing pancreatitis. Archives of surgery. 2007;142(12):1194-201.

[44] Friedland S, Kaltenbach T, Sugimoto M, Soetikno R. Endoscopic necrosectomy of organized pancreatic necrosis: a currently practiced NOTES procedure. Journal of hepato-biliary-pancreatic surgery. 2009;16(3):266-9.

[45] Bradley EL, 3rd, Dexter ND. Management of severe acute pancreatitis: a surgical odyssey. Annals of surgery. 2010;251(1):6-17.

[46] Bakker OJ, van Santvoort HC, van Brunschot S, Geskus RB, Besselink MG, Bollen TL, et al. Endoscopic transgastric vs surgical necrosectomy for infected necrotizing pancreatitis: a randomized trial. JAMA : the journal of the American Medical Association. 2012;307(10):1053-61.

[47]    Connor S, Ghaneh P, Raraty M, Sutton R, Rosso E, Garvey CJ, et al. Minimally inva-
        sive retroperitoneal pancreatic necrosectomy. Digestive surgery. 2003;20(4):270-7.

[48]    Carter CR, McKay CJ, Imrie CW. Percutaneous necrosectomy and sinus tract endos-
        copy in the management of infected pancreatic necrosis: an initial experience. Annals
        of surgery. 2000;232(2):175-80.

[49]    Seewald S, Groth S, Omar S, Imazu H, Seitz U, de Weerth A, et al. Aggressive endo-
        scopic therapy for pancreatic necrosis and pancreatic abscess: a new safe and effec-
        tive treatment algorithm (videos). Gastrointestinal endoscopy. 2005;62(1):92-100.

[50]    Lopes CV, Pesenti C, Bories E, Caillol F, Giovannini M. Endoscopic-ultrasound-guid-
        ed endoscopic transmural drainage of pancreatic pseudocysts and abscesses. Scandi-
        navian journal of gastroenterology. 2007;42(4):524-9.

[51]    Papachristou GI, Takahashi N, Chahal P, Sarr MG, Baron TH. Peroral endoscopic
        drainage/debridement of walled-off pancreatic necrosis. Annals of surgery.
        2007;245(6):943-51.

[52]    Seewald S, Ang TL, Teng KY, Groth S, Zhong Y, Richter H, et al. Endoscopic ultra-
        sound-guided drainage of abdominal abscesses and infected necrosis. Endoscopy.
        2009;41(2):166-74.

[53]    Haghshenasskashani A, Laurence JM, Kwan V, Johnston E, Hollands MJ, Richardson
        AJ, et al. Endoscopic necrosectomy of pancreatic necrosis: a systematic review. Surgi-
        cal endoscopy. 2011;25(12):3724-30.

[54]    van Santvoort HC, Besselink MG, Bakker OJ, Hofker HS, Boermeester MA, Dejong
        CH, et al. A step-up approach or open necrosectomy for necrotizing pancreatitis. The
        New England journal of medicine. 2010;362(16):1491-502.

[55]    Charnley RM, Lochan R, Gray H, O'Sullivan CB, Scott J, Oppong KE. Endoscopic ne-
        crosectomy as primary therapy in the management of infected pancreatic necrosis.
        Endoscopy. 2006;38(9):925-8.

[56]    Escourrou J, Shehab H, Buscail L, Bournet B, Andrau P, Moreau J, et al. Peroral trans-
        gastric/transduodenal necrosectomy: success in the treatment of infected pancreatic
        necrosis. Annals of surgery. 2008;248(6):1074-80.

[57]    Gardner TB, Chahal P, Papachristou GI, Vege SS, Petersen BT, Gostout CJ, et al. A
        comparison of direct endoscopic necrosectomy with transmural endoscopic drainage
        for the treatment of walled-off pancreatic necrosis. Gastrointestinal endoscopy.
        2009;69(6):1085-94.

[58]    Hocke M, Will U, Gottschalk P, Settmacher U, Stallmach A. Transgastral retroperito-
        neal endoscopy in septic patients with pancreatic necrosis or infected pancreatic
        pseudocysts. Zeitschrift fur Gastroenterologie. 2008;46(12):1363-8.

[59] Voermans RP, Veldkamp MC, Rauws EA, Bruno MJ, Fockens P. Endoscopic transmural debridement of symptomatic organized pancreatic necrosis (with videos). Gastrointestinal endoscopy. 2007;66(5):909-16.

[60] Coelho D, Ardengh JC, Eulalio JM, Manso JE, Monkemuller K, Coelho JF. Management of infected and sterile pancreatic necrosis by programmed endoscopic necrosectomy. Digestive diseases. 2008;26(4):364-9.

[61] Seifert H, Biermer M, Schmitt W, Jurgensen C, Will U, Gerlach R, et al. Transluminal endoscopic necrosectomy after acute pancreatitis: a multicentre study with long-term follow-up (the GEPARD Study). Gut. 2009;58(9):1260-6.

[62] Jurgensen C, Neser F, Boese-Landgraf J, Schuppan D, Stolzel U, Fritscher-Ravens A. Endoscopic ultrasound-guided endoscopic necrosectomy of the pancreas: is irrigation necessary? Surgical endoscopy. 2012;26(5):1359-63.

[63] Working Party of the British Society of G, Association of Surgeons of Great B, Ireland, Pancreatic Society of Great B, Ireland, Association of Upper GISoGB, et al. UK guidelines for the management of acute pancreatitis. Gut. 2005;54 Suppl 3:iii1-9.

[64] Uhl W, Warshaw A, Imrie C, Bassi C, McKay CJ, Lankisch PG, et al. IAP Guidelines for the Surgical Management of Acute Pancreatitis. Pancreatology : official journal of the International Association of Pancreatology. 2002;2(6):565-73.

[65] Connor S, Raraty MG, Neoptolemos JP, Layer P, Runzi M, Steinberg WM, et al. Does infected pancreatic necrosis require immediate or emergency debridement? Pancreas. 2006;33(2):128-34.

[66] Garg PK, Sharma M, Madan K, Sahni P, Banerjee D, Goyal R. Primary conservative treatment results in mortality comparable to surgery in patients with infected pancreatic necrosis. Clinical gastroenterology and hepatology : the official clinical practice journal of the American Gastroenterological Association. 2010;8(12):1089-94 e2.

[67] Lee JK, Kwak KK, Park JK, Yoon WJ, Lee SH, Ryu JK, et al. The efficacy of nonsurgical treatment of infected pancreatic necrosis. Pancreas. 2007;34(4):399-404.

[68] Runzi M, Niebel W, Goebell H, Gerken G, Layer P. Severe acute pancreatitis: nonsurgical treatment of infected necroses. Pancreas. 2005;30(3):195-9.

[69] Ramesh H, Prakash K, Lekha V, Jacob G, Venugopal A. Are some cases of infected pancreatic necrosis treatable without intervention? Digestive surgery. 2003;20(4): 296-9; discussion 300.

[70] Dubner H, Steinberg W, Hill M, Bassi C, Chardavoyne R, Bank S. Infected pancreatic necrosis and peripancreatic fluid collections: serendipitous response to antibiotics and medical therapy in three patients. Pancreas. 1996;12(3):298-302.

[71]  Adler DG, Chari ST, Dahl TJ, Farnell MB, Pearson RK. Conservative management of infected necrosis complicating severe acute pancreatitis. The American journal of gastroenterology. 2003;98(1):98-103.

[72]  Song JH, Seo DW, Byun SW, Koo DH, Bae JH, Lee SS, et al. [Outcome of intensive medical treatments in patients with infected severe necrotizing pancreatitis]. The Korean journal of gastroenterology=Taehan Sohwagi Hakhoe chi. 2006;48(5):337-43.

[73]  Zerem E, Imamovic G, Susic A, Haracic B. Step-up approach to infected necrotising pancreatitis: a 20-year experience of percutaneous drainage in a single centre. Digestive and liver disease : official journal of the Italian Society of Gastroenterology and the Italian Association for the Study of the Liver. 2011;43(6):478-83.

[74]  Gluck M, Ross A, Irani S, Lin O, Gan SI, Fotoohi M, et al. Dual modality drainage for symptomatic walled-off pancreatic necrosis reduces length of hospitalization, radiological procedures, and number of endoscopies compared to standard percutaneous drainage. Journal of gastrointestinal surgery : official journal of the Society for Surgery of the Alimentary Tract. 2012;16(2):248-56; discussion 56-7.

[75]  Alsfasser G, Schwandner F, Pertschy A, Hauenstein K, Foitzik T, Klar E. Treatment of necrotizing pancreatitis: redefining the role of surgery. World journal of surgery. 2012;36(5):1142-7.

[76]  Mouli VP, Sreenivas V, Garg PK. Efficacy of conservative treatment, without necrosectomy, for infected pancreatic necrosis: a systematic review and meta-analysis. Gastroenterology. 2013;144(2):333-40 e2.

[77]  Freeny PC, Hauptmann E, Althaus SJ, Traverso LW, Sinanan M. Percutaneous CT-guided catheter drainage of infected acute necrotizing pancreatitis: techniques and results. AJR American journal of roentgenology. 1998;170(4):969-75.

[78]  Navalho M, Pires F, Duarte A, Goncalves A, Alexandrino P, Tavora I. Percutaneous drainage of infected pancreatic fluid collections in critically ill patients: correlation with C-reactive protein values. Clinical imaging. 2006;30(2):114-9.

[79]  Bruennler T, Langgartner J, Lang S, Wrede CE, Klebl F, Zierhut S, et al. Outcome of patients with acute, necrotizing pancreatitis requiring drainage-does drainage size matter? World journal of gastroenterology : WJG. 2008;14(5):725-30.

[80]  Mortele KJ, Girshman J, Szejnfeld D, Ashley SW, Erturk SM, Banks PA, et al. CT-guided percutaneous catheter drainage of acute necrotizing pancreatitis: clinical experience and observations in patients with sterile and infected necrosis. AJR American journal of roentgenology. 2009;192(1):110-6.

[81]  Garg PK, Madan K, Pande GK, Khanna S, Sathyanarayan G, Bohidar NP, et al. Association of extent and infection of pancreatic necrosis with organ failure and death in acute necrotizing pancreatitis. Clinical gastroenterology and hepatology : the official

clinical practice journal of the American Gastroenterological Association. 2005;3(2): 159-66.

[82] Isenmann R, Rau B, Beger HG. Bacterial infection and extent of necrosis are determinants of organ failure in patients with acute necrotizing pancreatitis. The British journal of surgery. 1999;86(8):1020-4.

# 6

# Role of Surgery in the Treatment of Pancreatitis and Its Complications

Vincenzo Neri

## 1. Introduction

The nosography of pancreatitis has been modified because the established distinction between acute and chronic pancreatitis is under critical revision. In this argument there is a reduced availability or absence of histological data connected to a clinical picture; on the other hand the various classifications are based exclusively on clinical or laboratory data or on imaging exams [1]. Moreover, the extremely diversified territorial distribution of the various forms of pancreatitis generates uncertainties: this often provides different experiences to different observers. The rigorous distinction between acute and chronic pancreatitis has represented the basis of classifications in which there have been two distinct diseases. More recently, more comprehensive, prolonged and detailed clinical observations have enabled a more thorough knowledge of pancreatitis. These observations show that acute and chronic pancreatitis overlap [1]. According to these new perspectives, two clinical pictures should be reviewed and reconsidered: the onset and/or the acute manifestations of chronic pancreatitis due to severe tissue inflammation more evident than main/branch duct dilation; and acute pancreatitis that evolves anatomo-clinically towards chronic forms, because of the recurrence of acute episodes with evolution of inflammation in fibrosis, sclerosis and calcifications. The aim of the chapter is to evaluate surgical procedures with a minimally invasive approach as the preferred choice, demonstrating separately the diagnostic and therapeutic pathways for acute and chronic pancreatitis.

## 2. Acute pancreatitis

Acute pancreatitis is one of the most common gastrointestinal diseases. An increase in the annual incidence for acute pancreatitis has been reported in many countries. In the United

States, pancreatitis is among the most common gastrointestinal diseases requiring acute hospitalization [2,3]. The incidence of acute pancreatitis varies between 4.8 to 24.2 cases per population of 100,000 following data from England, Denmark and theUS, but has been also associated with an incidence of 40-50 cases per 100,000 habitants a year [4]. While part of this increase is certainly due to better clinical and diagnostic knowledge of these diseases, the possibility of a real increase cannot be ruled out [5]. Acute pancreatitis is a complex gastrointestinal disease with various aetiologies, most frequent biliary and alcoholic. Clinical presentation shows different degrees of severity with biphasic evolution. Acute pancreatitis is an inflammatory disease that can occur in an oedematous reversible form, most frequently, or in a necrotic one that is less frequent. Inflammatory diseases of the pancreas are characterized by autodigestion processes of the gland carried out by enzymes that have been inappropriately activated in the gland. Activation of trypsinogen into trypsin within the acinar cells is the starting event. The activation of other pancreatic proenzymes follows (proelastase, chymotrypsinogen, etc.). This autoactivation process of trypsin leads to pancreatic acinar cell damage with spillage of activated enzymes into the pancreatic and peripancreatic tissue [6-8].

## 2.1. Aetiological and nosographic assessment as a guide for surgery in therapeutic programmes

Many factors play an aetiological role in acute pancreatitis. In most countries biliary lithiasis and excessive alcohol consumption are the most frequent causes reaching a total incidence of 80%. Moreover, numerous other causes of pancreatitis are recognized that represent 20% of the total [9]. This remaining 20% constitutes a rather various group of causes of pancreatitis: hypercalcaemia, hypertriglyceridaemia, hereditary causes, sphincter of Oddi dysfunction, pancreas divisum, pancreatic neoplasms, medications, infections and parasitic agents, endoscopic retrograde cholangiopancreatography (ERCP) trauma (table. 1).

| Common causes | Uncommon causes | Rare causes |
| --- | --- | --- |
| Gallstones | Autoimmunity | Pancreas divisum |
| Alcoholism | Genetics | Annular pancreas |
| Hypertriglyceridaemia | Abdominal trauma | Scorpion venom |
| Post–endoscopic retrograde | Postoperative causes | Posterior penetrating ulcer |
| cholangiopancreatography | Sphincter of Oddi dysfunction | |
| Drug use | Ischaemia | |
| | Infections | |
| | Hypercalcaemiaand | |
| | hyperparathyroidism | |

Table 1. Aetiology of acute pancreatitis

Therefore pancreatitis can be considered diseases with different aetiological incidences in different countries based on environmental features and lifestyle.

In the current clinical appearance of acute pancreatitis the majority of patients (70-80%) present with a mild-moderate disease; however, approximately 20-30% run a severe course and require appropriate management in an intensive care unit. In the severe forms, in approximately 20% of cases, development of persistent organ failure and/or of infected pancreatic complications necessitates the definition of the most severe forms, identified as critical, early severe acute pancreatitis [10,11]. Critical forms are characterized by a short course, progressive multiple organ dysfunction, early hypoxaemia, high computed tomography severity index (CTSI), and increased incidences of necrosis, infection and abdominal compartment syndrome (ACS). Early severe acute pancreatitis mortality rate can be very high: 40% according to the literature. [12-16]

Severe acute pancreatitis can be seen as a biphasic disease, with the first two weeks phase characterized by early toxic-enzymatic injury (systemic inflammation response syndrome (SIRS)) and a late phase—in the third and fourth week—characterized by septic complications (infection of necrotic tissue and of peripancreatic fluid collection). Pancreatitis can present different severities in the first (toxic) phase: it can be self-limiting or quickly responsive to intensive care (especially rehydration), or it can quickly evolve into SIRS and multi-organ failure (MOF). The acute pancreatitis may progress and worsen from local disease to general involvement. The key of this evolution is the tissue response of the pancreas to acinous cell necrosis. Local actions of phlogosis lead to the activation of local macrophages and attraction of activated polymorphonuclear cells. General diffusion of phlogosis (SIRS) can develop from the passage of inflammatory mediators (pro-anti inflammatory mediators released from the splanchnic area) to systemic compartments by the lymphatic system, portal veins, and general circulation. Vascular alterations cause gut barrier failure with translocation by bacteria and endotoxin diffusion. The final results are distant organfailure (MOF) and generally later infection of fluid-necrotic pancreatic-peripancreatic gatherings [17-25].

The examination and evaluation of homogeneous clinical cases allows us to clarify the surgical options in the overall treatment programme. In our institution between 1998 to 2013 we observed and treated 304 pancreatitis cases, 294 acute biliary pancreatitis cases, and ten chronic alcoholic pancreatitis cases. The mean age was 49 years (range 30-86 years). Male:female ratio was 1:1.33 (table 2).

| 304 pancreatitis-mean age 49 yrs. (range 30-86 yrs.)- M:F ratio 1:1.33 | |
|---|---|
| Acute pancreatitis | Chronic pancreatitis |
| 294 | 10 |

Table 2. Demographic data, 304 pancreatitis.

An acute episode of pancreatitis was defined, at first assessment, on the basis of the clinical appearance of nausea, vomiting and abdominal pain in mesogastrium radiating through the back with abdominal wall tenderness (superficial/depth) and muscular rigidity of varying degrees, and laboratory data with almost twice the normal increase of the serum lipase and pancreatic amylase. This initial diagnostic phase was completed by evaluation of the involvement of general conditions and of the degree of pancreatic impairment by abdominal US.

Biliary aetiology was confirmed in 294 patients. This group included 93 patients with previous repeated episodes (31.63%). Among the 93 recurrent pancreatitis cases were also 20 patients, recently observed, with recurrent unexplained pancreatitis at first aetiological evaluation [26]. The biliary aetiology of pancreatitis has been established in a large majority of patients at initial etiological assessment by the research on abdominal US, gallbladder lithiasis, and/or gallstones, sludge, microlithiasis, etc. in the common bile duct (CBD), or also a dilation of the CBD (>8mm) with the addition of liver function tests, fasting serum calcium, and lipid profile (Tab 3). In 20% of these patients alcohol consumption slightly over the average has also been noted. Twenty patients (6.8%) have been diagnosed with recurrent unexplained forms at first-level aetiological assessment. The following diagnostic study, MRCP and/or endoscopic US, confirmed the biliary origin of pancreatitis in the majority of cases (14 patients). Only in six cases did the aetiology of pancreatitis remain unexplained. Following empirical criteria, four cholecystectomies and two ERCP/ES procedures were carried out in these six patients whose aetiology remained undefined and who had already undergone cholecystectomy.

| Dir Bil (0.02-0.30 mg/dL) <2 mg/dl | Dir Bil (0.02-0.30 mg/dL) 2 -5 mg/dl | AST/ALT X3 | g-GT (7-38 u/L) >200 u/L | |
|---|---|---|---|---|
| 61.2% | 38.8% | 29.4% | 63.4% | |
| Serum calcium (8.4-10.5 mg/dL) >10.5 mg/dL | Triglyceridaemia (40-170 mg/dL) >170 mg/dL | Cholecystic lithiasis/ sludge | CBD size (US) (8mm) | Undefined aetiology |
| 16% | 43% | 84% | 41.3% | 6.8% |

**Table 3.** 294 acute biliary pancreatitis: percentage incidence of biliary lithiasis and cholestasis indexes at first level aetiological assessment

Acute pancreatitis shows a wide range of disease, ranging from a mild form to a severe or early severe, rapidly progressive illness. The most common cause of acute pancreatitis is biliary lithiasis—almost the total number of cases in our experience. The majority of our patients had a mild-moderate disease. Mild acute pancreatitis takes a self-limiting form characterized by pancreatic or peripancreatic oedema and normal enhancement of pancreatic parenchyma on contrast-enhanced CT. Moderate pancreatitis develops early acute fluid collections located in or near the pancreas without a wall of fibrous tissue, almost always with spontaneous regression. These forms are not accompanied by impairment of the patient's general condition. In summary, regarding a first-line therapeutic approach, mild-moderate acute pancreatitis requires only supportive therapy and generally evolves towards a spontaneous recovery. Among 294 acute biliary pancreatitis cases we have observed and treated 167 (56.80%) mild-moderate forms, 61 (20.74%) moderate severe forms, 51 (17.34%) severe acute pancreatitis cases, and 15 (5.10%) early severe acute pancreatitis cases. Moderate-severe acute pancreatitis is characterized by large, broad peripancreatic and pancreatic involvement with fluid/necrotic collections but without impairment of general clinical conditions. Organ failure is transient or absent. Severe forms have diffuse or local areas of non-viable pancreatic parenchyma, peripancreatic fat necrosis, non-enhanced pancreatic parenchyma on contrast CT, and/or fluid-necrotic peripancreatic collections with persistent or transient organ failure [27-28]. Within the severe forms there are also critical or early severe forms with persistent or transient organ failure and infected pancreatic and peripancreatic collections. In our patients (294) we have applied CTSI with Balthazar scoring for the grading of acute pancreatitis and points for necrosis [29-31]. This classification is based on morphological and functional features: local or diffuse enlargement of the pancreas, pancreatic gland abnormalities, peripancreatic inflammation with pancreatic and peripancreatic fluid collections, and areas of non-enhanced parenchyma. In this morphologic assessment moderate (167), moderate-severe (61), severe (51) and early severe acute pancreatitis (15) cases have been included (table 4).

| | Grade B1 | 160 (54.42%) | |
|---|---|---|---|
| | Grade C2 | 68 (23.12%) | |
| | Grade D3 | 51 (17.34%) | |
| | Grade E4 | 15 (5.10%) | |
| | Pancreatic necrosis | | |
| 0 | None | | 228 |
| 2 | Less than/equal to 30% | | 49 |
| 4 | >30-50% | | 17 |
| 6 | >50% | | - |

**Table 4.** 294 acute biliary pancreatitis. CT severity index: CT grade point+point for necrosis (Balthazar)

The therapeutic approach of acute biliary pancreatitis usually develops in two phases following the evolution of the disease. The first phase in mild-moderate forms consists of simple fluid rehydration and control of abdominal pain. In severe acute pancreatitis the first phase is conventionally referred to the first two weeks from onset, and the initial approach is based on intensive care, initial aggressive fluid resuscitation, low dose steroids, anticoagulatory agents for anti-inflammatory properties, correction of hypoxaemia, enteral nutrition to preserve the intestinal wall integrity and antibiotic prophylaxis [32]. In this phase the most important purpose is to control and treat—by intensive care support—the impairment of the general conditions and single or multiple organ failure that can occur. Besides, the central key in the global therapeutic programme for acute biliary pancreatitis is the control and treatment of papillary patency. ERCP and endoscopic sphincterotomy (ES) can assure papillary flow and CBD cleaning if lithiasis obstacle, sludge, and microlithiasis are present. We scheduled ERCP/ES for within three to four days from onset in 217 patients (73.8%); three patients needed to be excluded because the procedure was not feasible. This therapeutic programme was performed in the following cases: 64 patients with severe and early severe acute pancreatitis, 60 with moderate-severe disease and 73 with recurrent pancreatitis, and finally in 17 with moderate pancreatitis. In these patients we achieved laboratoristic or US or MRCP confirmation of a papillary or CBD lithiasic obstacle. In seven patients with severe acute and moderate-severe pancreatitis ERCP/ES was delayed for ten days. Among 214 patients who underwent ERCP/ES, CBD cleaning was confirmed in 163 (76.16%). The therapeutic programme of acute biliary pancreatitis ends with videolaparocholecystectomy (VLC). The timing of the VLC is connected with the evolution of acute pancreatitis, waiting for the stabilization of the local phlogistic process, and of the general condition. In any case, in our opinion, the cholecystectomy should be performed in the same hospital stay [33,34]. The severe and early severe forms of acute biliary pancreatitis were evident for local and/or systemic complications. The degree of pancreas impairment with Balthazar score was five in severe acute pancreatitis (SAP), and eight in early severe acute pancreatitis (ESAP). Abdominal compartment syndrome (ACS) was demonstrated in only one patient with ESAP (1/15–6.6%), multiple organ dysfunction syndrome (MODS) in six patients with ESAP (6/15–40.46%), simple organ dysfunction in 26 patients with SAP (26/51–50.98%) versus eight patients with ESAP (8/15–53.33%), pancreatic sepsis in four patients with SAP (4/51-7.84%) versus three patients with ESAP (3/15-20%), hypoxaemia in 34 patients with SAP (34/51-66.66%) versus 11 patients with ESAP (11/15–73.33%). Mortality rate was 3.92% (2/51) (late) in SAP versus 13.33% in ESAP (2/15) (early). Mortality occurred early in patients with ACS (fifth postoperative day) and in patients with multiple organ dysfunction syndrome (first week from onset), and later in two patients who had not undergone surgical treatment, for prolonged organ dysfunction (third and fourth week) (table5).

|  | SAP | ESAP |
| --- | --- | --- |
| Impairment degree of pancreas (Balthazar CT score) | 5 | 8 |
| Abdominal compartment syndrome (ACS) (%) | - | 6.6% (1/15) |
| Multiple organ dysfunction syndrome | - | 40.46% (6/15) |
| Simple organ dysfunction | 50.98% (26/51) | 53.33% (8/15) |
| Pancreatic sepsis | 7.84% (4/51) | 20% (3/15) |
| Hypoxaemia | 66.66% (34/51) | 73.33% (11/15) |
| Mortality | 3.92% (2/51) late | 13.33% (2/15) early |

Table 5. Comparison of the clinical appearance of early severe acute pancreatitis (ESAP) and severe acute pancreatitis (SAP)

These forms required appropriate management in intensive care. In early severe forms there was a great compromise of general conditions by early toxic-enzymatic injury and high rate of early mortality (13.33%). The later phase of the disease (third and fourth week) was characterized by septic complications of pancreatic or peripancreatic fluid-necrotic collections.

The preferred approach to fluid and necrotic collections was US/CT guided percutaneous drainage. In our experience, considering 66 patients (51 SAP and 15 ESAP), we intervened only in eight patients: three US/CT guided percutaneous drainages of peripancreatic septic gatherings, two US/CT guided percutaneous drainages of fluid intrahepatic gatherings, and two US/CT guided percutaneous drainages of necrotic gatherings. These minimally invasive approaches were followed by clinical improvement without further intervention. We performed an open approach for decompression with midline laparotomy and immediate skin coverage in one patient with ACS. In the case of late evolution of acute pancreatitis we performed two pseudocyst-jejunostomies by an open procedure for acute postnecrotic pseudocysts.

Complications of ERCP/ES, including post-procedural pancreatitis, perforations, bleeding and infections are not unusual. The incidence of overall complications is evaluated to be about 10%, with a major morbidity of 1.5% and mortality less than 0.5% [35,36]. Recent data from the literature have shown an overall complication rate that is never negligible, but the majority of events are of mild-to-moderate severity [37]. In our experience, we registered two duodenal perforations (2/214-0.93%). One patient was treated with conservative therapy, and the other case was submitted to surgical intervention by cholecystectomy, duodenostomy and gastro-jejunal anastomosis. Severe post-procedural pancreatitis occurred in three patients (3/214-1.40%) and was treated with medical therapy followed by resolution with a prolonged hospital stay (ten days). We also observed two post-ERCP bleeding cases (2/214-0.93%) treated with an endoscopic approach (adrenalin infiltration). Minor complications such as mild pancreatitis with hyperamylasaemia alone and rapid self-limiting evolution were observed in 18 patients (18/214–8.41%). In this endoscopic procedure it is important to identify the risk factors in order to lower complication rates: physiopathological conditions such as Oddi sphincter dysfunction and biliary duct dilation, technical difficulties of the manoeuvres performed such as the use of a guide-wires, necessity to perform a pre-cut, and finally elderly high-risk patients.

A clinical and instrumental follow-up programme, three and six months after discharge, based on clinical control, laboratory tests and abdominal US has been planned for 294 patients with acute biliary pancreatitis. The follow-up programme has divided the patients of ERCP/ES (214/217 scheduled) from the patients not submitted to this therapeutic procedure (80), with mild-moderate forms of pancreatitis. Delayed control was carried out for 124 patients (124/214-57.94%) of the first group (submitted to ERCP/ES); 90 patients could not be reached. The results of the follow-up, at three and six months, showed the absence of critical episodes, and stable normalization of laboratory and instrumental cholestasis tests (table 6)

Four patients (4/124-3.22%) had a recurrence of a mild-moderate pancreatitis before the first control. The persistence of the papillary obstacle for incomplete sphincterotomywas assessed: the new sphincterotomy and medical therapy for resolution was performed. The same check was performed in 38 patients with mild-moderate pancreatitis not submitted to ERCP/ES (38/80-47.50%); 42 patients could not be reached. This control at three and six months from the

| | |
|---|---|
| Direct bilirubin (range 0,1-0,3 mg/dL) | 0.17 mg/dL |
| Gamma-GT (range 31-64 iU/L) | 52 iU/L |
| AST (range 22-57 iU/L) | 25 iU/L |
| ALT (range 25-64 iU/L) | 31 iU/L |
| Lipasaemia (range 120-221 iU/L) | 165 iU/L |
| Pancreatic amylasaemia (range 34-72 iU/L) | 47 iU/L |
| Alkaline phosphatase (range 67-220 iU/L) | 115 iU/L |
| CBD size (range 5-8 mm, Abdominal US) | 7 mm |
| Detection of CBD stones (Abdominal US) | - |

**Table 6.** 124 patients with acute biliary pancreatitis submitted to ERCP/ES. Follow-up at three to six months (mean of two controls)

discharge was normal. No patient had a relapse of the acute attack and the haematochemical values of cholestasis indexes and pancreatic enzymes were normal (table 7)

| | |
|---|---|
| Direct bilirubin (range 0,1-0,3 mg/dL) | 0.21 mg/dL |
| Gamma-GT (range 31-64 iU/L) | 48 iU/L |
| AST (range 22-57 iU/L) | 24 iU/L |
| ALT (range 25-64 iU/L) | 29 iU/L |
| Lipasaemia (range 120-221 iU/L) | 171 iU/L |
| Pancreatic amylasaemia (range 34-72 iU/L) | 42 iU/L |
| Alkaline phosphatase (range 67-220 iU/L) | 105 iU/L |
| CBD size (range 5-8 mm, Abdominal US) | 5 mm |
| Detection of CBD stones (Abdominal US) | - |

**Table 7.** 38 patients with acute biliary pancreatitis not submitted to ERCP/ES. Follow-up at three to six months (mean of two controls)

## 2.2. Role of surgery in the treatment of acute pancreatitis

General guidelines for surgical treatment can be found for acute pancreatitis, mainly with biliary pathogenesis,,which are clearly geared towards less aggression and minimally invasive approaches.

In mild-moderate acute biliary pancreatitis the minimally invasive therapeutic approach is the rule. The management programme includes the first-line diagnostic evaluation with the control of cholestasis laboratory tests and of CBD imaging (size, lithiasis, microlithiasis, sludge) by non-invasive instrumental exams (US). Usually the mild-moderate form undergoes a favourable self-limiting evolution; in fact, it needs only supportive therapy. In some patients the onset of moderate pancreatitis can be more aggressive but not with heavy impairment of general conditions. In these cases it is useful to direct intensive care with rehydration, control of abdominal pain, antibiotic prophylaxis, and enteral nutrition [38,39]. In patients with cholestasis index increases and/or dilation of the CBD, the MRCP should be mandatory. In patients with mild-moderate forms, without an increase of cholestasis indexes, and in the absence of a dilation of the intra-and extrahepatic biliary ducts, it is all the same useful to know if obstacles not clinically manifest are present in the CBD, and these patients should be submitted to an MRCP before cholecystectomy. In all these cases the extensive use of MRCP can be useful for a significant reduction in the number of non-therapeutic ERCP/ES incidences [40,41].

Therefore if a papillary or CBD lithiasic obstacle is demonstrated, the therapeutic programme includes assuring papillary patency and common bile duct cleaning with ERCP/ES [42-52]. In all patients with pancreatitis with biliary pathogenesis, submitted to ERCP/ES or not, it is necessary to perform laparoscopic cholecystectomy in the same hospital stay to complete the gallstone treatment. The timing of laparoscopic cholecystectomy is connected with acute pancreatitis evolution because it is preferable to wait for the stabilization and improvement of the general condition and of the phlogistic impairment of pancreatic and peripancreatic tissue.

In severe and early severe acute biliary pancreatitis the therapeutic minimally invasive approach is generally the procedure of choice. Severe and early severe acute pancreatitis can develop through an altered balance between the proinflammatory reaction to pancreatic necrosis in the peritoneal compartment (positive effect) and systemic circulation and diffusion of the high level of anti-inflammatory mediators (negative effect). This balance alteration can cause SIRS and MODS. The minimally invasive therapeutic programme of severe and early severe pancreatitis follows the biphasic development of the disease. The minimal invasiveness is necessary in the first phase because it promotes the control of the impairment of general conditions by means of systemic intensive therapies that encompass initial aggressive fluid resuscitation and support of vasopression (dopamine, vasopressin, etc.) [53]. In biliary severe acute pancreatitis, the papillary obstacle (lithiasis, microlithiasis, oddities) and choledocholi-thiasis can have a minimally invasive endolaparoscopic approach by ERCP/ES. In the later evolution (second phase), local complications, if not solved spontaneously, allow an efficacious minimally invasive approach to be preferred in patients in unstable conditions. Control and treatment of pancreatic peripancreatic gatherings (necrotic, fluid, infected) and control and treatment of belated acute postnecrotic pseudocysts should be planned.

In the very wide perspective of the role of the surgery in the treatment of acute pancreatitis, there are some points of discussion about the surgical therapeutic approach in various clinical appearances, difference for timing of presentation (early-late), and degree of severity.

The indications of emergency surgical procedures for severe and early severe acute pancreatitis are evident. This initial clinical event is placed at the onset of acute pancreatitis definitely comes outside of septic complications, which are on the contrary characteristics of the next evolution of the disease. In the first phase of severe acute pancreatitis the clinical scenario is dominated by the impairment of general conditions (toxic phase), emergency surgery has restricted indications such as ACS, and there exists cases of uncertainty of diagnosis that may persist even after imaging exams (US and/or CT). Aggressive fluid therapy is the rational treatment in the early phase of severe acute pancreatitis. This treatment allows the correction of hypovolaemia by third space fluid loss and a reduction of the high haematocrit that can serve as a marker of haemoconcentration, which is present in up to 60% of patients who develop organ failure. Aggressive fluid resuscitation with associated leaking capillaries can increase tissue oedema with concause intra-abdominal hypertension (IAH) and ACS [54,55]. Therefore, severe pancreatitis fluid resuscitation and capillary leakage can lead to intra-abdominal hypertension. For this reason monitoring of intra-abdominal pressure (IAP) is necessary for patients at risk of developing ACS. If IAP reaches 12 mmHg conservative methods such as appropriate restriction of intravenous fluids, gastrointestinal decompression by nasogastric tube, and drainage of ascites fluid should be applied to prevent the development of ACS. This conservative management can be successful. If ACS develops in spite of these procedures, surgical emergency decompression should be performed. The surgical procedures used in the treatment of ACS are very complex; they can be grouped under the definition of surgical decompression. The most commonly employed surgical procedure is the midline laparotomy. All the layers of the abdominal wall are divided by a xiphopubic vertical incision and complete exposition of the abdominal cavity. A similar result can be achieved with a transverse bilaterally extended incision few centimetres below the costal margins [56-57]. A reduction of IAP can be achieved with both techniques. The clinical scenarios of the management of the open abdomen are very difficult. The various methods to cover the abdominal viscera for the necessary time until ACS improvement—generally some days—include a plastic silo (Bogotà bag), vacuum-assisted wound closure, or a vacuum pack or self-made negative pressure dressing. Finally vacuum-assisted wound closure combined with a mesh-mediated fascial traction [58] has been proposed. After surgical decompression and ACS has been treated, the following step is the abdominal wall closure. The available techniques encompass the primary fascial closure or planned hernia with skin coverage and subsequent delayed abdominal wall reconstruction.

In our experience, urgent surgical decompression with midline laparotomy and immediate skin coverage has been useful in patients who have developed ACS. The uncertainty of the diagnosis in SAP is rather unusual because of the diagnostic efficiency of laboratory and instrumental exams. Furthermore in doubt of the acute abdomen the emergency laparotomy is mandatory. Outside of these aforementioned clinical situations, surgical procedures should be avoided in patients with severe pancreatitis due to the high death rate when performed within the first few days of onset.

Patient choice and the timing of ERCP/ES are a much-debated issue in the therapy of acute biliary pancreatitis. Papillary obstruction is widely recognized as the pathogenic factor of acute biliary pancreatitis. The role of papillary obstruction by stones, sludge, and microlithiasis migration to the CBD from the gallbladder with bile reflux into pancreatic ducts, was described by Opie in 1901 [59]. It must also be remembered that the obstacle can be transitory, with the spontaneous migration of the stones in the duodenum; in addition the transit of the stones may be followed by inflammation and papillary sclerosis. The diagnostic confirmation of acute biliary pancreatitis is almost always possible on the basis of clinical, laboratory and instrumental data. The severity of the disease can also be established by multifactorial scores (Ranson [60], Glasgow [61], Apache II [62]) at the point of admission and in the first 24-48 hours, by unifactorial markers (PCR, TAP [63], Procalcitonin [64], Hct), and subsequently by means of imaging (Balthazar score and CTSI). In severe or early severe acute pancreatitis the initial therapeutic approach, as mentioned, is based on aggressive fluid resuscitation, invasive hemodynamic monitoring, intensive care, correction of hypoxaemia, and enteral nutrition [65]. Next, the cornerstone of the therapeutic programme required, in the opinion of many authors [38-48], an urgent ERCP with endoscopic sphincterotomy. This is also in the absence of cholangitis and sometimes without the verification of cholestasis, because the papillary obstacle is the cause of pancreatitis. Recent evidences suggest that can useful to modify this therapeutic choice; ERCP/ES should be performed based on clinical-laboratory evidence of cholestasis and/or cholangitis or on demonstration of biliary or papillary obstacle by MRCP [38,49,66,67]. Furthermore, in the course of mild-moderate acute biliary pancreatitis the ERCP/ ES is reserved for cases with a documented papillary obstacle based on the increase of cholestasis indexes and/or of CBD size, or with obstacle presence (stones, odditis, etc.) in the CBD demonstrated by US/MRCP. On the other hand, only the therapeutic role of ERCP/ES has been established, while the diagnostic role for detection of CBD/papillary obstacles is played by MRCP.

There is a difficult decision to be made about the indication of ERCP/ES in a patient with acute pancreatitis with deterioration of general condition. Emergency ERCP in a patient submitted to intensive care, with the requirement of assisted ventilation, is a procedure with risk. In this clinical situation the therapeutic choice is not unanimously defined. In practice urgent ERCP/ ES (within three to four days from the onset) should be performed in severe and early severe acute pancreatitis with cholangitis, or cholestasis or jaundice with evidence of SIRS. In conclusion, there is no clear-cut answer to the question as to whether or not early ERCP/ES in cases of acute biliary pancreatitis (within 24-72 hours from onset) reduces the risk of progression of acute pancreatitis to severe disease (organ failure and/or necrosis). [38]

It is, however, determined in severe and early severe cases without evidence of cholestasis, in recurrent acute pancreatitis, in moderate-severe pancreatitis and in patients with mild-moderate forms, to be appropriate and useful to confirm papillary or CBD lithiasis obstacle by laboratory, US or MRCP before therapeutic ERCP/ES. In patients with mild-moderate pancreatitis without instrumental, clinical-laboratory demonstration of papillary-CBD obstruction, the ES is not indicated. This therapeutic choice is based on the consideration that in mild-moderate forms the papillary obstacle (without cholestasis) may be transient and the treatment is not required [49,51].

A flow-chart of ERCP/ES employment in acute biliary pancreatitis is shown in figure 1.

The management of acute severe necrotizing pancreatitis has been much modified over time. The prevalence of acute necrotizing pancreatitis is 15-20% and its pathological basis is the hypoperfusion of the parenchyma on a contrast-enhanced CT (Balthazar score) [31]. The necrotic process involves the pancreatic gland and the peripancreatic tissues with very variable extension. The extensive interstitial oedema is associated with pancreatic and peripancreatic necrosis in a short period of 48-72 hours after the onset of acute attack. These inflammatory,

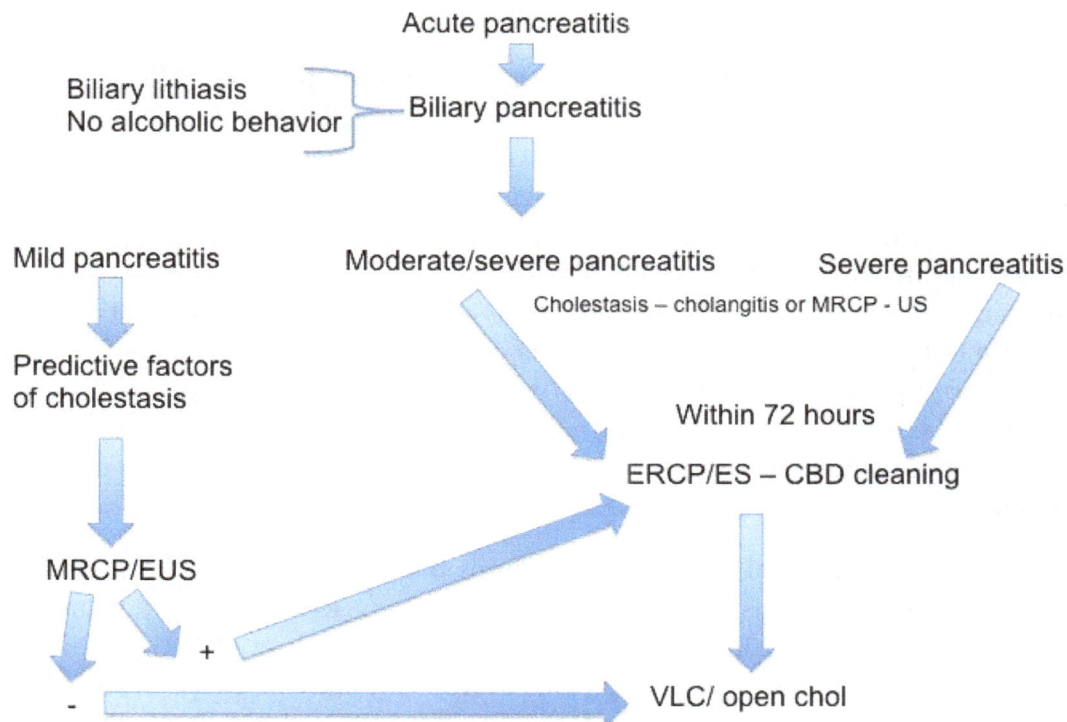

**Figure 1.** Flow-chart: ERCP/ES in acute biliary pancreatitis

necrotic tissues subsequently cause acute fluid collections with an amount of devitalized tissue. The further evolution of these fluid gatherings is characterized by demarcation between viable and necrotic tissue, and the limit is set with a wall of granulation tissue. The management of these pancreatic peripancreatic fluid-necrotic collections and their complications is the longest and most debated therapeutic problem.

Particularly in question are some specific surgical decisions: how long the control and observation of uncomplicated fluid-necrotic gatherings may be prolonged; which clinical, laboratory and instrumental data we must follow to differentiate between infected and sterile pancreatic necrosis; whether the intervention may be delayed for a few (four to eight) weeks in some patients with infected necrosis when the gathering has become walled off; and finally the choice of the best surgical approach for the treatment of fluid-necrotic complicated collections.

In severe acute pancreatitis (necrotizing) we can distinguish between two phases in the evolution of the disease, as is already reported; however, these two distinct phases can also be considered in relation to the surgical procedures. There is an early toxic phase (one to two weeks from the onset), characterized by the severe involvement of general conditions and the start of the dreaded SIRS: in this phase the main purpose is minimizing the mortality from MODS, and all surgical procedures should be avoided. The late phase (from the third week) is characterized by the fluid-necrotic collections with or without septic complications, such as infected pancreatic necrosis.

Uncomplicated fluid necrotic gatherings may be submitted to conservative procedures that can be extended for four to eight weeks, when persisting peripancreatic fluid collections are referred to as acute postnecrotic pseudocysts. If these gatherings in this phase are not symptomatic, surgical manoeuvres and percutaneous drainages should be avoided. Placement of a drain into a sterile necrotic collection can result in secondary infection, and prolonged drainage may increase the risk further [68,69]. Most patients with sterile necrosis show results with conservative non-surgical management. It is debatable as to which patients the surgical procedure to treat sterile pancreatic necrosis can be useful for. In the data from the literature there is no complete solution, but there is a suggestion that, in selected cases with persistent organ failure and severe impairment of general conditions despite intensive care unit therapy, surgery may be useful in sterile necrosis [70-72]. In our experience we have undergone US/CT guided percutaneous drainage in two patients with symptomatic fluid intrahepatic gatherings.

After diagnosis of pancreatic necrotic collections the next step is the differentiation between sterile and infected necrosis. This diagnostic data may be essential for the therapeutic choice. The exam of choice is the fine-needle aspiration for bacteriology (FNAB), which can usually be guided by CT and/or US. The suspicious of infection may be based on the demonstration by CECT of gas bubbles into the gatherings. Moreover, this should be performed in patients with evident pancreatic peripancreatic necrotic gatherings and clinical signs of sepsis. This diagnostic procedure is accurate and safe with a very low incidence of complications such as bleeding. If the clinical, laboratory, and instrumental data do not raise suspicion of sepsis in necrotic collections, the FNAB should not be performed, owing to a potential risk of secondary infection [73-76]. Surgical intervention is required in patients with fluid-necrotic septic collection, also because the septic condition worsens the impairment of general condition and organ failure On the other hand, not all patients with infected necrosis but without compromise of general conditions and/or organ dysfunction will require urgent intervention [77,78]. This therapeutic choice is based on the purpose to delay the surgical procedure for some weeks when the collection has become walled off [79].

## 2.3. Choice of surgical approach for gatherings

All therapeutic choices in acute pancreatitis should be connected with the evolution of the disease, which may be very complex. Organ failure (MODS) in the first phase of the disease is usually not related to infection but to SIRS. However, septic complications of disorganized necrotizing tissue can also occur in this phase, with further worsening of disease evolution [80]. The latter phase of the disease is characterized by a counteractive anti-inflammatory response syndrome (CARS). In this phase there is the risk of infected necrosis and organ failure related to infections. Gooszen et al. [81] report three scenarios in the late evolution of severe acute pancreatitis. First is improvement with intensive care after early onset organ failure, but this is followed by deterioration in the third or fourth week, often due to infection of necrosis. Another scenario is clinical impairment without distinct early organ failure, most likely to be caused by infected necrosis in the third or fourth week. In both cases further interventional procedures should be indicated. Finally, stable early onset organ failure without improvement is also indicated in the second to third week; in this case the verification of collection infection (FNAB, gas bubbles on CECT) can be useful for the programming of surgical intervention.

Sterile pancreatic peripancreatic fluid-necrotic collections require observation and conservative treatment. This choice is based on the physiopathological evolution of necrotizing pancreatitis. The principal characteristic that should be considered is the time of evolution of necrotizing pancreatic gatherings: this period is usually very long, from 24-36 hours up to 12 weeks. This evolution goes through three phases until the resolution or constitution of acute postnecrotic pseudocysts if the collection remains sterile [82]. In the first phase is true pancreatic necrosis with minimal separation of devitalized tissues, with a high solid/liquid ratio. Then comes the transitional pancreatic necrosis, also called the intermediate lesion. Infection can arise in every occurrence of this phase. The following phase is organized pancreatic necrosis with good separation of devitalized tissue within a fluid gathering, with development of a fibrous-granular wall. This last phase can be defined as a walled-off pancreatic necrosis. The acute postnecrotic pseudocyst is the final evolution characterized by the complete separation of the tissues, with a liquid content and fibrous wall. Therefore, in most cases the sterile asymptomatic pancreatic peripancreatic fluid-necrotic gatherings do not need treatment, instead requiring only clinical-instrumental observation by US-CT every 4 to 6 weeks, because the resolution can occur in 8 to 12 weeks in mean. There also exists in the literature extreme data up to 280 days [83] or one year [84]. In the phase of walled-off pancreatic necrosis, infected pancreatic peripancreatic necrotic fluid collections diagnosed by FNAB or gas bubbles on CECT, or suspected infection but with the impairment of general condition, has traditionally been considered an accepted indication for intervention. Based on the evolution of pancreatic peripancreatic necrosis the importance of choice on the timing of intervention is evident. From the data of the literature the almost unanimous conclusion is that the best choice is to delay intervention until the fluid-necrotic collections are encapsulated, and thus called walled-off necrosis. This process is usually completed in 4 to 6 weeks. If, during this evolution process of pancreatic peripancreatic necrosis, the deterioration of general conditions occurs, the administration of broad-spectrum antibiotics can prevent infections and it allows to delay of the surgical procedure. Surgery in the first two weeks from the onset—frequently necrosectomy for infected collections—has a mortality rate of 75% with a gradual decrease to 5% if performed later than four weeks from the onset. Compromise of general condition and multiple organ dysfunction causes a worsening of results [69,85-87]. In spite of the benefit of the postponing intervention, it is not always possible to delay surgery if the general condition of patient deteriorates, because infected collections can worsen organ failure in the first week of pancreatitis [88]. In summary, the better results in the surgical treatment of fluid-necrotic pancreatic gatherings are clearly connected to a suitable time interval—between the onset of symptoms and intervention—for encapsulation of collection and the recovery of general condition of the patient.

The surgical procedure employed in the treatment of pancreatic peripancreatic necrotic gatherings in the last decade showed a progressive evolution to minimally invasive procedures. Nevertheless, in this setting there are no unanimously standardized and accepted surgical procedures, and so overall there are no clearly defined indications for various surgical procedures. Until a short time ago, an open approach for infected necrotic collection (so called open necrosectomy) was the standard, first choice, surgical procedure. In this open procedure, the laparotomy is followed by complete debridement and necrosectomy and placement of a retroperitoneal lavage system and drains in the lesser sac. The mortality rate of this procedure, reported by Rau, is 25% [89]. Other open procedures are proposed but not commonly adopted, and have uncertain result, such as closed packing with referred mortality 11% [90], and the open abdomen strategy with planned relaparotomies, which has a very high mortality rate (70%) [81]. These results should be considered in a very severe disease scenario.

Recently necrosectomy by a minimally invasive procedure, such as percutaneous minimally invasive retroperitoneal necrosectomy, has been proposed [91]. Moreover the video-assisted retroperitoneal debridement (VARD) [92,93], by the minimally invasive surgical approach, aims to remove only some pieces of less adherent necrosis rather than all parts of the necrosis. In this way we can reduce the risk of bleeding, and the remnant necrotic tissue can be resorbed. This percutaneous procedure can be repeated, and drainage into cavity planned. Further minimally invasive procedures for the treatment of infected pancreatic necrotic collection include:

- Necrosectomy with minimally invasive step-up approach.

- Endoscopic transluminal necrosectomy (ETN).

- Percutaneous drainage.

The step-up approach has been proposed and compared with open necrosectomy in a Dutch multicentre randomised study on acute necrotizing pancreatitis [94]. The comparison showed minor complications with a step-up approach. This procedure consists of percutaneous or transgastric drainage, and then drain-guided necrosectomy if necessary. This procedure, which has been performed in some patients (35%), has achieved stable results only once.

In ETN the endoscopic access is usually transgastric. The procedure has a very low invasivity but there is the need for repeated procedures to remove the necrotic collection [95].

## 2.4. The global evaluation of this minimally invasive procedure is in progress.

Finally we have to consider the simple, basic percutaneous drainage of septic necrotic gatherings. The drainage is not necrosectomy but from the perspective of a minimally invasive approach, with a real possibility that the necrotic tissue can be resorbed, the percutaneous catheter drainage can be considered the first therapeutic approach in the case of (suspected or documented) infected necrotic pancreatic gatherings. Percutaneous drainage has been largely employed, but there is no complete therapeutic evaluation of this method. Recently many results of systematic reviews have become available [87]: the technical success rate was 99%, and the number of patients with necrotizing pancreatitis treated with percutaneous drainage alone was high (22-55%). In summary, we can accept that after the first step (percutaneous drainage) of a therapeutic programme for septic necrotic gatherings, if the drainage of the collection is incomplete, it should be necessary to perform a complete necrosectomy. Finally we can conclude that it is not clear what the best procedure is for the treatment of septic necrotic pancreatic collections. Open necrosectomy remains the last option after the failure of less invasive procedures. A flow-chart of the management of pancreatic peripancreatic gatherings is shown in figure 2.

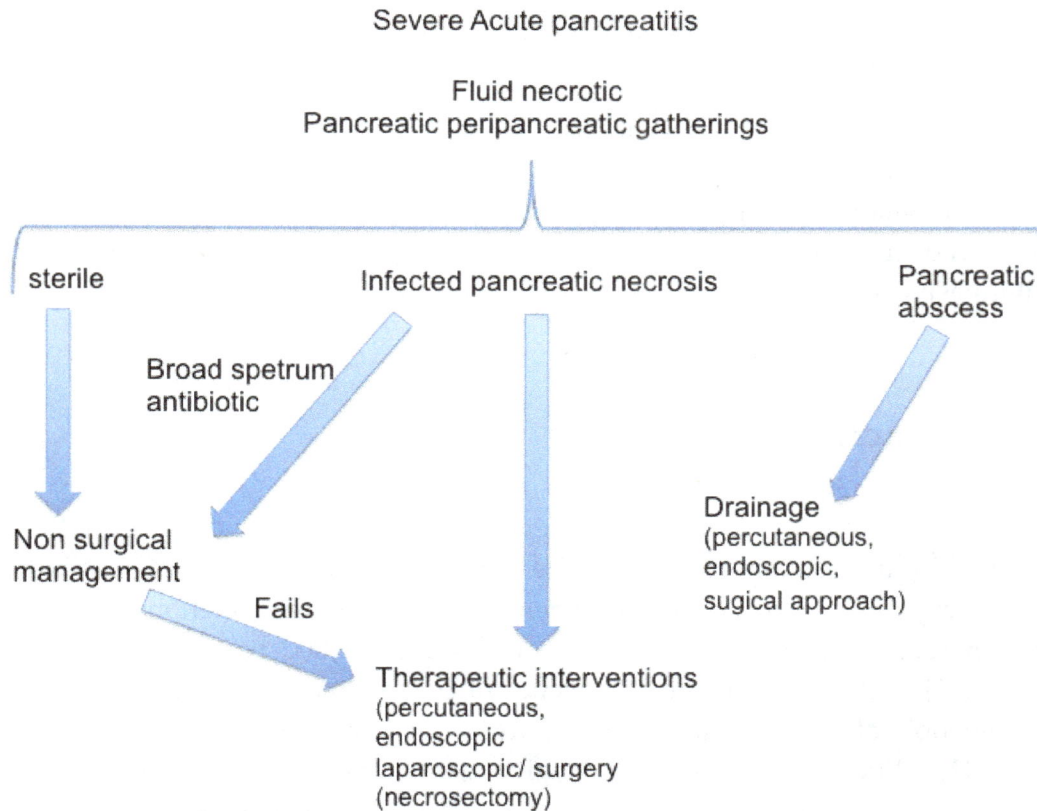

Severe Acute pancreatitis

Fluid necrotic
Pancreatic peripancreatic gatherings

sterile

Infected pancreatic necrosis

Pancreatic
abscess

Broad spetrum
antibiotic

Drainage
(percutaneous,
endoscopic,
sugical approach)

Non surgical
management

Fails

Therapeutic interventions
(percutaneous,
endoscopic
laparoscopic/ surgery
(necrosectomy)

**Figure 2.** Flow-chart: management of pancreatic-peripancreatic gatherings

Acute postnecrotic pseudocysts are the final evolution of necrotizing pancreatic gatherings, characterized by complete separation of the tissues, with liquid content and a fibrous wall. The incidence of acute pseudocysts is low, at 5-16% [82]. The evolution of a lesion with a fibrous wall can be complete in many weeks (12-16 weeks). Small cysts (<5-6 cm) can be observed for many months without clinical appearance. In some cases there is some spontaneous improvement until the resolution of the pseudocysts [96]. Treatment is required for a pseudocyst larger than 6-7 cm, or one that is symptomatic or persistent over many months. There are various surgical procedures for the treatment of pseudocysts. The pathological characteristic of acute pseudocysts is the connection with pancreatic ducts. In fact simple percutaneous US/CT guided drainage can be often followed by persistent leakage from the drain; other complications of this procedure include infections and the repeated changes required of the drain [97]. Based on the communication of the pseudocysts with pancreatic ducts, all surgical procedures should involve a cystodigestive prolonged connection (anastomosis, fistulas) for the steady drainage of pancreatic secretions. During its development, the pseudocysts establish a connection with adjacent intestinal organs to which the cyst is adherent: usually the stomach, small intestine, and duodenum. From this perspective there are various possible procedures. Drainage of the pseudocyst by endoscopic techniques has been proposed [98,99]: this is performed by creating a small opening between the cyst and stomach. The disadvantage of this technique is incomplete drainage with recurrence of pseudocysts and infection because the communication can be small and in site not declive. The surgical procedures use the adjacent intestinal organ (stomach, duodenum, small intestine) involved in each case for anastomosis with the cyst: cystogastrostomy, cystojejunostomy, cystoduodenostomy [96].

For cysts located in the body or tail of pancreas the cystojejunostomy or cystogastrostomy is performed depending the development of the cyst above or under the mesocolon. For pseudocysts developed in the head, cystoduodenostomy is usually performed. The same surgical procedures can be performed with a laparoscopic approach with the advantage of the minimal invasiveness.

## 3. Chronic pancreatitis

Chronic pancreatitis is a continuing, progressive inflammatory process of the pancreas, characterized by irreversible changes in the morphology of the gland. The gradual fibrosis of the parenchyma causes the loss of exocrine and endocrine functions. The incidence of chronic pancreatitis ranges from 1.6 to 23 cases per 100,000 population per year world-wide [100, 101]. The incidence and prevalence of chronic pancreatitis is low, and more than 50% are alcohol related. The incidence of the disease appeared to be increasing in past decades [102]. Whereas in acute pancreatitis tissue alteration may be reversible in the oedematous form, chronic pancreatitis is characterized by irreversible tissue changes and exocrine dysfunction. Chronic pancreatitis lies on a protracted inflammation of the pancreas characterized by the permanent alteration of the basic anatomical structure accompanied by functional deficits, even if the cause is eliminated. The cause of chronic disease is stable tissue inflammation by various causes. Therefore, there are multiple hypotheses as to the pathophysiology of chronic pancreatitis: necrosis-fibrosis, toxic-metabolic causes, plug and stone formation, duct obstruction, or sentinel acute pancreatitis event (SAPE) [100]. The pathological features are pancreatic parenchymal fibrosis, duct dilation, and pancreatic stones. Chronic abdominal pain characterizes the clinical appearance of the disease. Acute and chronic diseases are connected based on pathological features: both are characterized by a phlogistic process with autodigestive and/or ordinary varieties, interchangeable with each other but with different development processes [103,104]. Inflammatory processes of pancreatitis are generally characterized by autodigestion, but less frequently ordinary, uncharacteristic interstitial pancreatic phlogosis (as reaction to general disease) without signs of autodigestion can be observed. Both varieties of phlogosis can have an acute or chronic course. The ordinary variety of pancreatitis can transgress to an autodigestive or a chronic progressive variety at any time [105].

## 3.1. Aetiological and nosographic assessment as a guide for surgery in the therapeutic programmes

Chronic pancreatitis, in most cases caused by excessive alcohol consumption, is due to tissue injury by persistent inflammation based ontoxic-metabolic hypothesis [106]. The pathologic features are destruction of pancreatic parenchyma, substitution with large fibrosis, and infiltration of inflammatory cells in various degrees [107].

Generally the effect of alcohol is amplified by a high fat diet and smoking [108]. Smoking can be an independent risk factor for the development and progression of chronic pancreatitis. Smoking can have adverse effects on the secretion of pancreatic bicarbonate and water and causespancreatic calcifications through oxidative stress.. Other less common causes of chronic pancreatitis include autoimmune-immunologic causes in autoimmune diseases such as primary autoimmune pancreatitis or associated with Crohn's disease; genetic/hereditary pancreatitis with autosomal dominant or recessive mutations in the cationic trypsinogen gene (PRSSI-SPINK1); severe hypercalcaemia with protein plug obstructive hypothesis; obstructive chronic pancreatitis (pancreatic adenocarcinoma, neuroendocrine tumours, intrapapillary mucinous tumours, annular pancreas, pancreas divisum, etc.); nutritional factor deficiencies; and idiopathic causes (table 8).

| Common causes | Less common causes |
|---|---|
| Alcohol | Severe hypercalcaemia |
| Tobacco smoking | Autoimmune |
| | Genetic |
| | Duct obstruction |
| | Hyperlipidaemia |
| | Idiopathic |

**Table 8.** Aetiology of chronic pancreatitis

Recurrent episodes of heavy abdominal pain with back bilateral diffusion, but without compromise of general condition, and a history of abnormal alcohol consumption for many years, characterized the clinical appearance of ten patients with chronic pancreatitis. Our patients were subdivided into stage A and B of Amman's classification [109]: six patients in Stage A, initial, characterized by recurrent acute attacks, with mild impairment of pancreatic function; and four patients in Stage B, later, with increasing abdominal pain and more frequent acute attacks, with some complications such as chronic pseudocysts and main pancreatic duct dilation, and impaired pancreatic function. In end-stage disease (none of our patients were in this stage) there are decreases in acute attacks and abdominal pain intensity, and marked impairment of pancreatic function. The diagnosis of chronic pancreatitis is simple in the later stages, but difficult in the initial stages. Laboratory and instrumental (EUS, CT) examinations have confirmed the diagnosis following a EUS-based criterion. The new Rosemont classification [110] of chronic pancreatitis identifies major criteria such as main pancreatic duct calculi and lobularity with honeycombing and hyperechoic foci with shadowing. Minor criteria were cysts, dilated ducts >3.5 mm, irregular pancreatic duct contour, dilated side branches >1 mm, hyperechoic duct wall, and non-shadowing hyperechoic foci.

In our experience the diagnosis was based on imaging exams with confirmation of the main pancreatic duct and branch ducts being irregularity dilated or having stenosis and calcifications in some ducts. The common pancreatic function tests (focal elastase, fasting blood glucose/oral glucose tolerance tests) do not detect mild or moderate exocrine pancreatic insufficiency. Therefore these tests are subsidiary in the current clinical evaluation of chronic pancreatitis. In chronic pancreatitis the indication of the surgical approach comes after a long clinical evolution of the disease with a well-established diagnosis. In our experience chronic pancreatitis has been treated through an operative therapeutic approach in four patients: direct ductal-enteric drainage (Puestow procedure) in two patients; longitudinal pancreaticojejunostomy combined with a local pancreatic head resection (Frey procedure) in one patient; and pancreatoduodenectomy (Whipple procedure) in one patient. The remaining six patients have undergone conservative treatment that involves control and management of steatorrhoea, malnutrition and pain.

## 3.2. Role of surgery in the treatment of chronic pancreatitis

The pathological patterns of chronic pancreatitis are focused on inflammation and fibrosis of pancreatic parenchyma, stricture, and obstruction of the main and accessory ducts and intraductal calcification [111,112]. The particular histopathological characteristics are areas of acute inflammation and foci of pancreatic cell necrosis. The pain is connected with the foci of parenchymal inflammation and ductal hypertension. Also, the inflammatory damage of the sensory nerves of the pancreas can play a role in the development of the symptoms in chronic pancreatitis [113]. The first question concerns the indications for surgery in chronic pancreatitis: the principal symptom of chronic pancreatitis is abdominal pain. The most severe intractable pain is the cornerstone of surgical indication. The surgical treatment of chronic pancreatitis should be based on the clinical and pathological scenario: two types of surgical procedures are proposable. Decompression procedures with the aim of improving or eliminating ductal hypertension by intestinal anastomotic drainage can be performed. Resectional procedures aim to eliminate areas of chronic inflammation that are especially present in the head of the pancreas. There are also denervation procedures involving neurolysis of the celiac trunk and ganglia; the data from the literature report variable results [114]. The decompression procedure can involve the endoscopic treatment [115]. In the course of chronic pancreatitis, evident ductal dilation can develop as a late complication. The incidence of these chronic pseudocysts is high: 20-40% [85]. The endoscopic procedure aims to perform cystogastrostomy or duodenocystostomy following the development and anatomical connection between the pseudocyst and intestinal organ (stomach or duodenum) [116]. The morbidity of this procedure ranges from 3-11% with no mortality. The endoscopic approach can allow the treatment of the chronic pseudocyst by drainage through the duodenal papilla and ductal system. The procedure develops with selective endoscopic pancreatic sphincterotomy retrograde pancreatography and the positioning of the transpapillary endoprotesis as drainage. The morbidity ranges from 2-7% with no mortality [116]. If intraductal stones are present, this approach can allow transluminal stone removal and/or lithotripsy, followed by prolonged pancreatic duct stenting [115-117]. Unfortunately the endoscopic approaches are not always feasible because the anatomic difficulties such as location of the cysts, papillary patency, etc. The surgical management of pancreatic duct stones and stenosis has shown better results than endoscopic treatment [118,119]. The Puestow procedure [120] and its modification of Partington and Rochelle [121] are the standard surgical drainage methods in chronic pancreatitis with dilated ducts. In the original presentation there is the resection of the tail of pancreas, longitudinal incision of the main dilated duct along the body of the pancreas, and invaginating anastomosis with a Roux-en-Y loop of jejunum. The following modification is the elimination of the resection of the pancreatic tail. The immediate results of the procedure show very low mortality (less than 1%) and morbidity (less than 10%) [122]. Pain is relieved in 85-90% of patients; recurrent pain is observed in 30% [123-125].

In some patients with a dilated pancreatic duct, a fibrotic, inflammatory mass may be present in the head of the pancreas. In these patients, surgical approaches that couple drainage and resective procedures can be indicated. These interventions can be defined as 'hybrid' [125] and show numerous variants. In duodenum-preserving pancreatic head resection (DPPHR) proposed by Beger [126], the neck of the pancreas is divided, most of the head is resected sparing the CBD and duodenum, and the procedure is completed by side-to-side pancreato-jejunostomy (Roux-en-Y). Berne modification of DPPHR consists of excavation of the head of the pancreas, without division of the pancreatic neck, completed by pancreaticojejunostomy (Roux-en-Y) [127]. Frey described the local resection of the head of the pancreas and longitudinal pancreatico-jejunostomy (LR-LPJ) [128]. Subsequently local resection of the pancreatic head with longitudinal pancreaticojejunostomy (Roux-en-Y) by Frey Hamburg modification [129], with the inclusion of the excavation of the central portion of uncinate process, in continuity with the V-shaped excavation of the body along the main pancreatic duct, has been proposed. All these hybrid surgical procedures give results that overlap, with a very low mortality (less than 1%) and a rate of morbidity from 20-30% [125]. Pain relief occurs in 80-85% of patients, also in late control [130].

The resective procedures had a general indication for the prevalence of the chronic phlogistic process in the pancreas parenchyma with lesser duct dilations. Pancreatoduodenectomy, generally called the Whipple procedure, is effective in managing pain in 70-90% of patients. The mortality is less than 5% but the morbidity can reach 40% [131]. Similar results are obtained with pylorus-preserving pancreatoduodenectomy (PPPD). The major problem of these surgical resective procedures is the pancreatic anastomotic leak that can occur with a variable incidence range from 10-30% or more. Although the pancreatic parenchyma in chronic disease generally has a hard consistency, the size of the main duct in the gland with diffuse sclerosis can be very small, at around 2-3 mm, and consequently difficult for anastomosis. Other resectional procedures are also proposed. Distal pancreatectomy, for example, has been proposed for the patients in whom the fibrotic process of the pancreas is located in the body and tail. These procedures have had medium results, resulting in pain relief in 60% of patients [132]. Almost total distal pancreatectomyand total pancreatectomy achieve good relief of abdominal pain but the metabolic consequences are an adverse result [133]. Pancreatectomy with islet auto-transplantation has been proposed [134] with interesting results but its use is limited by diffusion. A flow-chart of therapeutic management in chronic pancreatitis is shown in figure 3.

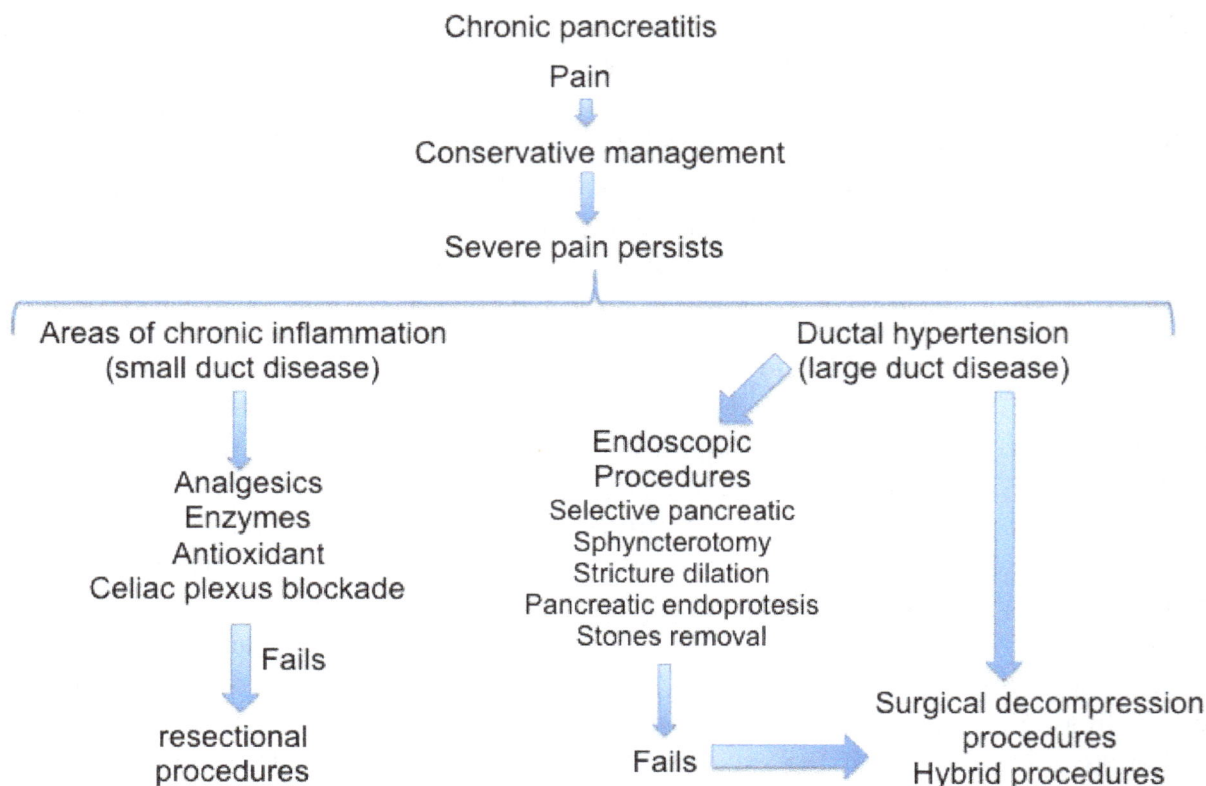

Chronic pancreatitis
Pain

Conservative management

Severe pain persists

Areas of chronic inflammation
(small duct disease)

Ductal hypertension
(large duct disease)

Analgesics
Enzymes
Antioxidant
Celiac plexus blockade

Endoscopic
Procedures
Selective pancreatic
Sphyncterotomy
Stricture dilation
Pancreatic endoprotesis
Stones removal

Fails

resectional
procedures

Fails

Surgical decompression
procedures
Hybrid procedures

**Figure 3.** Flow-chart: management of chronic pancreatitis

## 4. Conclusions

The management of severe acute pancreatitis requires a radical revision. The role of the surgery should be limited to percutaneous drainage of septic-necrotic collections, a procedure that in most cases could reduce the need for surgical intervention. If major surgical interventions are required, these should be as conservative as possible, and minimally invasive approaches are preferred [135].

In summary, chronic pancreatitis with duct obstruction, stones and protein plugs, chronic pseudocysts and abdominal pain exacerbation may be treated with drainage operations. Major resection procedures have infrequent indications based on prevalent phlogistic involvement of pancreatic parenchyma, non-dilated pancreatic ducts, and enlarged pancreatic head.

In conclusion, based on pathological and clinical observations, we can believe that the surgical interventions that couple the drainage of the distal pancreas and resection of the core of the head are procedures with acceptable results in the treatment of chronic pancreatitis.

## Author details

Vincenzo Neri[*]

Address all correspondence to: vincenzo.neri@unifg.it

General Surgery-Dept. of Medical and Surgical Sciences-University of Foggia, Italy

## References

[1] Bassi C, Butturini G. Definition and classification of pancreatitis. In: Blumgart LH et al. (eds). Surgery of the liver, biliary tract and pancreas. Saunders Elsevier Philadelphia; 2007:1. p. 685-699.

[2] Fagenholz PJ, Fernandez del Castillo C, Harris NS et al. Direct medical costs of acute pancreatitis hospitalizations in the United States. Pancreas 2007 (4): 302-307.

[3] Shaheen NJ, Hansen RA, Morgan DR et al. The burden of gastrointestinal and liver diseases. Am J Gastroenterol 2006; 101(9): 2128-2138.

[4] Go VLW, Everhart JE. Pancreatitis in Everhart JE, ed. Digestive disease in United States: epidemiology and impact. Washington DC: US Department of Health and Human Services, Public Health Service, National Institutes of Health, National Institute of Diabetes and Digestive and Kidney Diseases; 1994 p. 693. NIH publ. no 94 1447.

[5] Gullo L, Migliori M, Olah A et al. Acute pancreatitis in five European countries: aetiology and mortality. Pancreas 2002; 24:223-227.

[6] Banks PA, Conwell DL, Toskes PP. The management of acute and chronic pancreatitis. Gastroenterol Hepatol 2010; 6:1-16.

[7] Al Mofleh IA. Severe acute pancreatitis: pathogenetic aspects and prognostic factors. World J Gastroenterol 2008; 14(5): 675-84.

[8] Wang GJ, Gao CF, Wei D et al. Acute pancreatitis: aetiology and common pathogenesis. World J Gastroenterol 2009. 15, 1427-1430.

[9] Lankisch PG, Brener N, Burns A et al. Natural history of acute pancreatitis: a long-term population-based study. Am J Gastroenterol 2009; 104:2797-2805.

[10] Yadav D, O'Connel M, Papachriston GJ. Natural history following the first attack of acute pancreatitis. Am J Gastroenterol 2012; 107:1096-1103.

[11] Banks PA, Bollen TL, Dervenis C, Gooszen HG et al. Classification of acute pancreatitis-2012: revision of the Atlanta classification and definitions by international consensus. Gut 2013; 62 (1):102-111.

[12] Bassi C, Falconi M, Butturini G et al. Early complications of severe acute pancreatitis. In Holzheimer RG, Mannick JA (eds). Surgical treatment: evidence-based and problem-oriented. Munick Zuckschwerdt 2001. http://www.ncbi.nlm.nih.gov/books/NBK6978.

[13] Petrov MS, Windsor JA. Classification of the severity of acute pancreatitis: how many categories make sense? Am J Gastroenterol 2010;105:75-76.

[14] Di Fabio F, Abu Hilal M, Johnson CD. Acute pancreatitis: mild, severe or potentially fatal. Pancreatology 2011;11:373-375.

[15] Dellinger EP, Forsmark CE, Layer P et al. Determinant-based classification of acute pancreatitis severity. An international multidisciplinary consultation. Ann Surg 2012;256:875-880.

[16] Sarr MG. 2012 revision of the Atlanta classification of acute pancreatitis. Polskie Archiwuum Medyeyny Wewnetnzne J 2013;123 (3): 118-123.

[17] Dugernier TL, Laterre PF, Wittebole X et al. Compartimentalization of the inflammatory response during acute pancreatitis: correlation with local and systemic complications. Am J Respir Crit Care Med 2003; 168:148-157.

[18] Mayer J, Rau B, Gansauge F et al. Inflammatory mediators in human acute pancreatitis: clinical and pathophysiological implications. Gut 2000; 47:546-552.

[19] Makhija R, Kingsnorth AN. Cytokine storm in acute pancreatitis. J Hepatobiliary Pancreat Surg 2002; 9:401-410.

[20] Lipsett PA. Serum cytokines, proteins, and receptors in acute pancreatitis: mediators, markers, or more of the same? Crit Care Med 2001; 29:1642-1644.

[21] Pezzilli R, Maldini K, Morselli-Labate AM et al. Early activation of peripheral lymphocytes in human acute pancreatitis. J Clin Gastroenterol 2003; 36: 360-363.

[22] Poch B, Gansauge F, Rau B et al. The role of polymorphonuclear leukocytes and oxygen-derived free radicals in experimental acute pancreatitis: mediators of local destruction and activators of inflammation. FEBS Letters 1999; 461: 268-272.

[23] Sakai Y, Masamune A, Satoh A et al. Macrophage migration inhibitory factor is a critical mediator of severe acute pancreatitis. Gastroenterology 2003; 124:725-736.

[24] Guzman EA, Rudnicki M. Intricacies of host response in acute pancreatitis. J Am Coll Surg 2006; 202:509-519.

[25] Deitch EA, Xu DZ, Qi L, et al. Bacterial translocation from the gut impairs systemic immunity. Surgery 1991; 109: 269-276.

[26] Neri V, Lapolla F, Di Lascia A et al. Defining a therapeutic program for recurrent acute pancreatitis patients with unknown etiology. Clinical Med Insights: Gastroenterology 2014; 7: 1-7.

[27] Heider TR, Brown AB, Grimm IS et al. Endoscopic sphincterotomy permits internal laparoscopic cholecystectomy in patients with moderately severe gallstone pancreatitis. J Gastro Surg 2006; 10: 1-5.

[28] Nealon WH, Bawdamiak J, Walser EM. Appropriate timing of cholecystectomy in patients who present with moderate to severe gallstone pancreatitis associated acute pancreatitis with peripancreatic fluid collections. Ann Surg 2004; 239: 741-751.

[29] Balthazar EJ, Robinson DL, Megibow AJ et al. Acute pancreatitis: value of CT in establishing prognosis. Radiology 1990; 174: 331-336.

[30] Balthazar EJ, Freeny PC, Vansonnenberg E. Imaging and intervention in acute pancreatitis. Radiology 1994; 193 (2): 297-306.

[31] Balthazar EJ. Acute pancreatitis: assessment of severity with clinical and CT evaluation. Radiology 2002; 223: 603-613.

[32] Beger HG, Rau BM. Severe acute pancreatitis: clinical course and management. World J Gastroenterol 2007; 13 (38): 5043-5051.

[33] Van Baal MC, Besselink MG, Bakker OJ et al. Timing of cholecystectomy after mild biliary pancreatitis. A systematic review. Ann Surg 2012; 255: 860-866.

[34] Neri V. Mild biliary pancreatitis: interval (delayed) cholecystectomy is associated with readmission for recurrent biliary events. Evid Based Med 2013; 18:e11-doi: 10,1136/eb-2012-100847.

[35] Freeman ML. Adverse outcomes of endoscopic retrograde cholangiopancreatography. Rev Gastroenteral Disord 2002; 2: 147-168.

[36] Davis WZ, Cotton PB, Arias R et al. ERCP and sphincterotomy in the context of laparoscopic cholecystectomy: academic and community practice patterns and results. Am J Gastroenterol 1997; 92(4): 597-601.

[37] Andriulli A, Loperfido S, Napolitano G et al. Incidence rates of post-ERCP complications: a systematic survey of prospective studies. Am J Gastroenterol 2007; 102 (8): 1781-1788.

[38] Tenner S, Bailie J, Dewitt J et al. American College of Gastroenterology guidelines: management of acute pancreatitis. Am J Gastroenterol Jul. 30 2013; 1-16 doi: 10.1038/ajg2013.218.

[39]  Haydock MD, Mittal A, Van den Heever M et al. National survey of fluid therapy in acute pancreatitis. Current practice lacks a sound evidence base. World J Surg Oct 2013; vol./is.37/10(2428-35),0364-2313.

[40]  Neri V, Fersini A, Ambrosi A. et al. Mild-moderate acute biliary pancreatitis: role of magnetic resonance cholangiopancreatography in preparation of cholecystectomy. Pancreas 2009; 38(6): 717.

[41]  Neri V, Fersini A, Ambrosi A et al. Diagnostic evaluation prior to cholecystectomy in mild-moderate acute biliary pancreatitis. Ann It Chir 2009; 80: 363-367.

[42]  Fan ST, Lai EC, Mok FP et al. Early treatment of acute biliary pancreatitis by endoscopic papillotomy. N Engl J Med 1993; 328(4): 228-32.

[43]  Folsch UR, Nitsche R, Ludtke R et al. Early ERCP and papillotomy compared with conservative treatment of acute biliary pancreatitis. The German Study Group on Acute Biliary Pancreatitis. N Engl J Med 1997; 336(4):237-242.

[44]  Neoptolemos JP, Carr-Locke DL, London NJ et al. Controlled trial of urgent endoscopic retrograde cholangiopancreatography and endoscopic sphincterotomy versus conservative treatment of acute pancreatitis due to gallstones. Lancet 1988; 2(8618): 979-983.

[45]  Kroh M, Chand B. Choledocholithiasis, endoscopic retrograde cholangiopancreatography, and laparoscopic common bile duct exploration. Surg Clin North Am 2008; 88(5):1019-1031.

[46]  Petrov MS. Early use of ERCP in acute biliary pancreatitis without jaundice: an unjaundiced view. JOP 2009; 10(1):1-7.

[47]  Kopetanos DJ. ERCP in acute biliary pancreatitis. Word J Gastrointest Endosc 2010; 2(1):25-28.

[48]  Vitale GC, Davis BR, Zavaleta C et al. Endoscopic retrograde cholangiopancreatography and histopathology correlation for chronic pancreatitis. Am Surg 2009; 75(8): 649-653.

[49]  Petrov MS, van Santvoort HC, Besselink MG et al. Early endoscopic retrograde cholangiopancreatography versus conservative management in acute biliary pancreatitis without cholangitis: a meta-analysis of randomized trials. Ann Surg 2008; 247(2): 250-257.

[50]  Moretti A, Papi C, Aratari A et al. Is early endoscopic retrograde cholangiopancreatography useful in the management of acute biliary pancreatitis? A meta-analysis of randomized controlled trials. Dig Liver Dis 2008; 40(5):379-385.

[51]  Acosta JM, Katkhouda N, Debian KA et al. Early ductal decompression versus conservative management for gallstones pancreatitis with ampullary obstruction: a prospective randomize clinical trial. Ann Surg 2006; 243(1): 33-40.

[52] van Santvoort HC, Besselink MG, de Vries AC et al. Early endoscopic retrograde cholangiopancreatography in predicted severe acute biliary pancreatitis: a prospective multicenter study. Ann Surg 2009; 250(1):68-75.

[53] Gardner TB, Vege SS, Pearson RK et al. Fluid resuscitation in acute pancreatitis. Clin. Gastroenterol. Hepatol. 2008; 6:1070-1076.

[54] Leppaniemi A. Surgical management of abdominal compartment syndrome; indications and techniques. Scandinavian journal of trauma, resuscitation and emergency medicine 2009;17:17-21.

[55] Mentula P, Leppaniemi A. Timely interventions in severe acute pancreatitis are crucial for survival. World Journal of Emergency Surgery 2014; 9:15-24.

[56] De Waele JJ, Hoste EA, Malbrain ML. Decompressive laparotomy for abdominal compartment syndrome. A critical analysis. Crit. Care 2006; 10:R51.

[57] Leppaniemi A, Mentula P, Hienonen P et al. Transverse laparostomy is feasible and effective in the treatment of abdominal compartment syndrome in severe acute pancreatitis. World J Emerg Surg 2008; 3:6.

[58] Petersson U, Acosta S, Bjorck M. Vacuum assisted wound closure and mesh-mediated fascial traction. A novel technique for late closure of the open abdomen. World J Surg 2007;31:2133-2137.

[59] Opie EL. The aetiology of acute hemorrhagic pancreatitis. Bull Johns Hopkins Hosp 1901: 12; 182-188.

[60] Ranson JH, Pasternack BS. Statistical methods for quantifying the severity of clinical acute pancreatitis. J Surg Res 1977; 22:79-91.

[61] Blamey SL, Imrie CW, O'Neill J et al. Prognostic factors in acute pancreatitis. GUT 1984;25:1340-1346.

[62] Knans WA, Draper EA, Wagner DP et al. APACHE II: a severity of disease classification system. Crit Care Med 1985;13:818-829.

[63] Neoptolemos JP, Kemppainen EA, Mayer JM et al. Early prediction of severity in acute pancreatitis by urinary trypsinogen activation peptide: a multicenter study. Lancet 2000; 355: 1955-1960.

[64] Viedma JA, Perez-Mateo M, Agullo J et al. Inflammatory response in the early prediction of severity in human acute pancreatitis. Gut 1994; 35: 822-827.

[65] De Madeira E, Soler Sola G, Sancez-Paya J et al. Influence of fluid therapy on the prognosis of acute pancreatitis: a prospective cohort study. Am J Gastroenterol 2011; 106:1843-1850.

[66] Van Santvoort HC, Besselink MG, De Vries AC et al. Early endoscopic retrograde cholangiopancreatography in predicted severe acute biliary pancreatitis: a prospective multicenter study. Ann Surg 2009; 250:68-75.

[67] Howard TJ. Acute and chronic pancreatitis in Gastrointestinal tract and abdomen ACS Surgery: principles and practice 2013; 11/13. Decker Intellectual Properties doi 10.2310/7800.1151.

[68] Walser EM, Nealon WH, Marrognin S et al. Sterile fluid collections in acute pancreatitis: catheter drainage versus simple aspiration. Cardiovasc Intervent Radiol 2006; 29(1): 102-107.

[69] Zerem E, Imamovic G, Omerovic S et al. Randomized controlled trial on sterile fluid collections management in acute pancreatitis: should they be removed? Surg Endosc 2009; 23(12): 2770-2777.

[70] Karimgani J, Porter KA, Langevin RE, Banks PA. Prognostic factors in sterile pancreatic necrosis. Gastroenterology 1992;103:1636-1640.

[71] Beger HG, Buchler M, Bittner R et al. Necrosectomy and postoperative local lavage in necrotizing pancreatitis. Br J Surg 1988; 75: 207-212.

[72] Tsiotos GG, Luque Le, Sorcide JA et al. Management of necrotizing pancreatitis by repeated operative necrosectomy using a zipper technique. Am J Surg 1998; 175: 91-98.

[73] Rau B, Pralle Y, Mayer JM et al. Role of ultrasonography guided fine-needle aspiration cytology in the diagnosis of infected pancreatic necrosis. Br J Surg 1998;85:179-184.

[74] Gerzof SG, Banks PA, Robbins AH et al. Early diagnosis of pancreatic infection by computed tomography-guided aspiration. Gastroenterology 1987; 93:1315-1320.

[75] Banks PA, Gerzof SG, Langevin RE et al. CT-guided aspiration of suspected pancreatic infection: bacteriology and clinical outcome. Int J pancreatol 1995;18:265-270.

[76] Hiatt JR, Fink AS, King W et al. Percutaneous aspiration of peripancreatic fluid collections: a safe method to detect infection. Surgery 1987; 101: 523-530.

[77] Buter A, Imrie CW, Carter CR et al. Dynamic nature of early organ dysfunction determines outcome in acute pancreatitis. Br J Surg 2002; 89:298-302.

[78] McKay CJ, Imrie CW. The continuing challenge of early mortality in acute pancreatitis. Br J Surg 2004; 91:1243-1244.

[79] Carter CR, McKay CJ. Management in necrotizing pancreatitis. In:KJ Bland et al. (eds). Surgery of the pancreas and spleen Springer Verlag London Limited; 2001. p 3-15.

[80] Petrov MS, Shanbhag S, Chakreborty M et al. Organ failure and infection of pancreatic necrosis as determinants of mortality in patients with acute pancreatitis. Gastroenterology 2010; 139:813-820

[81] Gooszen HG, Besselink MG, van Santvoort HC et al. Surgical treatment of acute pancreatitis. Langerbecks Arch Surg 2013; 398:799-806.

[82] Carter CR. Percutaneous management of necrotizing pancreatitis. HPB 2007; 9(3): 235-239.

[83] Dulcenserie R, Yzet T, Ducroix JP. Prophylactic antibiotics in treatment of severe acute alcoholic pancreatitis. Pancreas 1996;13:198-201.

[84] Maringhini A, Uomo G, Patti R et al. Pseudocysts in acute nonalcoholic pancreatitis: incidence and natural history. Dig Dis Sci 1999; 44(8):1669-1673.

[85] Mier J, Luque-de Leon E, Castillo A et al. Early versus late necrosectomy in severe pancreatitis. Am J Surg 1997; 173 (2): 71-75.

[86] Besselink MG, van Santvoort HC, Bakker OJ et al. Draining sterile fluid collections in acute pancreatitis? Primum non nocere. Surg Endosc 2010;25(1):331-332.

[87] Van Baal Mc, van Santvoort HC, Bollen TL et al. Systematic review of percutaneous catheter drainage as primary treatment for necrotizing pancreatitis. Brit J Surg 2011; 98(1): 18-27.

[88] Besselink MG, van Santvoort HC, Boermeester MA et al. Timing and impact of infections in acute pancreatitis. Br J Surg 2009;96 (3):267-273.

[89] Rau B, Bothe A, Beger HG. Surgical treatment of necrotizing pancreatitis by necrosectomy and closed lavage: changing patient characteristics and outcome in a 19-year,single center series. Surgery 2005; 138 (1):28-39.

[90] Rodriguez JR, Razo AO, Targarona J et al.Debridement and closed packing for sterile or infected necrotizing pancreatitis: insights into indications and outcomes in 167 patients. Ann Surg 2008; 247(2): 294-299.

[91] Raraty MG, Halloran CM, Dodd S et al. Minimal access retroperitoneal pancreatic necrosectomy: improvement in morbidity and mortality with a less invasive approach. Ann Surg 2010; 251(5): 787-793.

[92] Horvath K, Freeny P, Escallon J et al. Safety and efficacy of video-assisted retroperitoneal debridement for infected pancreatic collections: a multicenter, prospective, single-arm phase 2 study. Arch Surg 2010; 145(9): 817-825.

[93] van Santvoort HC, Besselink MG, Horvath KD et al. Videoscopic assisted retroperitoneal debridement in infected necrotizing pancreatitis. HPB 2007; 9(2): 156-159.

[94] van Santvoort HC, Besselink MG, Bakker OJ et al. A step-up approach or open necrosectomy for necrotizing pancreatitis. N Engl J Med 2010; 362 (16): 1491-1502.

[95]   Bakker OJ, van Santvoort HC, van Brunschot S et al. Endoscopic transgastric vs surgical necrosectomy for infected necrotizing pancreatitis: a randomized trial. JAMA 2012; 307 (10): 1053-1061.

[96]   Werner J, Warshaw A. Cystic disease of the pancreas pseudocysts, postinflammatory cystic fluid collections and other non-neoplastic cysts. In: Trede M, Carter D (eds) Surgery of the pancreas. 2nd Ed. Churchill Livingstone New York ; 1997. p. 405-415.

[97]   Nealon W, Walser E. Main pancreatic duct anatomy can direct choice of modality for treating pancreatic pseudocysts. Ann Surg 2002; 235:751-758.

[98]   Ferrucci J, Muller P: Interventional approach to pancreatic fluid collections. Radiol Clin North Ann 2003; 41:1217-1226.

[99]   Naoum E, Zavos A, Goudis K et al. Pancreatic pseudocysts: 10 years of experience. J Hepatobil Pancreat Surg 2003; 10: 373-376.

[100]  Whitcomb DC. Hereditary pancreatitis: a model for understanding the genetic basis of acute and chronic pancreatitis. Pancreatology 2001; 1:565-570.

[101]  Schneider A, Whitcomb DC. Hereditary pancreatitis: a model for inflammatory diseases of the pancreas. Best Pract Res Clin Gastroenterol 2002; 16 (3) : 347-363.

[102]  Yadav D, Timmons L, Benson JT et al. Incidence, prevalence and survival of chronic pancreatitis: a population based study. Am J Gastroenterol 2011; 106 (12): 2209.

[103]  Bassi C, Butturini G. Definition and classification of pancreatitis. In: Blumgart LH et al. (eds). Surgery of the Liver, biliary tract and pancreas. Saunders Elsevier Philadelphia; 2007:1. p. 685-699.

[104]  Noigaard C, Becker U, Matzen P et al. Progression from acute to chronic pancreatitis: prognostic factors, mortality and natural course. Pancreas 2011; 40: 1195-1200.

[105]  Remmele W. Exokrines Pankreas. In: W Remmele (Hrsg). Pathologie Springer Verlag Berlin; 1997. p. 335-390.

[106]  Ammann RW. The natural history of alcoholic chronic pancreatitis. Intern Med 2001; 40: 368-375.

[107]  Witt H, Apte MV, Keim V et al. Chronic pancreatitis: challenges and advances in pathogenesis, genetics, diagnosis and therapy. Gastroenterology 2007; 132:1557-1573.

[108]  Yadav D, Whitcomb DC. The role of alcohol and smoking in pancreatitis. Nat Rev Gastroenterol Hepatol 2010; 7(3):131-145).

[109]  Amman RW. A clinically based classification system for alcoholic chronic pancreatitis: summary of an international workshop on chronic pancreatitis. Pancreas 1997; 14: 215-221.

[110] Catalano MF, Sahai A, Levy M et al. EUS-based criteria for the diagnosis of chronic pancreatitis: the Rosemont classification. Gastrointestinal endoscopy 2009; 69 (7): 1251-1261.

[111] Fisher WE, Andersen DK, Bell RH Jr. The Pancreas. In: Brunicardi FC, Andersen Dk, Billian TR et al.(eds) Schwatz's Principles of Surgery 8th Ed. McGraw-Hill New York; NY 2005. p.1221-1296.

[112] Proca DM, Ellison EC, Hibbert D et al. Major pancreatic resections for chronic pancreatitis. Arch Pathol Lab Med 2001; 125: 1051-1054.

[113] Bockman DE, Buchler M. Pain mechanisms. In: Beger HG, Warshaw AL, Buchler MW (eds). The Pancreas. Blackwell-Science London; 1998. p.698.

[114] Gress F, Schmitt C, Scherman S et al. A prospective randomized comparison of endoscopic ultrasound and computed tomography guided celiac plexus block for managing chronic pancreatitis pain. Am J Gastroenterol 1999; 94:900-905.

[115] Elefthieriadis N, Dinu F, Delhaye M. Long-term outcome after pancreatic stenting in severe chronic pancreatitis. Endoscopy 2005; 37:223-230.

[116] Binmoeller KF, Sochendra N. Endoscopic ultrasonography in the diagnosis and treatment of pancreatic pseudocysts. Gastrointest Endosc Clin N Am 1995; 5: 805-816.

[117] Vitale GC, Cothron K, Vitale EA et al. Role of pancreatic duct stenting in the treatment of chronic pancreatitis. Surg Endosc 2004; 18: 1431-1434.

[118] Dite P, Ruzicka M, Zboril V et al. A prospective, randomized trial comparing endoscopic and surgical therapy of chronic pancreatitis. Endoscopy 2003; 35: 553-558.

[119] Cahen DL, Gouma Dj, Nio Y et al. Endoscopic versus surgical drainage of the pancreatic duct in chronic pancreatitis. N Engl J Med 2007;356: 676-684.

[120] Puestow CB, Gillesby WJ. Retrograde surgical drainage of pancreas for chronic relapsing pancreatitis. AMA Arch Surg 1958; 76:898-907.

[121] Partington PF, Rochelle RE. Modified Puestow procedure for retrograde drainage of the pancreas duct. Ann Surg 1960; 152:1037-1043.

[122] Izbiki JR et al. Surgical treatment of chronic pancreatitis and quality of life after operation. Surg Clin North Am 1999, 79:913-944.

[123] Brandley EC III. Long term results of pancreatojejunostomy in patients with chronic pancreatitis. Am J Surg 1987; 153:207-213.

[124] Mannel A, Adson MA, Mc Ierath DC et al. Surgical management of chronic pancreatitis: long-term results in 141 patients. Br J Surg 1988; 75:467-472.

[125] Andersen DK, Frey CF. The evolution of the surgical treatment of chronic pancreatitis. Ann Surg 2010; 251:18-32.

[126] Beger HG, Schlosser W, Friess HM et al. Duodenum preserving head resection in chronic pancreatitis changes the natural course of the disease: a single center 26 year experience. Ann Surg 1999; 230:512-519.

[127] Gloor B, Friess H, Uhl W et al. A modified technique of the Beger and Frey procedure in patients with chronic pancreatitis. Dig Surg 2001; 18:21-25.

[128] Frey CF, Smith GJ. Description and rationale of a new operation for chronic pancreatitis. Pancreas 1997; 2:701-707.

[129] Izbiki JR, Bloechle C, Broering DC et al. Longitudinal V-shaped excision of the ventral pancreas for small duct disease in severe chronic pancreatitis: prospective evaluation of a new surgical procedure. Ann Surg 1998; 227:213-219

[130] Strate T, Taherpour Z, Bloechle C et al. Long-term follow up of a randomized trial comparing the Beger and Frey procedures for patients suffering from chronic pancreatitis. Ann Surg 2005;241:591-598.

[131] Russell RC, Theis BA. Pancreatoduodenectomy in the treatment of chronic pancreatitis. World J Surg 2003; 27:1203-1210.

[132] Brancatisano RP, Williamson RL. Distal pancreatectomy with or without splenectomy. In: Beger HG, Warshaw AL, Buchler MN (eds) The Pancreas. Blackwell-Science London; 1998. p. 854.

[133] Andersen DK. Mechanisms and emerging treatments of the metabolic complications of chronic pancreatitis. Pancreas 2007; 35:1-15.

[134] Najarian JS, Sutherland DE, Baumgartner D et al. Total or near total pancreatectomy and islet autotransplantation for the treatment of chronic pancreatitis. Am Surg 1980; 192:526-542

[135] Dutch Pancreatitis Study Group, van Santvoort HC, Bakker OJ et al. A conservative and minimally invasive approach to necrotizing pancreatitis improves outcome. Gastroenterology 2011; 141 (4): 1254-1263.

# 7

# Haemosuccus Pancreaticus in Chronic Pancreatitis — Diagnosis and Treatment

Hirotaka Okamoto and Hideki Fujii

## 1. Introduction

Obscure gastrointestinal bleeding (OGBI) has been defined as persistent or recurrent bleeding from the gastrointestinal tract, even though initial gastrointestinal- and colon-endoscopy or small bowel radiological imaging were performed for initial evaluation [1].

In 10-20% of cases of patients who present with gastrointestinal bleeding, the underlying etiology may not be evident on initial evaluation. About half of these patients were observed in recurrent or persistent bleeding and had to need the further challenge to both diagnosis and management. The underlying etiology often remains difficult to define, despite extensive examinations. This fact results in recurrent hospitalization and multiple blood transfusions [2, 3].

Hemosuccus Pancreaticus is known to be a cause of OGIB. Lower and Farrel first reported that blood was expelled into the duodenum via the main pancreatic duct [4]. The term 'hemosuccus pancreaticus' was coined by Sandblom in 1970 [5]. Hemoductal pancreaticus was proposed by Longmire and Rose in 1973 [6]. These terms describe the emission of red blood cells along pancreatic ducts through the papilla.

Diagnosis of hemosuccus pancreaticus is often difficult because the condition involves intermittent gastrointestinal bleeding. In this paper, we describe two rare cases of hemosuccus pancreaticus from our clinical experience and discuss the diagnosis and pathogenesis of this disease with a review of the literature.

## 2. Case reports

### 2.1. Case report 1

A 47-year-old Japanese male had a past history of peritoneal drainage for acute necrotizing pancreatitis at 23 years of age and a lateral pancreaticojejunostomy (Puestow procedure) for chronic pancreatitis at age 31. The patient experienced several episodes of tarry stools following the Puestow operation. Physical examination on admission revealed severe conjunctiva pallor and tarry stools.

Emergent gastrointestinal fiberscopy was performed, and no abnormal lesions were found in the stomach or duodenum. Hemorrhagic scintigraphy and abdominal computed tomography (CT) were also carried out, but no hemorrhagic lesions were found. After blood transfusion, total colonoscopy was performed via insertion up to the terminal ileum, which also revealed no abnormal lesions. Although interventional radiology was considered as a treatment option, hemostasis seemed possible through conservative therapy alone. The bleeding point was assumed to be in the upper jejunum, including the reconstructed jejunum.

Two week later, more tarry stools occurred, the patient went into hemodynamic shock and subsequently underwent laparotomy without delay. After inspection of the whole abdomen, the intestine was found to contain coagulated blood in the upper jejunum. Intra-operative endoscopy through an incision in the reconstructed jejunal loop at the close proximal end revealed massive bleeding. After suction of the bleeding and coagulation clots, an active bleeding site from the side-to-side anastomotic pancreatic duct became clear (Fig. A). Longitudinal jejunotomy was performed, and the bleeding point was sutured and ligated [7].

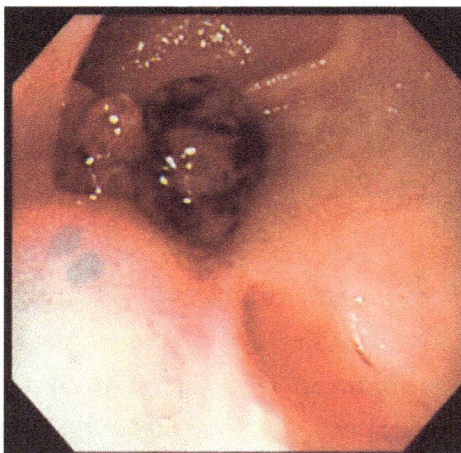

**Figure 1.** Active bleeding from side-to-side pancreaticojejunostomy

### 2.2. Case report 2

A 45-year-old Japanese male had been treated by medication for chronic pancreatitis and gastroduodenal peptic ulcer. The patient had a complaint of hematomesis and emergent gastrointestinal endoscopy revealed massive duodenal bleeding. Emergent distal gastrectomy was performed. After discharge, he had epigastric pain and was re-admitted with a diagnosis of chronic pancreatitis. Abdominal CT revealed splenomegaly and a pancreatic cyst in the pancreatic tail. Angiography revealed aneurysm of the distal pancreatic artery. Distal pancreatectomy and splenectomy were performed. The resected specimen included was a pseudocyst filled with a blood clot in the pancreatic tail, and it communicated with the main pancreatic duct. Furthermore, the splenic artery had ruptured into the pseudocyst [8].

# 3. Diagnosis

## 3.1. Symptoms

The usual presentation of hemosuccus pancreaticus is the development of symptoms of upper or lower gastrointestinal bleeding, such as hematomesis, vomiting of bloody contents, melena, tarry stool, hematochezia, or fresh rectal bleeding. The feature of gastrointestinal bleeding is that it is intermittent, waxing and waning. The bleeding source is not determined by standard endoscopic technique as usual. The symptoms of this condition are categorized as a cause of obscure overt gastrointestinal hemorrhage. Obscure gastrointestinal bleeding (OGBI) has been defined as persistent or recurrent gastrointestinal bleeding, after negative initial examinations.

More than one half patients with hemosuccus pancreaticus also have symptoms as abdominal pain, usually located in the epigastric lesion or upper part of the abdomen. The characteristics of the pain is like being crescendo-decrescendo in nature, meaning that it slowly increases and decreases in intensity with time. This symptom is thought to be due to transient blockage and increasing pressure of the pancreatic duct from the source of bleeding or clots [9].

| | |
|---|---|
| Upper abdominal pain | intermitted |
| | crescendo-decrescendo |
| Upper gastrointestinal bleeding | hematomesis |
| | vomiting of bloody contents |
| Lower gastrointestinal bleeding | melena |
| | tarry stool |
| | hematochezia |
| | fresh rectal bleeding |

**Table 1.** Symptom of Hemosuccus Pancreaticus

## 3.2. OGIB: Obscure Gastrointestinal Bleeding

Obscure gastrointestinal bleeding (OGBI) has been defined as persistent or recurrent gastrointestinal bleeding after negative initial evaluation by pan-endoscope and radiological small intestinal imaging [9]. On initial endoscopic evaluation with standard endoscopy, such as esophago-gastroduodenoscopy and colonoscopy, as well as the limited capacity of endoscopy to examine the small bowel the main challenges related to the evaluation of OGBI include the high miss rate for lesions. Therefore, the management of these patients has traditionally required invasive procedures such as intra-operative enteroscopy and exploratory laparotomy. The technological advances such as the introduction of video capsule endoscopy, single and double balloon enteroscopy, spiral enteroscopy, CT enterography can overcome the limitation of old diagnostic modalities.

### 3.3. Diagnostic features

Hemosuccus pancreaticus is known to be a cause of OGIB. It is often difficult to diagnose hemosuccus pancreaticus because the bleeding is usually intermittent. Endoscopy represents the first diagnostic step in patients with upper gastrointestinal bleeding. Although it is essential to rule out other causes of bleeding such as peptic ulcers, esophageal, and gastric varices, endoscopy rarely identifies blood in the ampulla of Vater. Pancreatic pseudocysts or aneurysms of peripancreatic arteries can be visualize by ultrasonography. Doppler ultrasound and dynamic ultrasound have been also reported to be useful diagnostic modalities [10, 11]. And contrast-enhanced CT is an further excellent modality for demonstrating the feature of chronic pancreatitis, pseudocysts and pseudoaneurysm [12, 13]. Selective angiography of the celiac axis and the superior mesenteric artery provides formal proof of hemosuccus pancreaticus by opacifying the main pancreatic duct, the presence of an aneurysm or pseudo-aneurysm with a high sensitivity [14].(Table 2) Diagnosis of hemosuccus pancreaticus accomplished by advanced technologies such as video capsule endoscopy, single-and double-balloon enteroscopy, spiral enteroscopy, and computed tomography enterography has not been reported until now. These advanced technologies provide vital information for the diagnosis of hemosuccus pancreaticus.

---

Esophago-gastro-duodenoscopy
Side-viewing upper gastrointestinal endoscopy
Doppler or dynamic ultrasound
Contrast-enhanced CT
Angiography

---

**Table 2.** Diagnostic Modalities of Hemosuccus Pancreaticus

# 4. Pathogenesis and etiology

Hemosuccus pancreaticus complicates an underlying pancreatic disease in 80% of cases and vascular anomaly in 20% of cases [15]. Chronic pancreatitis is the cause of about 90% of pancreatic diseases [15, 16]. Several mechanisms are thought to be involved. A pseudocyst is thought to be one of causes of hemosuccus pancreaticus, because of hemorrhagic pseudocyst or communication of cyst to pericystic artery. Arterial aneurysm and pseudo-aneurysm are also known to be a cause of hemosuccus pancreaticus. These aneurysms are frequent in about 10 % in chronic pancreatitis. Vascular ulceration by pancreatic intraductal stone is also thought to be a cause of hemosuccus pancreaticus [10, 18]. Although aneurysm and chronic pancreatitis are often associated, there is no clear causal relationship. Other causes of hemosuccus pancreaticus are rare: neuroendocrine tumor [15], intraductal papillary-mucinous carcinoma [19], ectopic pancreas [20], pancreas divisum [21], and Puestow procedure [7]. Finally, hemosuccus pancreaticus can result from a post ERCP (endoscopic retrograde cholangiopancreatography) complication. As for acute pancreatitis, hemosuccus pancreaticus can occur after necrosis of the adjacent arterial wall such as gastroduodenal artery, splenic artery, pancreaticoduodenal arcade. The pathogenesis and etiology are summarized in Table 3.

| |
| --- |
| Chronic pancreatitis |
| Acute pancreatitis |
| Pancreatic cysts |
| Pancreatic tumor |
| Ectopic pancreas |
| Pancreas divisum |
| Arterial aneurysm or pseudoaneuysm |
| Iatrogenic, (ERCP, operation) |

**Table 3.** Pathogenesis and Etiology of Hemosuccus Pancreaticus

## 5. Management and treatment

The management for hemosuccus pancreaticus should be aimed at completely eradicating the source of bleeding. Three therapeutic options are considered for this disorder: endoscopic treatment, angiographic embolization, and surgery have been documented. Endoscopic treatment was used in a rare case in which hemosuccus pancreaticus caused by post ERCP pancreatitis was treated by endoscopic stent tree tamponade [22]. Interventional radiographic methods are chosen for initial treatment when the hemodynamic situations is under control. The treatment response rate was 67% to 100% of cases [23-25]. Most hemosuccus pancreaticus cases can receive angiography. If the source of hemorrhage is found by angiography, interventional radiological therapy should be done following this examination. Interventional radiological therapy by implantation of an uncoated metal Palmaz stent across the aneurysmal segment of splenic artery is also reported [26]. Transcatheter arterial embolization was reported to be effective for hemosuccus pancreaticus treatment [27-29]. However, ischemia also can develop in the tissue supplied by the artery if the collateral circulation is not sufficient, and other complications of aneurysm infection and splenic infarction may arise. Sources bleeding from a pseudoaneurysm were reported to arise from the splenic artery in most cases but also the gastroduodenal artery, from the branch of the superior pancreaticoduodenal artery, from the branch of the inferior pancreaticoduodenal artery, from the superior mesenteric artery or vein, and from an unnamed intracystic artery [30]. Some authors documented that recurrent bleeding rates were about 30% [12]. Thus, arterial embolization is recommended as the initial therapeutic method, either to stabilize the patient to perform elective surgery or as a definitive treatment where possible [31, 32].

Surgical treatment is indicated in uncontrolled hemorrhage, persistent shock, where embolization is not feasible or when embolization fails. Ligation of the pancreatic duct is one of the surgical approaches, but results are unsatisfactory because the causal lesion remains intact. Ligation of the causal artery is more effective but does not remove the risk of recurrence. Pancreatic resection such as distal pancreatectomy, central pancreatectomy, or pancreatico-dudenectomy treats both the pancreatic and the arterial diseases. Distal pancreatectomy is indicative for bleeding pseudoaneurysms in the body or tail of the pancreas. When the location of the pseudoaneurysm is the head of the pancreas, pancreaticoduodenectomy is chosen. However, increased mortality and morbidity have been reported, and consequently angioembolization alone has been proposed as the recommended treatment modality [25, 26, 31, 32]. Bleeding from the pancreaticoduodenal artery has a higher mortality rate than bleeding from the splenic or gastroduodenal artery [31, 32]. Most patients suffer from chronic pancreatitis so the potential perioperative complications and postoperative pancreatic insufficiency should be noted. Most surgical series have documented success rates of 70% to 85% with mortality rates of 20% to 25% and rebleeding rates of 0% to 5% [31-34]. The treatment options are summarized in Table 4.

| |
|---|
| Endoscopic therapy |
| Stent tamponade |
| Angioembolization |
| Surgery |
| Ligation of bleeding vessel |
| Pancreaticoduodenectomy |
| Central pancreatectomy |
| Distal pancreatectomy |

Table 4. Treatment of Hemosuccus Pancreaticus

# 6. Conclusion

A flow chart for management of hemosuccus pancreaticus is shown in Figure 1. Hemosuccus pancreaticus is a rare and potentially life threatening clinical entity. It is the least frequent cause of upper gastrointestinal bleeding and is most often caused by chronic pancreatitis. Its diagnosis is difficult because of its rarity and its anatomical location as well as its intermitted bleeding. During the intermitted phase, it cannot be diagnosed by the upper gastrointestinal endoscope. The timely diagnosis is often delayed because of the intermitted nature of bleeding. Therapeutic options consist of embolization, stenting, endoscopic stenting, and surgery. Endovascular therapy by embolization is effective in most patients, although to achieve a complete cure there is no consensus on the need for surgery. Embolization can control unstable haemodynamics. Emergent surgery is required in patients with recurrent bleeding or failed first-line therapies such as embolization or stenting.

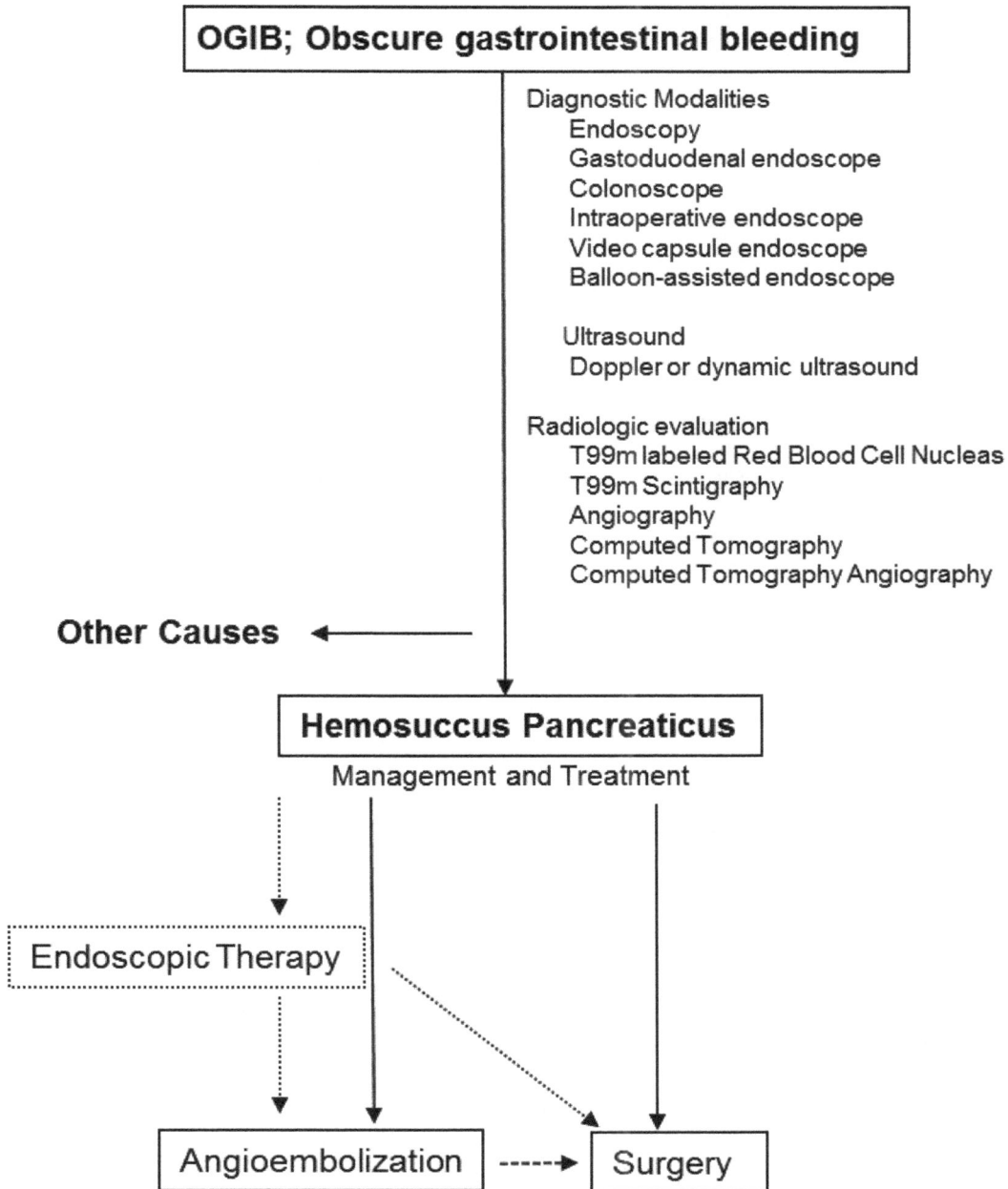

**OGIB; Obscure gastrointestinal bleeding**

Diagnostic Modalities
    Endoscopy
    Gastoduodenal endoscope
    Colonoscope
    Intraoperative endoscope
    Video capsule endoscope
    Balloon-assisted endoscope

Ultrasound
    Doppler or dynamic ultrasound

Radiologic evaluation
    T99m labeled Red Blood Cell Nucleas
    T99m Scintigraphy
    Angiography
    Computed Tomography
    Computed Tomography Angiography

**Other Causes** ←

**Hemosuccus Pancreaticus**

Management and Treatment

Endoscopic Therapy

Angioembolization ----→ Surgery

**Figure 2.** Flowchart for the management of hemosuccus pancreaticus

## Author details

Hirotaka Okamoto[1,2*] and Hideki Fujii[2]

*Address all correspondence to: hirotaka@yamanashi.ac.jp

1 Department of Surgery, Tsuru Municipal Hospital, Japan

2 Department of Gastrointestinal, Breast & Endocrine Surgery, Faculty of Medicine, University of Yamanashi, Japan

## References

[1] Raju GS, Gerson L, Das A, Lewis B. American Gastroenteroogical Association (AGA) Institute technical review on obscure gastrointestinal bleeding. *Gastroenterology.* 2007;133:1697-1717.

[2] Thompson JN, Salem RR, Hemingway AP, Rees HC, Hodgson HJ, et al. Specialist investigation of obscure gastrointestinal bleeding. *Gut.* 1987;28:47-51.

[3] Lin S, Rockey DC. Obscure gastrointestinal bleeding. *Gastoenterol Clin North Am.* 2005;34:679-698.

[4] Lower WE, Farred JJ: Aneurysm of the splenic artery. Report of a case and review of literature. *Arch Surg.* 1931;23:182-190.

[5] Sandblom P:Gastrointestinal hemorrhage through the pancreatic duct. *Ann Surg.* 1970;171:61-66.

[6] Longmire WP, Rose AS. Hemoductal pancreatitis. *Surg Gynecol Obstet.* 1973;136:246-250.

[7] Okamoto H, Miura K, Fujii H. Hemosuccus pancreaticus following a Puestow procedure in a patient with chronic pancreatitis. *Case Rep Gastroenterol.* 2011;5:452-456.

[8] Iino H, Shirasu T, Karikome K, et al. A case of chronic pancreatitis with hemosuccus pancreaticus and left-sided portal hypertension. *Jpn J Gastroenterol Surg.* 1994;27:2461-2465.

[9] Clay R, Farnell M, Lancaster J, Weiland L, Gostout C. Hemosuccus pancreaticus. An usual cause of upper gastrointestinal bleeding. *Ann Surg* 1985;202:75-79

[10] Risti B, Marineck B, Jost R, et al. Hemosuccus pancreaticus as a source of obscure upper gastrointestinal bleeding: three cases and literature of review. *Am J Gastroenterol.* 1995; 90:1878-1880.

[11] Benz CA, Jakob P, Jakobs R, et al. Hemosuccus pancreaticus-a rare cause of gastrointestinal bleeding: diagnosis and interventional radiological therapy. *Endoscopy.* 2000;32:428-431.

[12] de Perrot M, Berney T, Buhler L, et al. Management of bleeding pseudoaneurysms in patients with pancreatitis. *Br J Surg.* 1999;86:29-32.

[13] Koizumi J, Inoue S, Yonekawa H e al. Hemosuccus pancreaticus: diagnosis with CT and MRI and treatment with transcatheter embolization. *Abdom Imaging.* 2002;27:77-81.

[14] Bergert H, Hnterseher I, Kersting S, et al. Management and outcome of hemorrhage due to arterial pseudoaneurysms in pancreatisis. *Surgery.* 2005;137:323-328.

[15] Peroux JL, Arput JP, Saint-Paul MC, et al. Wirsungorragie compliquant une pancréatite chronique associée á une neuroendocrine du pancréas. *Gastroenterol Clin Biol.* 1994;18:1142-1145.

[16] Emilie E, Regenet N, Tuech JJ, Pessaux P, Meurette G, et al. Diagnosis and treatment of hemosuccus pamcreaticus. *Pancreas* 2007;34:229-232.

[17] Arnaud JP, Bergamashi RR, Serra-Maudet V, et al. Pancreatoduodenectomy for hemosuccus pancreaticus in silent chronic pancreatitis. *Arch Surg.* 1994;129:333-334.

[18] el Hamel A, Parc R, Adda G, et al. Bleeding pseudocysts and pseudoaneurysms in chronic pancreatitis. *Br J Surg.* 1991;78:1059-1063.

[19] Kuruma S, Kamisawa T, Tu Y, et al. Hemosuccus pancreaticus due to intraductal papillary-mucinous carcinoma of the pancreas. *Clin J Gastroenterol.* 2009;2:27-29.

[20] Meneu JA, Fernandes-Cebrian JM, Alvarez-Baleriola I, et al. Hemosuccus pancreaticus in a heterotopic jejuna pancreas. *Hepatogastroenterology.* 1999;46:177-179.

[21] Vasquez-Iglesias JL, durana JA, Yanez J et al. Santorinrrhage: hemosuccus pancreaticus in pancreas divisum. *Am J Gastroenterol.* 1988;83:876-878.

[22] Gutkin E, Kim SH. A novel endoscopic treatment of hemosuccus pancreaticus: A stent tree tamponade. *JOP. J Pancreas* 2012;13:312-313.

[23] Stabile BE, Wilson SE, Debas HT. Reduced mortality from bleeding pseudocysts and pseudoaneurysms caused by pancreatitis. *Arch Surg.* 1983;118:45-51.

[24] Kahn LA, Kamen C, McNamara MP Jr. Variable color Doppler appearance of pseudoaneurysm in pancreatitis. *AJR Am J Roentgenol.* 1994;162:187-188.

[25] Gambiez LP, Emst OJ, Merlier OA, et al. Arterial embolization for bleeding pseudocysts complicating chronic pancreatitis. *Arch Surg.* 1997;132:1016-1021.

[26] Akpinar H, Dicle O, Ellidokuz, et al. Hemosuccus pancreaticus treated by transvascular selective arterial embolization. *Endoscopy.* 1999;31:213-214.

[27]  Sugiki T, Hatori T, Imaizumi T, Harada N, Fukuda A, et al. Two cases of hemosuccus pancreaticus in which hemostasis was achieved by transcatheter arterial embolization. *J Hepatobiliary Pancreat Surg.* 2003;10:450-454.

[28]  Naitoh I, Ando T, Shimohira M, Nakazawa T, Hayashi K, et al. Hemosuccus pancreaticus associated with segmental arterial mediolysis successfully treated by transarterial embolization. *JOP. J Pancreas* 2010;11:625-29.

[29]  Ray S, Das K, Ray S, Khamrui S, Ahammed M, et al. Hemosuccus pancreaticus associated with severe acute pancreatitis and pseudoaneurysms: A report of two cases. *JOP. J Pancreas* 2011;12:469-472.

[30]  Rammohan A, Palaniappan R, Ramaswami S, Perumal SK, Lakshmanan A, et al. Hemosuccus pancreaticus: 15-year experience from a territory care GI bleed centre. *ISRN Radiology* 2013, ID 191794, 1-6.

[31]  Bender JS, Bouwman DL, Levison MA, et al. Pseudocysts and pseudoaneurysms:Surgical strategy. *Pancreas* 1995;10:143-147.

[32]  Heath DI, Reid AW, Murray WR. Bleeding pseudocysts and pseudoaneurysms in chronic pancreatitis. *Br J Surg.* 1992;79:281.

[33]  Udd M, Leppaniemi AK, Bidel S, et al. Treatment of bleeding pseudoaneurysms in patients with chronic pancreatitis. *World J of Surg.* 2007;31:504-510.

[34]  Waltman AC, Luers PR, Athanasoulis, et al. Complementary roles of surgery and transcatherter occlusive techniques. Arch Surg. 1986;121:439-443.

# 8

# The Role of EUS — Diagnosis and Therapeutic Interventions in Patients with Acute Pancreatitis

José Celso Ardengh, Eder Rios de Lima Filho, Rafael Kemp and
José Sebastião dos Santos

## 1. Introduction

Acute pancreatitis (AP) is defined as an acute inflammatory process involving the pancreatic gland with variable involvement of other adjacent or distant organs. Its incidence ranges from 2 to 50/100.000 habitants and seems to have grown from the 80s, probably due to increased alcohol consumption among young people and the formation of gallstones in some specific areas [1, 2].

These two etiologies account for about 80% of all cases of AP. Fortunately, most cases are mild and self-limiting [3-5]. However about 30% manifest as a severe form. Necrotizing acute pancreatitis (nAP) is a severe condition and is associated with local or systemic complications and can be fatal [6-8]. Many causes have been attributed to AP, but in some episodes, they are difficult to be identified [9, 10]. When some etiological factors can be identified and eliminated, prognosis is better and new outbreaks can be prevented.

The abuse of alcohol and gallstones are common causes of AP and account for 50-80% of cases [11]. The first is more frequent in males and the latest in women. These conditions can be easily identified by the patient's history (alcohol use) or by abdominal ultrasound (US) in cholelithiasis [12].

Gallstones are responsible for approximately 60% of all cases of AP due theoretically, to a transitory impaction of gallstones through the duodenal papilla. Indeed, biliary stones are often found in the gallbladder and common bile duct during surgical exploration in patients with AP are also found in more than 90% of all cases, after wet sieving of stools in the first 24 hours of the acute episode [13-17].

When analyzing all the episodes of biliary AP, gallstones are identified in 80% by US after the resolution of the attack [18]; 10% are visualized by endoscopic retrograde cholangiopancreatography (ERCP) [19] and/or Magnetic Resonance Cholangiopancreatography (MRCP) [20, 21] and the remaining gallstones are detected during laparotomy or postmortem examination [14, 22, 23]. Six to 8% of individuals with gallstones present episodes of AP [24] and in those with microlithiasis the rate of AP reach 22% [25]. In some patients, the outbreak of AP is relate to hypertriglyceridemia, hypercalcemia, reactions to drugs, abdominal trauma, surgery, or ERCP [26].

## 2. The role of EUS diagnosis in acute pancreatitis

EUS can be used in two situations: for diagnosis of parenchymal abnormalities in AP [27] or used for determining the etiologic diagnosis in cases of UAP [28-30].

### 2.1. Unexplained Acute Pancreatitis (UAP)

Notwithstanding the foregoing, in many episodes of AP the cause is not identified, even after a clinical history, physical examination and laboratory tests such as US, serum triglycerides and calcium which reveal normal. Such episodes are labeled as having "no apparent cause" [26]. Despite the propaedeutic methods available, the frequency of UAP is around 10% to 30% and 25-50% will present recurrence two years after the first episode [31, 32]. UAP has a high rate of morbidity and mortality due to the tendency for recurrence [33, 34]. It is important to establish the etiology of AP, not only for its prognostic implications, but to adopt the appropriate treatment, enhancing patient outcome and reducing the risk of recurrence [35, 36].

Ranson [37], Miquel et al. [38] and Tarnasky & Hawes [26] showed that approximately 30% of UAP are secondary to undiagnosed microlithiasis of the gallbladder (GML). They easily tend to migrate through the cystic duct [39] with impaction in the duodenal papilla [13] and causing biliary colic, jaundice and AP [40]. Therefore, endoscopic ultrasound (EUS) is very useful in these patients.

### 2.1.1. Microlithiasis and biliary sludge

Some peculiarities of Microlithiasis such as radiolucency [41] and small size (maximum size 3 mm) [42], make it difficult to identify by conventional image methods such as US, CT, ERCP, MRCP [41]. According to these authors, stones presenting these characteristics constitute microlithiasis (Figure 1 and 2).

Biliary sludge appears in ultrasound or EUS as multiple hyperechoic mobile signals, without acoustic shadow, forming levels within the gallbladder and are labeled as microlithiasis (Figure 3 and 4) [43, 44].

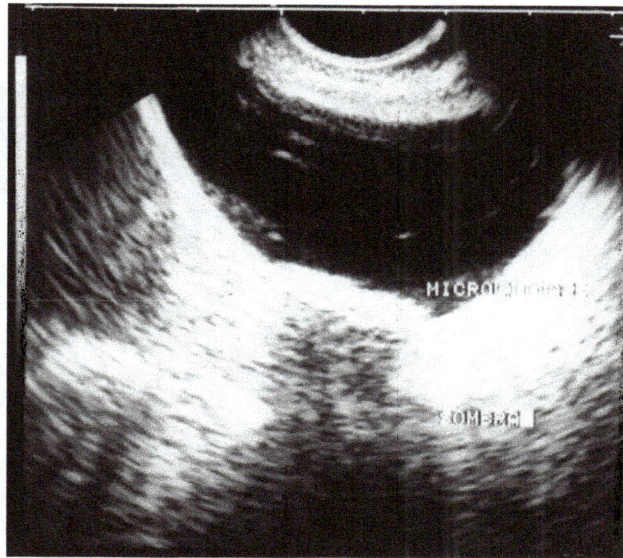

**Figure 1.** Electronic sectorial EUS. Hyperechoic image forming level, with the presence of acoustic shadow of gallbladder body in a patient with multiple episodes of AP.

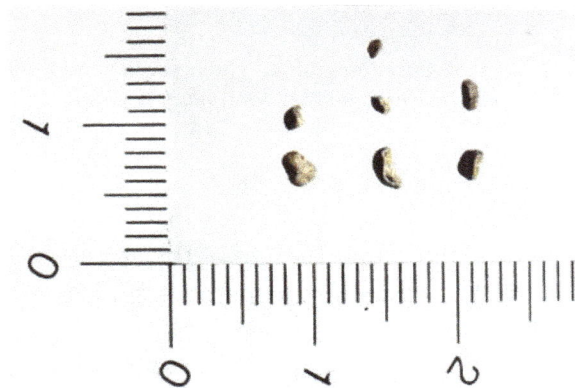

**Figure 2.** Small stones (less than 3 mm), causing episodes of AP. Stones up to 3 mm, found in the surgical specimen are also included.

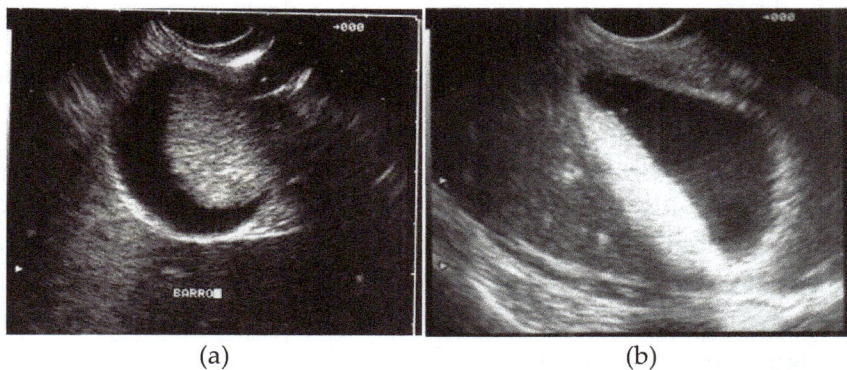

| (a) | (b) |

**Figure 3.** EUS images (a e b) shows mobile multiple hyperechoic signals, without acoustic shadow, forming levels within the gallbladder.

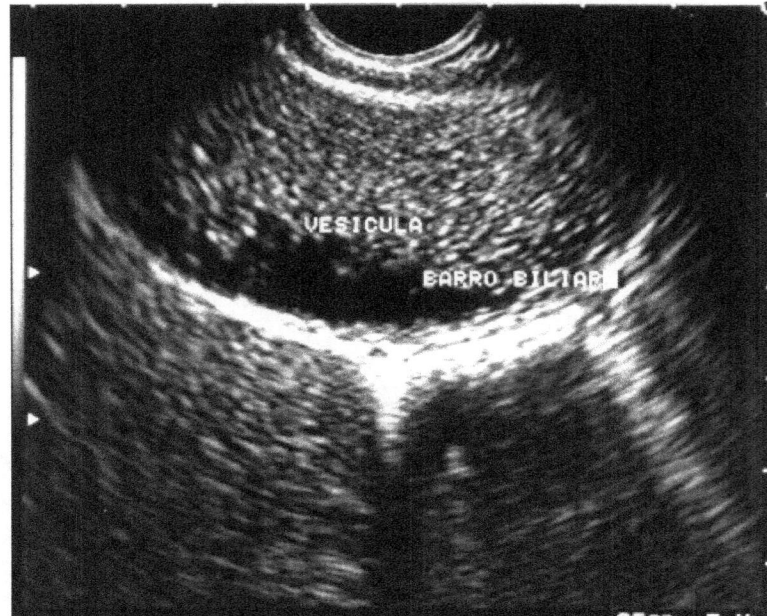

**Figure 4.** Electronic sectorial EUS shows wall thickening (acute cholecystitis) and multiple hyperechoic mobile signals without acoustic shadow, producing level within the gallbladder (biliary sludge).

### 2.1.2. Genesis of the episode of AP in patients with GML

The risk of AP in these patients is related to the size of the stones, the caliber of the cystic duct and the size and length of the Oddi's sphincter. Armstrong et al. demonstrated, in a prospective study, that the diameter of the cystic duct was 4.94 + 2.3 mm in patients with AP, in contrast to a shorter diameter found in those patients without AP (control group) [24]. Additionally, revealed that in 64.5% of patients with GML, the passage through the cystic duct was easy, while in the control group the passage of GML occurred in only 22.4% due to the smaller diameter of the cystic duct. A mechanical important factor is the diameter of the Oddi's sphincter, which ranges from 2 + 1 mm, constituting an obstacle to the passage of stones, which could cause AP [45].

The length of the common bile duct seems to be involved in the genesis of the outbreaks of AP as it is much larger in these patients than in those without the condition [24]. Starting from this premise, it is inferred the importance of this anatomical condition which increases the migration time of microlithiasis [24, 45]. Such concepts strongly advocated a theory that patients with AP have anatomical conditions that facilitate the migration of gallbladder microlithiasis (GML) to the common bile duct and whose expulsion is delayed due to a longer route to reach duodenum [24, 45]. Another author showed that besides the larger diameter of the cystic duct, the number of stones is higher in patients with AP [23]. This finding was confirmed in our study where all patients with GML showed multiple stones (Figures 1, 2, 3, 4 and 5) [46].

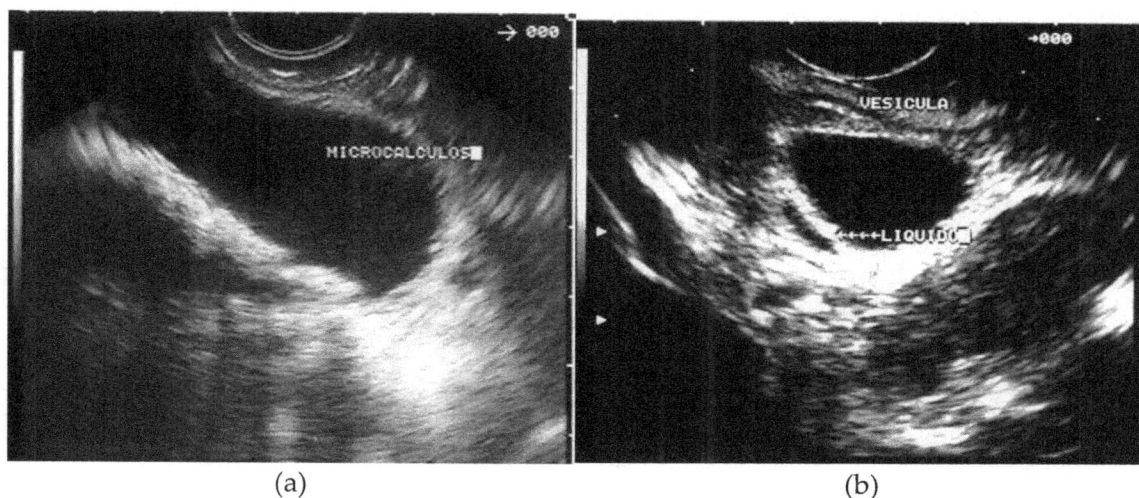

(a)          (b)

**Figure 5.** EUS Images obtained from patients with UAP. (a) Multiple hyperechoic echoes, some of them showing acoustic shadow. Histologic examination of the surgical specimen revealed cholesterolosis. (b) Gallbladder image shows perivesicular fluid. Surgical procedure revealed the presence of microlithiasis undetected by EUS e o pathological examination of the surgical specimen revealed cholesterolosis.

### 2.1.3. Diagnosis

#### 2.1.3.1. Parenchymal changes in AP

Sugiyama et al. used EUS in 23 patients with AP (16 mild AP and 7 nAP). The following criteria were observed: focal or diffuse parenchymal increasing and pancreatic echotexture ranging from normal (compared to the liver), diffusely hypoechoic, focal intrapancreatic masses (well-defined hypoechoic areas and hyperechoic dots). They observed an increase in pancreatic parenchyma in edematous form in 62.5% and in all patients with nAP. Echotexture was normal in 25% of patients with nAP and diffusely hypoechoic in the other 75%. Among the 7 patients with nAP, 5 (71.4%) had well-defined hypoechoic areas and 2 (28.6%) showed hypoechoic areas with hyperechoic dots. The location and size of focal masses corresponded to areas of pancreatic necrosis seen on CT. The main pancreatic duct (MPD) was considered normal (up to 2mm) in 11 patients and slightly dilated (2-4mm) in 7. Extrapancreatic extension was identified as hypoechoic areas. EUS was able to identify all cases of fluid collection in cul de sac. Retroperitoneal involvement was observed in 77.7% (7 of 9 patients). In this situation the extrapancreatic extension was limited according to the range of transducer (5-7cm). Subsequently, the hypoechoic areas with hyperechoic dots progressed to pancreatic abscesses [27].

In another study involving 36 patients with biliary AP (mild and necrotizing), Chak et al evaluated the following parameters: increasing of the pancreatic parenchyma, peripancreatic fluid, echogenicity, echotexture and heterogeneity, and edema of the gastroduodenal wall, correlating them with the hospitalization time until clinical condition improves [47]. Understandably, patients with peripancreatic fluid collection present a longer hospital stay. However, the authors were unable to explain the correlation between the coarse echotexture and a longer hospital stay [47]. We agree it would be very difficult to explain.

## 2.1.4. Biliary etiology

### 2.1.4.1. Choledocholithiasis

According to Sugiyama et al [27], mentioned above, EUS sensitivity for diagnosis of choledocholithiasis was 100% against 43% and 57%, for US and CT respectively. The US sensitivity for diagnosis of gallstones varies between 87 and 98% [48] and for choledocholithiasis between 22 and 75% [49]. Table 1 shows the results of several studies evaluating US, CT, and EUS findings, in the diagnosis of choledocholithiasis.

| Author, year | n | Method | Sensitivity% | Specificity% | VP+% | VP-% | Accuracy% |
|---|---|---|---|---|---|---|---|
| Amuoyal, 1994 [49] | 62 | US | 25 | 100 | 100 | 56 | - |
|  |  | CT | 75 | 94 | 92 | 78 | - |
|  |  | EUS | 97 | 100 | 100 | 97 | - |
| Sugiyama, 1995 [27] | 23 | US | 43 | - | - | - | - |
|  |  | CT | 57 | - | - | - | - |
|  |  | EUS | 100 | 100 | - | - | 100 |
| Sugiyama, 1997* [50] | 142 | US | 63 | 95 | - | - | 83 |
|  |  | CT | 71 | 97 | - | - | 87 |
|  |  | EUS | 96 | 100 | - | - | 99 |
| Sugiyama, 1998[51] | 35 | US | 47 | 90 |  |  | 71 |
|  |  | CT | 47 | 95 |  |  | 74 |
|  |  | EUS | 100 | 100 |  |  | 100 |
| Chak, 1999 [47] | 36 | US | 50 | 100 | 100 | 74 | 83 |
|  |  | ERCP | 92 | 87 | 79 | 94 | 89 |
|  |  | EUS | 91 | 100 | 100 | 95 | 97 |
| Ardengh, 2000 [52] ** | 22 | ERCP | 53.3 | 100 | 100 | 50 | 68.2 |
|  |  | EUS | 86.7 | 80 | 92.9 | 66.7 | 77.3 |
| Liu, 2001 [29] | 100 | US | 26 | 100 | - | - | 75 |
|  |  | ERCP | 97 | 95 | - | - | 96 |
|  |  | EUS | 97 | 98 | - | - | 98 |

*patients with or without history of AP

**choledochal microlithiasis

**Table 1.** Results of different image methods in the diagnosis of choledocholithiasis.

In our experience, we evaluated 22 patients with suspected choledochal microlithiasis during outbreaks of AP. We found that EUS identified the presence of stones in 86.7% of cases (mean stone size: 5mm), when compared to ERCP (sensitivity of 53.3%). The common bile duct was studied in all patients. No procedure-related complications were observed. We conclude that EUS is able to identify small stones and biliary dilatation, and should be considered as a diagnostic alternative in patients with suspected choledochal stones (Figure 6) [52].

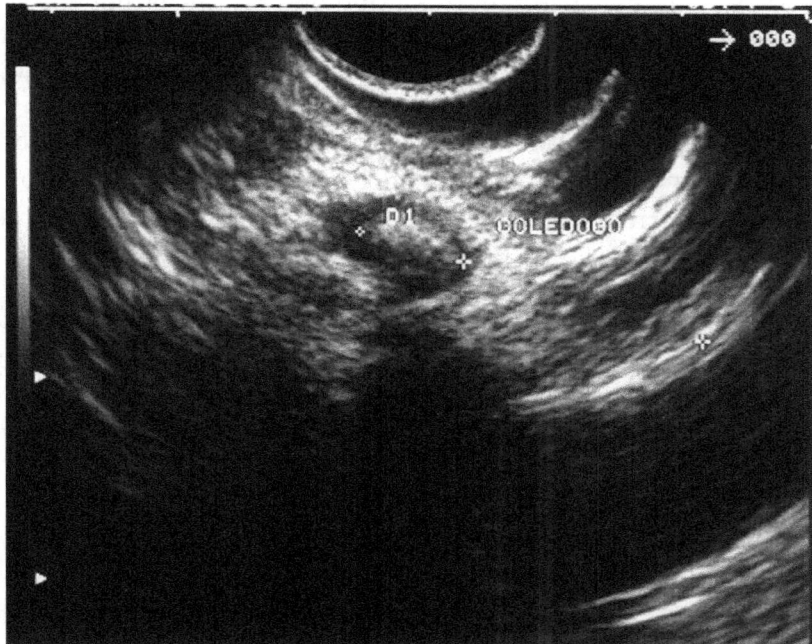

**Figure 6.** EUS image shows hyperechoic arciform area, with acoustic shadow, within choledocolithiasis in a patient with UAP. This finding was confirmed by ERCP.

### 2.1.4.2. Microlithiasis

After systematic diagnostic investigation (clinical, biochemical and by imaging methods) to identify the etiology of AP, about 10% to 30% of patients have no known cause and were labeled as UAP [53, 54]. It is at least controversial the assertion that if the etiology of an episode of AP remains unclear, after detailed endoscopic investigation (ERCP or ERCP + bile collection), this condition should be labeled as "idiopathic" [26, 32].

The identification of patients with microlithiasis arouses great interest due to the possibility of recurrent outbreaks of AP, and allowing early treatment, especially when the disease is silent or little symptomatic [25, 36, 55]. For this reason, the introduction of sensitive diagnostic and minimally invasive methods, and the resurgence of old methods (collection of bile for crystals search) became attractive along with more invasive methods such as endoscopic manometry [56].

About this point of view, seem to loom in importance the advanced endoscopic techniques: ERCP, ERCP with bile collection, for research of crystals [81, 82] and EUS in order to detect GML [57-62]. Thus, the diagnosis of stones less than 3 mm (ML) is of fundamental importance for the adoption of an appropriate therapeutic measure.

The radiological demonstration of biliary stones depends on the difference of tone between the stone and the environment that surrounds it [63]. Patients with migrant and radiolucent stones have episodes of biliary colic, AP recurrence and transient jaundice [14], despite normal appearance of the biliary tract seen in MRCP, ERCP, and US. We consider the biliary sludge (Figures 3, 4 and 5a) as ML, because biliary sludge and stones larger than 4 mm diameter, present acoustic shadow, can be identified by the US, [64], and being confused "in vivo" according to Simeone et al. [65] and can be differentiated "in vitro" according to Filly et al. [43].

Simeone et al. [65] showed the presence of microlithiasis in 8.3% of patients with "biliary sludge" undergoing surgery. Filly et al. [43] concluded that the presence of "biliary sludge" should be considered abnormal because there may be calcium bilirubinate or cholesterol precipitates (ML).

The possibility of finding GML in a patient with gallstones detected by imaging methods, according to the concept of less than or equal to 3 mm diameter size, is around 25% [25, 42]. This rate increases to 40% when the stone changes from 3 mm to 5 mm. When the criterion of radiolucency is used, it drops to 10% [66, 67].

Thus, due to the small size, stones smaller or equal to 3 mm are difficult to identify by MRCP, ERCP, and US, remaining a diagnostic challenge, especially for the latter, due to possible confusion with biliary sludge. Patients with AP recurrence that have no changes in US may present stones during surgery. The size and density of the stones are the most important factors in the occurrence of false results [68].

The ERCP is used in the etiological diagnosis of patients with UAP, identifying potentially treatable conditions in 30% to 70% of cases and stones (Figure 7) between 4% to 15% [56, 57]. But one must keep in mind that this test is able to raise the levels of amylase in 30% to 75% of asymptomatic patients, and that AP is the most frequent complication after this procedure, ranging from 0.5% to 17% [69]. Thoeni et al reported CT signs varying from mAP to nAP in 28% of patients undergoing diagnostic ERCP [70].

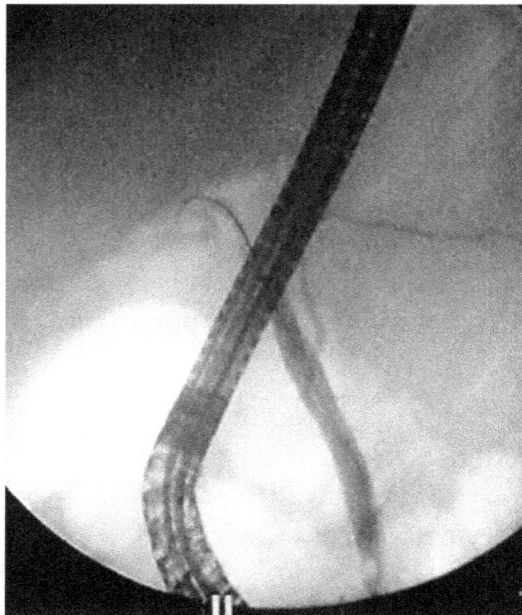

**Figure 7.** ERCP image showing microlithiasis within the bile duct without dilatation.

Dahan et al, in a prospective study, compared the accuracy of EUS and collecting bile for detecting biliary crystals in patients with suspected biliary etiology. They had symptoms of AP, transient jaundice and cramping in the right upper quadrant, and a negative US for biliary stones. The study included 45 patients, 24 with gallstones confirmed by surgery. The sensitivity, specificity, positive and negative predictive values for EUS were, 96%, 86%, 89% and 95% and for the collection of bile, 67%, 91%, 89% and 70%, respectively. The major problem related to EUS was the existence of 3 false positives. According to this author the images taken as stones were due to acoustic reverberation produced by the movement of the gallbladder wall, forming artifacts confused with ML [71].

In our study involving 36 patients with UAP, sensitivity was 92.6% and positive predictive value was 86.2%, for identifying GML. Based on these data, it appears that EUS is safe and provides good diagnostic accuracy. The probable responsible factors for a high rate of GML detection include the proximity of gallbladder related to stomach and duodenal wall; the reduced distance (0.5 mm) between the EUS transducer and the gallbladder compared to the US abdominal transducer. Besides that the facility to obtain the ideal focal point to produce undistorted images; the study of the entire gallbladder (infundibulum, body, and fundus) and cystic duct, even in patients with nAP and the use of frequencies of 5.0, 7.5 and 12 MHz, producing detailed images [72].

Moreover, specificity and negative predictive value were 55.6% and 71.4%, respectively. These data are questionable and imprecise. The main responsible factors for these rates, to a greater or lesser degree include a very small sample of individuals without the disease and the greater likelihood of patients included in the study having biliary etiology as the cause of episodes of AP [72].

In a study involving 168 patients with UAP, Frossard et al using EUS could identify the presence of gallstones in 103 (61%) cholelithiasis or microlithiasis in 52, biliary sludge in 12 choledocholithiasis in 10, and more than one of these findings in 29. Ruling out other causes (chronic pancreatitis, tumors, etc.), only 37 remained with unchanged diagnosed [58]. A similar study using EUS in 44 patients with UAP, Norton & Alderson found a definite cause for AP in 18 patients (41%) and a probable etiology in 14 (31.8%). Only 9 had no diagnosis. EUS showed 2 false-positive results, and due to technical problems in 1 patient it was not possible to do the procedure [48].

Liu et al prospectively studied 89 patients with UAP. All of them underwent CT, ERCP, and US up to 24 hours from hospital admission. After these procedures, 18 patients were labeled as having UAP. All underwent EUS, which revealed GML in 14 (77.7%) and 3 had concomitant stones in the common bile duct (21.4%). These findings suggest that a patient with AP should not be labeled as UAP before underwent EUS [73].

Tandon & Topazian evaluated the role of EUS in etiological diagnosis of UAP episodes. In 21/31 patients (68%) EUS revealed the etiologic factor. Biliary stones in 14%, initial chronic pancreatitis in 45%, pancreas divisum in 6.5%, and tumor in 3.2%. In 32% of cases, EUS was normal and could not identify the cause. The results of this study show that EUS is less invasive than ERCP, effectively demonstrating the etiology of AP in more than two thirds of cases [30].

In biliary AP, EUS performed before ERCP helps in selecting patients requiring endoscopic therapy, reducing the need for diagnostic cholangiography (and its potential risks) in about 50% of them [51].

Levy et al in a multicenter study evaluated various factors to predict biliary etiology of AP. In 213 patients with AP, biliary etiology was present in 62%, alcohol in 35% and other causes in 13%. In 15% of patients with biliary etiology, only EUS was able to make diagnosis. The other tests were negative. The authors conclude that EUS is useful to confirm or exclude biliary stones, as a source of AP, and the age, sex and alanine transaminase obtained during admission are the only predictive factors in favor of biliary origin [73].

Shimpi et al demonstrated the diagnostic accuracy of EUS and ERCP in patients with UAP. EUS revealed the diagnosis in 44% [28/63] of patients, whereas ERCP made the diagnosis in 71% [45/63]. The rate of occurrence of AP after ERCP and manometry was 17%. There was no adverse event related to EUS and EUS-FNA in two patients. The authors conclude that EUS has an important role in diagnosis of UAP etiology [56].

### 2.1.4.3. Personal casuistic

From 1999 to 2006, we studied prospectively 143 patients (76 women) with a mean age of 51 years (8-84y). According to ultimate etiology, the causes included biliary, parenchymal and/or ductal, vesicular and neoplasm. We compared the results of EUS and surgery in 103 patients. Forty patients had a mean follow up of 36 months (13-56m). The final diagnosis was obtained by EUS [72], surgery [16], EUS-FNA [12] and ERCP [9]. EUS detected changes in 101 patients (70%). The cause of AP was biliary in 68 patients, parenchymal and/or ductal in 14, neoplastic in 14, vesicular in 9, and no cause in 37. When compared to a multidisciplinary investigation, EUS (diagnosis of biliary, parenchymal, neoplastic, and vesicular etiologies) we found these rates for diagnostic accuracy: 89.7%, 64%, 44% and 86.6%, respectively. EUS clarified the etiology of AP in 89.7%. Therefore, EUS is of great value in identifying the etiology of patients with UAP. This diagnosis should be made after EUS evaluation.

Moreover, EUS-FNA can help diagnose of UAP episodes. In the former group, 16 patients underwent EUS-FNA. Previously, all had undergone at least to US and CT, which revealed no biliary-pancreatic alterations, and 64% of patients had more than one episode of AP. EUS findings, up to 1 week of the outbreak, found solid [11] and cystic lesions [5]. The final diagnosis of malignancy [11] and benign lesion [5] was confirmed in 15 cases by surgery and in 1 by clinical follow-up. We compared the results of EUS-FNA with surgical findings and follow-up. In this population of patients with UAP [143], the finding of tumors occurred in 9.8%. The final etiologic diagnosis was ductal adenocarcinoma [7], intraductal mucin-producing neoplasm [3], cystadenocarcinoma [2], inflammation of the common bile duct with stenosis [2], mucinous cystadenoma [1] and neuroendocrine tumor [1]. Isolated EUS and EUS-FNA showed sensitivity, specificity, positive and negative predictive values, and accuracy for diagnosis of malignancy of 92.3% and 80%, 33.3% and 100%, 85.7% and 100 %, 50% and 75%, 81.3% and 87.5%, respectively. In this series, no adverse events occurred. EUS-FNA is safe and effective for diagnosing of neoplastic etiology in patients with UAP, and should be performed in suspected tumors, because it increases the specificity and negative predictive value.

## 3. The role of EUS-therapeutic intervention in acute pancreatitis

The pancreatic fluid collections (PFC) develop by fluid extravasation or from liquefaction of pancreatic necrosis after an episode of AP, chronic pancreatitis (CP), surgery or abdominal trauma. The Atlanta classification defined the nomenclature of PFC. The presence of underlying ductal injury; the severity of AP and the maturation of PFC relative to the beginning of AP are factors that influence formation and composition of a PFC (Figure 8) [74, 75].

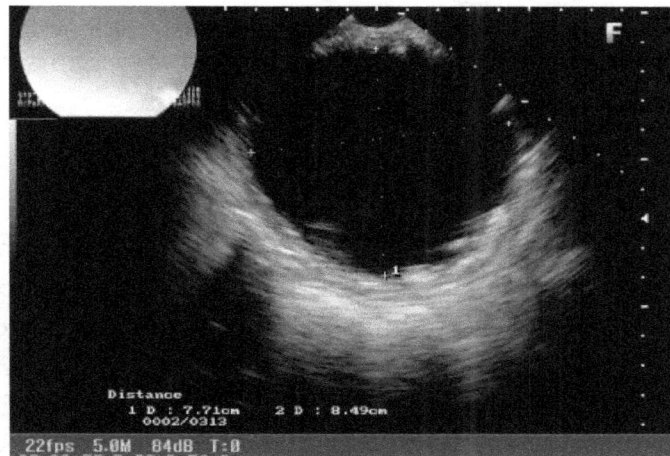

**Figure 8.** Pancreatic fluid collection without debris after 8 weeks from acute pancreatitis.

### 3.1. Pseudocyst (PSC)

PSC is the most common cystic lesion of the pancreas. By definition it is a localized fluid collection, rich in pancreatic secretions, within or adjacent to the gland, surrounded by a non-epithelial wall, which results from an episode of AP or CP, pancreatic ductal obstruction or trauma. The pancreatic secretion leakage causes an inflammatory response, resulting in a cystic wall formation composed by fibrotic tissue, granulation tissue, which appears weeks after the clinical onset. The development of a well-defined wall of granulation tissue differentiates a PSC from an acute fluid collection and thus facilitates the therapeutic approach [74].

The term PSC emphasizes the non-neoplastic origin of this encapsulated collection, which should be differentiated from pancreatic cystic neoplasm (PCN), which contains an epithelial lining [76, 77]. Moreover, they must be distinguished from other forms of evanescent fluid collections often seen by imaging. The most important are the acute fluid collections that occur in more than 50% of patients with moderate or severe AP. These collections should not be confused with PSC, as over 50% resolve spontaneously. They generally occur near the pancreas and have no granulation tissue wall. They represent an exudative reaction to a pancreatic injury, with inflammation, and have no communication with the MPD. Pancreatic enzymes are present in low concentrations, being similar to plasma fluid. Seen by image methods, these collections are irregular in shape and have no interface with the adjacent organs (Table 2) [76, 77]. Therefore, PSC is a cystic cavity lined by the pancreas and inflammatory epithelium [78].

| Acute fluid collections | Pseudocysts |
|---|---|
| Moderate / severe AP | CP, ductal obstruction or trauma |
| About 65% have spontaneous resolution | Located liquid Collection |
| No well-defined wall | Well defined wall without epithelial lining |
| Irregular Shape | Rounded or oval |
| May be multiple | Located, adjacent to the pancreas |
| No communication with the pancreatic duct | Frequent communication with the duct |
| Can turn into PSC | Spontaneous resolution in 30% |

**Table 2.** Fluid collection within or adjacent to pancreas in AP [2, 6, 7].

### 3.1.1. Incidence and etiology

The incidence of PSC varies from 1.6 to 69% [75, 78, 79]. This wide variation is due to the diagnostic method used. In the past, studies based on contrast radiography of the esophagus, stomach and duodenum reported very low incidences (1-3%) [80]. From the 70s, with the advent of US and CT, its diagnosis has become more frequent [81-83]. They appear as a complication of AP in 10 to 50% of cases, and 20 to 40% appear after CP, which is the most common etiology. PSC accounts for approximately 75% of pancreatic cystic lesions. Retention cysts account for 10% of the cystic lesions, and represent a MPD dilatation near a local obstruction, caused by CP or carcinoma. Other cystic lesions include congenital cysts (5%) and PCN (10%) [77, 81, 83]. PSC is associated to AP and is frequently seen in patients between 30 and 50 years old. Chronic pancreatitis (CP) secondary to alcoholism seems to be the main cause in most studies, accounting for 59-78% of cases [77, 81, 83]. However, most of these studies are retrospective. In a French study, chronic PSC was associated with chronic alcoholic pancreatitis in 94% of cases, and acute PSC was associated with cholelithiasis in 45% [84].

### 3.1.2. Differential diagnosis

Approximately 90% of pancreatic (or peripancreatic) cystic lesions are PSC (Figure 9). The remaining 10% are due to others disorders [83]. The differentiation between PSC and PCN is essential in determining the best therapeutic approach, especially before draining. In a prospective study based on clinical and radiological criteria Sand et al. considered a cystic lesion as a PSC when it occurs after AP of known cause, preceded by CP of known cause, or when ERCP showed changes compatible with CP. The cystic lesion was considered as a probable PCN when there was no history of AP or CP or when ERCP showed a normal pancreatography [85]. However, Warshaw et al did not show any reliable clinical or radiological criteria for the differentiation of cystic lesions (Figure 10) [86]. In this context, EUS is an excellent method for diagnosis of PCN, which can identify structural details (wall and contents) [12, 29, 44, 45]. Mucin producers PCNs (intraductal papillary neoplasms) shows similar appearance to PCS when delineated by CT and US. Mucinous PCN frequently are complex cysts with thick walls and irregular internal septa (Figure 11) [29].

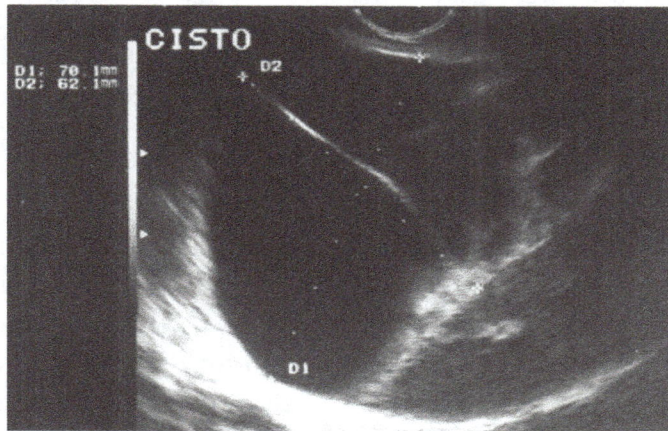

**Figure 9.** EUS Image of a pancreatic pseudocyst. Note the debris inside, which can be confused with PCN.

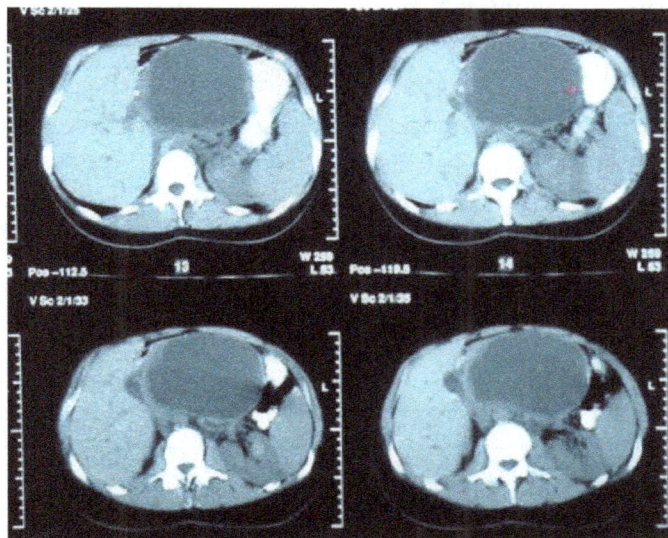

**Figure 10.** Tomographic image of alleged pancreatic pseudocyst. Note the thickness of the cyst wall located in the body of pancreas.

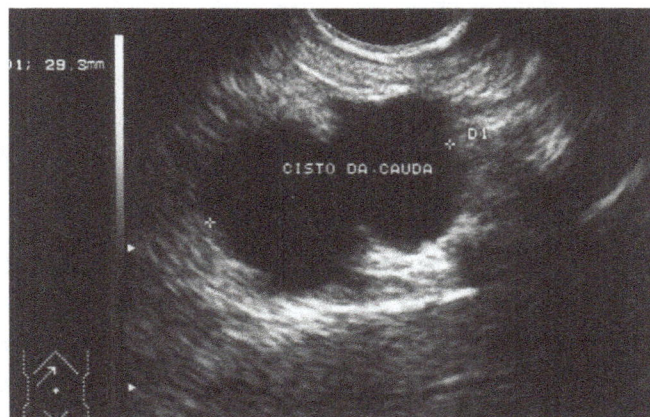

**Figure 11.** EUS image shows a 2.9 cm anechoic area, bilobed, and homogenous. This lesion was located in the tail. The pathologic study revealed a mucinous cystadenoma.

Solid components inside and calcifications in the walls can also be found. EUS images can often differentiate mucinous cystadenomas from mucinous cystadenocarcinoma and mucin producing intraductal neoplasms. These tumors may present regional MPD dilatation, with elevated areas and mass inside. Pancreatic parenchyma may be normal or shows atrophy, without calcifications and / or fibrosis. Intraductal tumors are premalignant lesions. EUS can identify focal mass [87].

Serous cystadenomas appear as large solid-cystic masses with predominantly microcysts, but macrocystic serous cystadenomas may cause confusion with PCS. These cysts contain fluid without "debris" inside. These lesions are not associated with mass or changes in MPD, but may show calcifications inside. The accuracy of EUS for differentiate serous and mucinous cystadenoma is around 84% and is superior to helical CT. EUS associated with fine needle aspiration (EUS-FNA) has been used to differentiate PSC and PCN. The fluid analysis includes the determination of amylase, CA19-9, CEA, and microhistopathology (Table 3) [88-90]. Although PSC shows low levels of CEA, high values may occasionally be found, especially in infected PSC. The tumor marker CA 19-9 is commonly elevated in inflammatory conditions and is not specific for malignancy. There is some concern about the possibility of infection after diagnostic puncture of a pancreatic lesion [91]. Wiersema et al observed infectious complications in 14% of patients with cystic lesions underwent puncture, well above the 0.5% after punctures of solid masses. In addition, a negative puncture does not completely rule out the presence of PCN. For these reasons, some authors do not advocate routine puncture in all cystic lesions [91, 92].

|  | PSC | Serous cystadenoma | Mucinous Neoplasia | Cystadenocarcinoma |
|---|---|---|---|---|
| Viscosity | low | Low | Often High | High |
| Amylase | High | Variable | Variable | Variable |
| CEA* | Low | Low | High | High |
| CA 19-9 | Variable | Variable | Variable | Variable |
| Cytology | Inflammatory | Cells rich in glycogen | Mucinous cells | Mucinous cells |

* Carcinoembryonic antigen

Table 3. Tumor Markers in fluid aspirated from pancreatic cystic lesions [46-49].

## 3.2. Endoscopic and EUS-guided Management

### 3.2.1. Which PSC need drainage?

In a review of published articles, Andren-Sandberg & Dervinis [93], showed a wide variation in spontaneous resolution of PSC range from 20% to 70%. Bradley et al. [94] followed 31 patients with PSC after AP and 62 after CP. The spontaneous resolution has occurred in 10/24 patients (42%) in PSC occurring in less than 6 weeks. However, only 1/23 (8%) of PSC which persisted for 7 to 12 weeks had spontaneous resolution. None of the remaining 12 PSC resolved during 18 months of follow-up. Vitas & Sarr [95] followed 68 patients with spontaneous resolution in 57% of 24 patients with satisfactory radiological follow up. In 38% resolution time was longer than 6 months. Maringhini et al [96] reported that 65% of PSC resolved until 1 year after diagnosis, and those less than 5 cm resolved more quickly than larger ones. Aranha et al [97] show that only 4/26 PSC greater than 6 cm resolved spontaneously. The average PSC, which resolved spontaneously had 4 cm compared to 9 cm with no resolution.

Thus, we think there are still some conflicting data about PSC drainage, although there is a greater tendency for resolution in those less than 6 cm and in asymptomatic cysts. Until recently, surgical treatment was the only approach, with mortality rates of 5-12% and morbidity of 21-50%. Due to these data and with the advancement of imaging methods and treatment, other modalities have been adopted [98].

### 3.2.1.1. Endoscopic drainage

The endoscopic treatment of PSC can be accomplished in two ways: transpapillary or transmural (cystogastrostomy or cystoduodenostomy) approach [99]. Success rates and recurrence are similar to open surgery [100]. However, in experienced hands, endoscopic therapy has significantly lower morbidity and mortality. In a literature review encompassing 437 patients undergoing endoscopic drainage, Lo et al found initial success in 94%, with resolution of PCS in 90%, recurrence in 16%, and 20% morbidity and mortality in 0.23% of cases [101].

**Transpapillary drainage**

It is possible only in cases where there is a communication between PSC and the MPD which occurs in 55-80% of cases, more commonly CP (49%) against 20% in AP [75, 102]. The procedure starts with pancreatography for delineate MPD communication. Then, a guide wire is inserted into MPD, reaching PSC cavity. A pancreatic sphincterotomy (optional) is performed, followed by insertion of a 5 or 7 plastic stent over the guide wire. Some authors advocate advancing the prosthesis through PSC, while others claim a transpapillary prosthesis, or a simple sphincterotomy are sufficient if there is no ductal stenosis [74]. The prosthesis stays for an average period of 2-3 months [103]. About 6% of patients experience pain or pancreatitis by occlusion of transpapillary prosthesis [104]. Removal or exchange must be done after 4-6 weeks due to high occlusion rate after this period, reaching 100% after 9 weeks. Due to the possibility of infection, antibiotic prophylaxis is always indicated.

Transpapillary drainage was successful in 84% of 117 patients treated by Beckingham et al [98] with recurrence in 9% and complications in 12%. There were no deaths. The most frequent complication was mild and self-limiting AP (6 patients), followed by infection (3 patients), treated with prosthesis replacement. The presence of a stent within MPD duct can lead to irregularities, similar to those found in CP, in 50% of patients. For this reason, some authors prefer a transmural approach or simple pancreatic sphincterotomy in patients with acute PSC and normal pancreatography. The success is higher for drainage in cephalic portion. In caudal portion, success is lower because MPD diameter diminish as it progresses from proximal to distal gland.

**Transmural drainage**

Transmural endoscopic therapy, by either cystogastrostomy or cystoduodenostomy, is only possible if there is a clear bulging of gastrointestinal wall. Furthermore, the distance between the lumen of the digestive system and the cyst should not exceed 10 mm by CT and/or EUS [105, 106]. When gastroduodenal bulging is not well defined or absent, during the endoscopic examination, the chance of perforation is 10%. In these patients, in particular, EUS can identify the best site for puncture and drainage [107].

Some authors advocate enlarging the hole of puncture with a balloon dilation, thus reducing the risk of bleeding [107-109]. Others prefer to puncture the cyst with a needle, injecting contrast material and aspirating cyst to reduce the possibility of hemorrhage. Cremer [110] has shown success in cystogastrostomy and cystoduodenostomy in 100% and 96%, and recurrence in 18% and 9%, respectively. Complications are rare in cystoduodenostomy, but significant in cystogastrostomy (18%). A review covering 50 patients, showed success of cystogastrostomy in 82%, with recurrence in 18%. There were no deaths. However, 8% had bleeding and 8% had perforation. In 71 patients undergoing cystoduodenostomy, the success rate was 89%, with recurrence in only 6%. Severe bleeding and perforation were observed in 4% of cases [82]. Based on these data, endoscopic drainage of PCS is considered one of the greatest risk endoscopic procedures [111].

In some cases, transmural and transpapillary drainage can be combined. This combination should be reserved for very large cysts associated with MPD stenosis, particularly if the cyst present very dense material or "debris". In a retrospective study comparing surgery and endoscopy (between 1985 and 1990), Froeschle et al [112] observed similar results after a follow up period of 33 months (50% improvement after surgery and 52% after endoscopic treatment). Similar results were observed by Barthet et al [113] in 143 patients. In summary, the guidelines for endoscopic drainage of PSC are listed in Table 4.

| |
|---|
| 1. Wait enough time until PCS become "mature" |
| 2. Identify pseudoaneurysm |
| 3. Evaluate the presence of portal hypertension and gastric varices |
| 4. Ensure proximity between the cyst and gastric / duodenal wall |
| 5. Perform a pancreatography before draining |
| 6. Identify the presence of "debris" in PSC |
| 7. Use the transpapillary route whenever possible |
| 8. Use a needle to test the drainage site before puncture (hemorrhage seems to be avoided) |
| 9. Clinical findings should confirm the nature of PSC |
| 10. If there is some doubt between a PSCS and PCN, use EUS-FNA and collect material before the procedure |

Table 4. Guidelines for safe endoscopic drainage of PSC.

### 3.2.2. EUS-guided drainage of PSC

EUS is a "weapon" available to endoscopists for approaching PSC, as it can obtain high quality pancreatic images. It is considered useful in the detection and treatment of PSC, and can be used prior to drainage, acting as a complement to conventional endoscopy or can be used for treatment itself. EUS meets several principles listed in Table 5 and for this reason, several authors recommend its use in the treatment of this disease. The main advantages of EUS are listed in Table 5 [108, 111].

| |
|---|
| 1. Safely measure the distance between PCS and the gastrointestinal wall |
| 2. Identifies gastric varices (high sensitivity) |
| 3. Detects gastric submucosal vessels |
| 4. Identifies pseudoaneurysm |
| 5. Identifies "debris" inside the cystic cavity |
| 6. Differentiates between PCS and PCN |
| 7. Shows the puncture site in the absence of bulging [29, 86] |
| 8. Allows drainage of PCS in a single procedure |

**Table 5.** Applications of EUS- guided drainage in PSC.

The development of therapeutic echoendoscopes with an operative channel of large diameter represented a great technological advancement in the treatment of PCS. The passage of large caliber prostheses can be achieved without the necessity to replace the device (for a duodenoscope) and no fluoroscopy is used [107]. Wiersema et al [114] reported the first case of drainage performed entirely by EUS in 1996 using a Pentax FG 36UX device. Vilmann et al [115] described a new method of EUS-guided drainage ("one step"), using the Pentax FG 38UX device. Regardless of some small technical variations of EUS-guided PSC drainage includes the following steps:

1. location of the cyst and the contact zone between it and the gastric / duodenal wall;

2. evaluation of gastric/duodenal wall with Doppler to rule out the presence of large vessels;

3. puncture of the cyst, which can be performed in two ways:

4. with a 19G needle,

5. with a cistostomo catheter

6. removing the "needle-knife" wire, and using the teflon sheath

7. passage of a guidewire (0.035 inch) through the teflon sheath up to the cyst;

8. enlarge the tract by balloon dilatation (up to 20mm) and

9. exploration of the cystic cavity with endoscopic ultrasound device and

10. introducing one or two "pig tail" prostheses over the guidewire to maintain the hole.

Some studies show the effectiveness of this technique. Giovannini et al [116] conducted drainage of 15 patients with PSC and of 20 with pancreatic abscess. Thirty-three patients underwent cystogastrostomy and 2 were submitted to cystoduodenostomy. Endoscopy revealed gastric bulging in only 1 patient. Plastic stents of 8.5 F or 7 F nasocystic drains were placed. The drainage was successful in 33 of 35 patients (failure in 2 cases of abscess), with only one episode of pneumoperitoneum, treated by clinical measures. One patient had recurrence of PSC (treated with new puncture) and 2 had recurrence of abscesses. Four patients with abscess underwent surgery (final successful 31/35 to 88.5%). No bleeding was observed. A potential disadvantage of this approach is not performing a pancreatography, thus the identification of stenosis or disruption of the MPD is not possible. In theory, this limitation may lead to a higher rate of relapse.

Ardengh et al [117]treated 12 patients with PSC without bulging (8 drainages and 4 aspirations), all by EUS. After a 12 months follow up, 10 had complete resolution, 1 recurred and undergone a new EUS-guided drainage, and 1 required surgical treatment. This technique allows the insertion of prostheses in unusual locations such as PSC in the uncinate process and tail, placement of drains near the esophageal hiatus, and allow drainage of PSC without bulging of the wall of the digestive system (Figure 12). In an attempt to reduce the rates of complications related to endoscopic drainage, some authors advocate the use of EUS, and compared it with the traditional technique. Poley et al [118] performed 53 drainages in 49 patients with PSC. Twenty-five submitted to the endoscopic drainage and 28 EUS-guided drainage. In the first technique there were fewer cases of abscess and infected necrosis compared to EUS group (p = 0.016). The success of EUS group was 96% [27/28] versus 56% [14/25] for endoscopic group (p <0.001). A higher number of prostheses was insert in the EUS group compared to endoscopic (average of 3 to 1 with p <0.001). The long-term results were superior to patients undergoing EUS: 81% [22/27] versus 42% [10/22] for endoscopic group (p = 0.003). More complications occurred in this group: 28% [7/25] vs. 7% [2/28] for those undergoing EUS (p = 0.04). In this work, although some cases has been analyzed retrospectively, has a great impact and endorses the opinion of these authors that the EUS-guided drainage of PSC should be the method of choice when endoscopic techinique is the best way of proceeding.

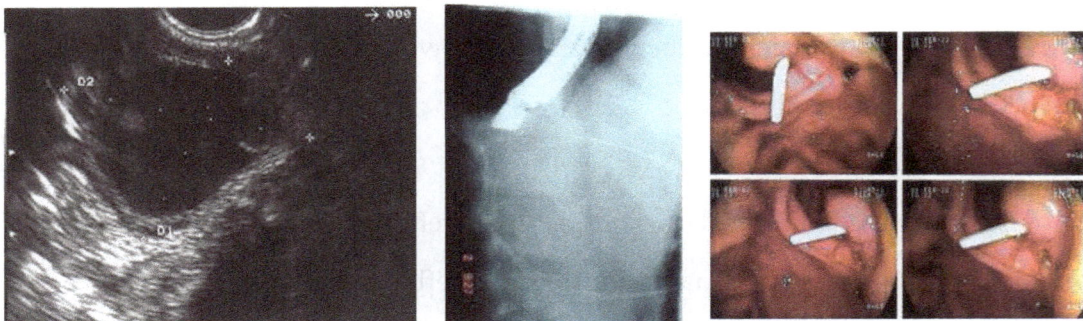

**Figure 12.** Steps of a PCS echo-guided drainage without bulging the wall. A) Identification of PCS. b) Fluoroscopic control of guide wire insertion and c) endoscopic view of prosthesis positioned in duodenal wall.

Lopes et al [119] demonstrated that EUS-guided drainage is a minimally invasive, safe and effective procedure for patients with PSC or abscesses. The authors retrospectively studied 51 patients who underwent 62 EUS-guided procedures. This procedure was successful in 94% of patients; 3 patients were referred to surgery. There were two minor complications treated medically and recurrence at 39 weeks was 17.7%. There was no mortality in this series. The insertion of a nasocystic drain for treat abscesses did not reduce the possibility of complications, but the insertion of two prosthesis diminished the number of complications.

We studied 77 patients with sterile non-necrotic pancreatic or peripancreatic collections. Patients were referred for echoendoscopic evaluation after CT scans [75], MRI [29] and ERCP [47]. None had a bulging or communication with MPD according to endoscopic pancreatography or MRI. Thus, transpapillary or endoscopic transmural drainage (cystoduodenostomy or cystogastrostomy) was not feasible. All patients had some type of symptom such as persistent abdominal pain or cholestasis. Simple EUS-guided aspiration was indicated in the following situations: patients with PSC without debris or visible wall, parenchymal collection, when the gap between the gastric wall and cyst was greater than 2.0 cm, and for cysts up to 3.0 cm in diameter. Thirty-three underwent EUS-guided aspiration using a 19G needle (Group II) and 44 were treated by transmural EUS-guided drainage and prosthesis placement (Group I). The vast majority of patients was treated (90.6%). A complete cyst aspiration occurred in all cases (100%) and transmural EUS-guided drainage, based on intention to treat, occurred in 83.3%. No complications occurred in group II. In group I occurred 3 complications (4.4%). These results reveal that EUS-guided drainage is possible in most patients with PSC. Those who underwent aspiration showed a high relapse rate. Thus, EUS-guided aspiration is an alternative in cases where EUS-guided transmural drainage is difficult.

## 3.3. Abscess

### 3.3.1. Definition, incidence and etiology

Defined by the Atlanta classification as a "circumscribed collection of pus containing little or no necrotic pancreatic tissue, which arises as a consequence of AP or trauma [120]. Its incidence has been estimated at around 1% to 5% [121] with mortality rates around 20% to 60% in some studies [122]. As a large proportion of patients are affected by episodes of severe AP, a greater number have developed this condition secondary to pancreatic infections. The search for a correct nomenclature has created discussions in the literature. Several reports in the literature between the years 60-80, named pancreatic abscess as an "infected pancreatic necrosis". With a better understanding of the pathophysiology of AP we know that infectious complications occur early in the course of AP resulting in infected pancreatic necrosis [123].

The difference between the natural history of pancreatic abscess and infected pancreatic necrosis and the management of these conditions has been better understood over time. In a series of 1,200 patients, Lumsden & Bradley [124] reported that alcohol is the main etiological factor (34%), followed by lithiasis (25%), postoperative complications (22%), idiopathic (10%), trauma (3%), and post-endoscopic retrograde cholangiopancreatography (ERCP) in 8%. The average time between the episode of AP and pancreatic abscess formation has been reported. Analyzing the literature reviews, Widdison et al. [125], showed that 50% of patients developed pancreatic abscess two weeks after the episode of AP. Kaushik et al. [126] reported an average period of 3-60 days. Warshaw & Jin [127] reported an average time of 32 days, and, in 58% of patients, the onset occurred in 2 weeks.

### 3.3.2. Diagnosis

Laboratory tests are nonspecific for this clinical condition, but leukocytosis with left shift may be an important factor. The abdominal X-ray shows the presence of gases, fluid level, and aspect of soap bubble or speckled gas in up to 35% of cases. Chest X-ray may show pleural effusion. CT and US allow not only defining the exact location of abscess as well as its follow-up during treatment. Magnetic resonance imaging (MRI) offers no advantage besides having a higher cost. EUS allows locating, characterizing, and draining it (Figures 13 e 14).

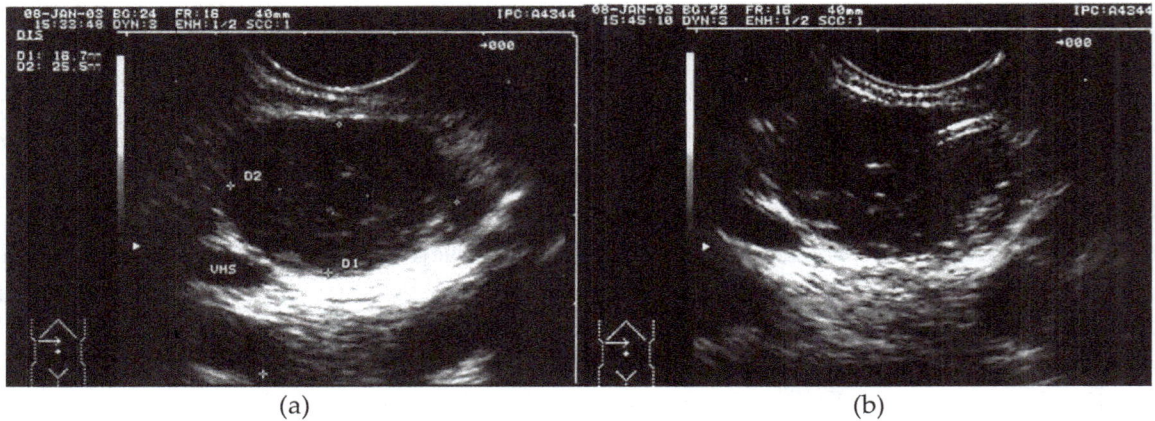

(a)                                                                    (b)

**Figure 13.** (a) echoendoscopic aspect of infected pancreatic collection. Note the numerous debris scattered throughout the content, which is not homogeneous. (b) echo-guided aspirative puncture performed at Intensive Care Unit for confirming the type of bacteria and then echo-guided drainage was performed using a plastic stent.

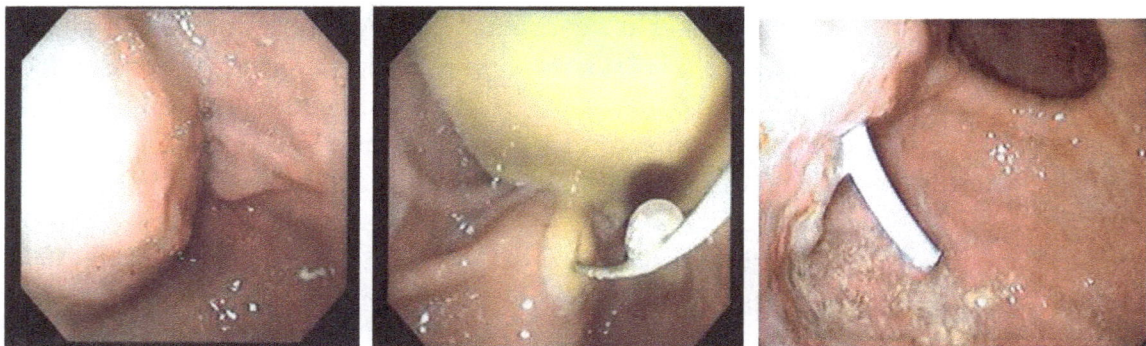

**Figure 14.** Endoscopic drainage of pancreatic abscess. A) Note an enormous bulging on the gastric wall. B) After puncturing the bulge, a guide wire is insert. C) Then the placement of a prosthesis.

### 3.3.3. Treatment

The best treatment is surgery. CT-guided percutaneous drainage has become an option, but is still a controversial method. Sunday et al. [128] reported bad a success rate of around 25% in patients with infected pancreatic collections when submitted to CT-guided drainage. Steiner et al [129] showed the results in 25 patients with pancreatic abscess. Nineteen were initially treated by percutaneous drainage and 6 required surgery after percutaneous drainage due to the presence of residual collection. Among 19, eight were cured, 1 died and the remaining 10 required surgery for proper drainage. In the group of 6 patients who underwent surgery after percutaneous drainage, all had a good outcome. We conclude that percutaneous drainage alone is not effective as an initial method, but that may be a good option for treating residual collections. However, other studies show conflicting results; Baril et al [130] evaluated 42 patients with positive culture of peripancreatic abscess, or collection. Among these, 25 were initially treated with percutaneous drainage and 6 required surgery after this drainage due to the presence of residual collection. None among these six required percutaneous drainage for a residual collection after surgery. In this six patients the surgical indication was: 3 with persistent sepsis, 1 with colon perforation after percutaneous drainage, 1 with thrombosis of the splenic vein evolving to variceal bleeding and 1 underwent surgical intervention due to a worsening in clinical condition. Of the 19 initially underwent percutaneous drainage, 18 were cured and 1 died, with success of 72% in this group. Van Sonnenberg et al [131] reported 86% success with percutaneous drainage in 59 patients with pancreatic abscess.

Endoscopic therapy also has its place. Park et al [132] drained 11 pancreatic abscess compressing the stomach, duodenum, or both through the creation of a fistula between the abscess and the digestive wall, washing the abscess cavity and stenting. The resolution was considered complete in the absence of symptoms and by CT imaging. Ten abscesses resolved within 32 days after placement of prosthesis. In 2 there was a need to put a nasocystic drain for washing and cleaning the abscess cavity of debris. Bleeding and relapse occurred in 1% and 13%, respectively, after a period of 18 months.

In recent years, EUS has gained acceptance in the therapeutic armamentarium for pancreatic abscesses. Giovannini et al [116] drained PSC and abscesses in 35 patients with an average size of 7.8 cm. A 7 F nasocystic drainage was successfully located in 18/20 cases of pancreatic abscess. The surgery was performed in 2 other patients. Drainage of PSC with 8.5 F prosthetic was successfully in 10 patients. The overall success of EUS was 31/35 patients (88.5%), and only 4 patients with abscess required surgery. Seewald et al [133] drained 13 patients with pancreatic necrosis and abscess, avoiding an emergency surgery. Transpapillary drainage was carried out by ERCP and transmural drainage was performed by EUS. Surgery was avoided in 9 patients with a mean follow up of 8.3 months. Surgery was combined with endoscopy in 1 case because of the extension of the abscess. Lopes et al [119] demonstrated that DEE is feasible and safe and that nasocystic drain did not reduce the possibility of complications, but the insertion of two prosthesis reduced the number of complications.

Our experience includes 12 patients. All had a strong suspicion of pancreatic abscess and were referred for an attempt to EUS-guided drainage. The presence of abscess was confirmed in 100%. Ten were drained successfully by EUS with 10 F prosthesis interposition and 2 underwent aspiration to confirm the presence of infection. Once confirmed, we opted for surgical treatment. There was no mortality in this series. None of the patients had bulging of the wall of the digestive system. In 3 cases surgical intervention was necessary because EUS-guided drainage was not sufficient. These results demonstrate that EUS-guided is a good method for the treatment of pancreatic abscess.

### 3.4. Walled off pancreatic necrosis

#### 3.4.1. EUS-guided necrosectomy

The Atlanta classification defines pancreatic necrosis as focal or diffuse areas of non-viable pancreatic parenchyma, typically associated with peripancreatic fat necrosis, and sometimes accompanied by the development of severe pancreatic duct disruption. During several weeks, an initial focus of necrosis can expand and may contain liquid and/or solid residues. In many cases, pancreatic necrosis progresses, reaching the retroperitoneal space with corrosion of retroperitoneal vessels. The radiological iconography of organized pancreatic necrosis (OPN) may be similar to an acute pseudocyst by CT. Radiographically, some characteristics help to identify the presence of solid residues. These include significant necrosis of the gland and large filling defects seen during contrast injection in CT and MRI, which indicates the presence of solid residues. Pancreatic abscess is defined as an intrabdominal circumscribed purulent collection, usually located near the pancreas, containing little or no necrosis. It has a well-defined wall, can be multilocular and is prone to rupture [123, 134].

The surgery is the preferred treatment to pancreatic necrosis and abscess, however, this modality is associated with high rate morbimortality. In selected patients the CT-guided percutaneous drainage may be effective but this method is not effective, when the fluid is thick and contains purulent debris. Furthermore, a catheter is invariably associated with bacterial colonization and fistula formation of difficult treatment. Endoscopic drainage of pancreatic fluid collections has been performed for more than two decades. It is noteworthy that pancreatic necrosis and abscesses are the biggest challenges to deal rationally and consciously! The development of EUS has expanded the indications for transmural drainage of collections without bulging the wall of the digestive system and allows the treatment of high risk fluid collections. Endoscopic therapy involves in most cases: ERCP/pancreatic sphincterotomy, transmural stent, EUS-guided puncture, dilation and drainage, endoscopic necrosectomy and exhaustive washing associated with a gastrocystic/duodenocystic fistula [135].

#### 3.4.2. Technique and accessories

The procedure starts with a puncture 19 G needle, through which can be passed a 0.035-inch terumo or Teflon type guide wire. The fistulous tract should be enlarged with a 20 mm (Maxforce; Microvasive) wire guided balloon. Another attractive accessory for necrosectomy are the 10F or 6.5F cistostomy catheters (EndoFlex, Voerde, Germany) used before insertion of one or more double pigtail" stents. An appropriate "input window" is necessary before start drainage, to define the patient's anatomy and to distinguish whether the content is a simple fluid, or complex, with solid debris. Most expert authors using this technique recommend assessing the integrity of the main pancreatic duct by endoscopic retrograde pancreatography. We are included this salutary practice.

The decision to the endoscopic intervention in patients with WOPN should be carefully discussed, because it is not easy to decide the moment of intervention. This technique, although safe, has high rate of adverse events, and involves patients in poor condition. Generally it should be performed when the collection is already organized, a fact that occurs after the fourth week of the initial episode. On the other hand if identified infected collection should be treated immediately. A pancreatic abscess is already infected by definition, requiring a faster approach. The absence of bulging of a pancreatic collection in the wall of the digestive system, the presence of portal hypertension, which carries a high likelihood of bleeding, failure of transmural endoscopic therapy and the need to exclude a cystic neoplasm, are reasonable arguments to priority the use of EUS as an approach for endoscopic drainage. Only skilled endoscopists in ERCP and EUS should perform these procedures. Moreover, it should be done in a tertiary hospital where pancreatobiliary surgeons and interventional radiologists are able to deal with an eventual complication.

## 3.5. Patient preparation

Endoscopic drainage is a lengthy and technically difficult procedure involving the use of fluoroscopy and ultrasound in several stages. Therefore, the aid of anesthesia is recommended. All patients should receive antibiotics before and during the procedure.

## 3.6. Evaluation prior to drainage

### 3.6.1. Description of the procedure

As described by Baron, transmural drainage is the preferred method for such collections. After entering the collection through the stomach or duodenal wall, the hole is enlarged to 15 mm, allowing the output of solid material around the endoprosthesis (generally two pigtail 10 F stents). A 7 F tube located inside the retrogastric space for irrigation and removal of solid debris is realized (Figure 15) [136]. Initially, up to 200 or 400 ml of saline is infused through the tube every 4-6 h. Preventive antibiotics should be administered. After irrigation, patients should be hospitalized for observation. Antibiotics and irrigation should be continued until latent serial imaging revealed complete resolution of the collection. Thus, internal drains can be removed endoscopically (Figure 16).

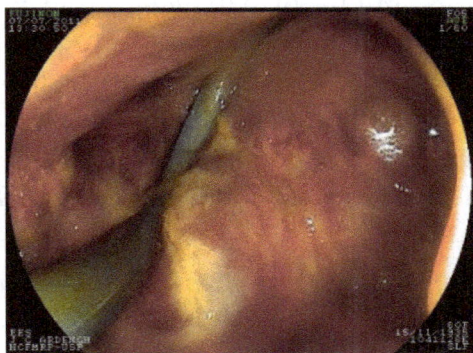

**Figure 15.** Note the 10 F-pigtail prosthesis inside the cavity with debris. Frontal vision endoscope shows the gastrocystic fistula.

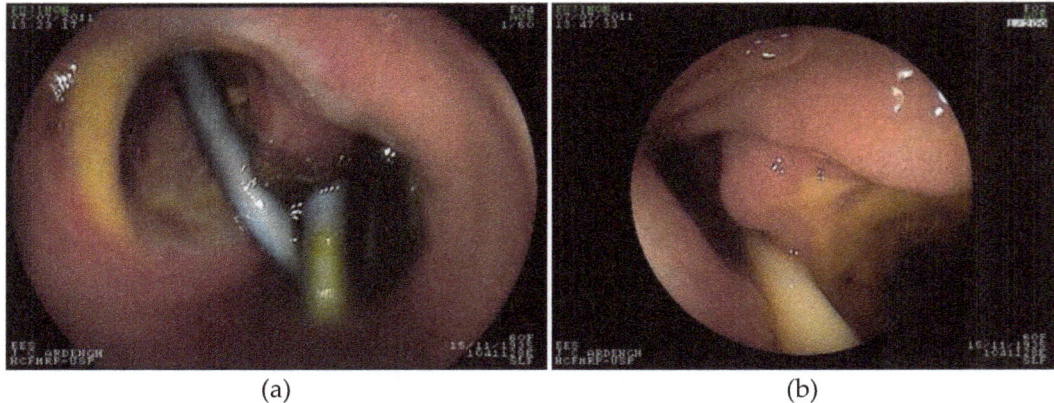

(a) (b)

**Figure 16.** The same patient shown in the previous figure. Note another prosthesis "pig tail" passing through duodeno-cystic fistula (a). (b) Note the introduction of a Dobbhoff feeding tube passing near another duodenocystic fistula, located in the second portion of duodenum, below the papilla.

As described by Seewald, the procedure involves a aggressive algorithm. The first session includes ERCP with transpapillary sphincterotomy, then, EUS-guided transmural access, with balloon dilatation of the fistulous tract and after this procedure is followed by repetitive necrosectomy for washing [137]. The technique of endoscopic necrosectomy is performed day-by-day until full evacuation of liquid and purulent necrosis. A basket or a rat tooth forceps can be used to remove necrotic material. Endoscopic wash is performed using a 10 F spray catheter connected to a Water-Jet Endo system. After MPD has been evaluated, if there is a communication between that and the cavity, a 7 F teflon nasopancreatic catheter should be placed over the guide wire after pancreatic sphincterotomy.

Coelho & Ardengh [135] described an aggressive algorithm similar to those described by Sewald et al In patients with WOPN the first session includes the following sequence: ERCP with detailed assessment of the pancreatic duct, and then, EUS. Depending on the aspect of MPD, according to Takishima classification, we choose the type of drainage (transpapillary, transmural or combined). If there is bulging a necrosectomy is made without performing an EUS, but if the bulging is not evident an endoscopic ultrasound is performed for approaching necrosis (Figures 15 and 16). If we opt for EUS to make a transmural access, a 20 mm balloon is used for dilation, and then a front-view endoscope is introduced for suction of liquid content and mobilization of solid residues. This procedure is performed every 7 days until the apparent improvement in the patient's condition. The technique of EUS-guided necrosectomy is performed every 7 days until complete evacuation of fluid and purulent necrosis. A basket (FG-18Q-1, Olympus, Tokyo, Japan) or rat tooth forceps can be used to remove necrotic material.

## 4. Literature review of EUS-guided necrosectomy

In 2002, Baron et al, compared the results of endoscopic drainage for acute pancreatic necrosis, pseudocysts, and chronic pancreatic pseudocysts. In this retrospective study, patients with necrosis and chronic pseudocysts showed no satisfactory resolution after endoscopic drainage with rates ranging from 72% to 74%, respectively. These rates were lower than the resolution rate of 92% for the drainage of acute pseudocysts. In patients with necrosis the complications were more frequent (37%) than patients with acute pseudocysts (19%), or chronic pseudocysts (17%). Recurrence of collections occurs more frequently in patients with necrosis (29%) than in patients with acute (9%) or chronic pseudocysts (12%) [74].

Park et al [132] assessed 11 pancreatic abscesses in nine patients drained endoscopically. Ten abscesses (91%) completely disappeared after stenting during 32 days. In two patients, one nasopancreatic catheter was necessary for irrigation, dilution of thick pus and disintegration of necrotic residues. There was one case of uncomplicated bleeding. The recurrence rate was 13% during a median follow-up of 18 months.

In 2000, Venu, et al [138], have shown similar results using the transpapillary approach. In this study, 11 patients underwent endoscopic transpapillary drainage with technical success in 10 patients (90%). Eight (74%) had resolution of pancreatic abscess. The installation of an intracavitary nasopancreatic drain and instillation of gentamicin were used in two patients. The patient who presented failure of endoscopic treatment underwent percutaneous drainage successfully.

In 2000, Seifert et al [139] were the first to describe the use of EUS for transmural approach in necrotizing pancreatitis or abscess, followed by dilation of the fistula created to perform an endoscopic direct debridement of the retrogastric space. The gastric fenestration and debridement of infected necrosis by pneumoretroperitonioscopy was performed in three patients. This method obtained rapid clinical improvement and no adverse events.

Other study with EUS-guided drainage of PSC and abscesses in 35 patients (20 abscesses). The drainage was successful in 18/20 patients with a 7F nasocystic drain. Two patients required surgery, and a median follow-up of 27 months two relapses were observed [116].

Another retrospective study with a EUS-guided procedure associated or not with transpapillary drainage, and followed by balloon dilatation of the fistula (cystogastrostomy or cystoduodenostomy), was done in patients with WOPN and abscess. Endoscopic necrosectomy were performed daily. In 13 consecutive patients, 5 with infected necrosis, and 8 with abscesses. This technique was successful in solving the infection in 12/13 patients during a mean follow-up of 9.5 months. One patient required a surgical treatment for necrosis resection in paracolic space. Two patients with ductal rupture developed recurrent collections after 2 and 4 months. These patients required resection of the pancreatic head. Three episodes of locally controlled hemorrhage were reported. The average number of necrosectomies was 7 [133].

In 2006, Hookey et al [140] evaluated the results of endoscopic drainage for pancreatic collections in 116 patients. Eighty had necrosis and 9 had pancreatic abscess. In this study, drainage of organized necrosis showed failure rates significantly greater than in other collections. The clinical and technical success of necrosis drainage was only 25% and 50%, respectively. Six of the eight undergone to a nasocavitary catheter insertion and one had recurrence. There were two complications related to the procedure in this subgroup. Nine patients underwent endoscopic drainage of pancreatic abscess. Seven/9 were treated by nasocavitary catheter. All procedures were successful, and 8/9 (88.9%) patients had clinical success. One had abscess relapse and there was no procedure-related complications.

In 2007 Papachristou et al [141] performed a retrospective analysis of 53 patients underwent endoscopic transmural drainage/debridement of sterile collection (27 patients) and infected WOPN (26 patients). An average of three sessions per patient were performed. The result after the initial endoscopic intervention proved successful in 81% (43 patients) and persistence of organized pancreatic necrosis in 19% (10 patients). Twenty-one patients (40%) required simultaneous radiologic/echo-guided drainage, and 12 patients (23%) required open surgery, due to the persistence of organized pancreatic necrosis [3], recurrence [2], fistula formation [2], technical failure [1], persistent pain [1], colonic obstruction [1], perforation [1], and abscess [1].

Coelho & Ardengh treated 56 patients with WOPN. 49/56 (87%) patients were successfully treated by 20 mm balloon dilation in serial sessions every 7 days. During this period, we had 3 cases of recurrence and no case of death. Ardengh et al in the DDW 2013 presented the results of programmed EUS-guided necrosectomy in patients with severe necrotizing acute pancreatitis. The programmed EUS-guided necrosectomy allows created multiple transluminal gateways to improve transmural removal of necrosis. We treated 17 patients with infected WOPN with this technique. One or more transmural fistulas were performed. The necrosectomy was performed and after a plastic pigtail stents were placed. The average sessions was 2.5 [1-6]. Successful resolution of WOPN occurred in 15/17 (88.2%) patients. Plastic pigtail were placed in 12, self-expandable metallic stents (SEMS) in 3, and in 2 patients no stents were placed. Three patients experienced bleeding (entry side [2], inside cavity [1]) and worsening of infection (33.3%), all of which were successfully treated endoscopically by another session of EUS-N. The mortality rate was (11.7%). One underwent surgery (5.8%) and other patient died due to poor medical conditions. The mean duration of hospital stay was 19 days (6-48 days). We concluded that the programmed EUS-N is an effective option for the treatment of infected WOPN because it eliminates the need for surgery and can be performed in the absence of a visible bulging [142].

One of the biggest challenges during EUS-guided drainage was the sequential transgastric stent placement and positioning of nasocystic drain, which can be difficult due to a reduced visual field. Abundant fluid, the tangential axis of puncture, and the presence of solid residues makes the passage of a catheter up to cavity, a difficult maneuver. The use of conventional plastic stents for drainage of necrosectomies is troublesome. The insertion of a removable self-expandable metallic stent, maybe facilitate drainage of infected pancreatic necrosis after several unconventional necrosectomies, but this approach needs to be better evaluated [143].

# 5. Conclusion

PSC, WOPN and abscess are the most serious adverse eventss of acute pancreatitis. The endoscopic approach for these problems has developed and, more recently, we have seen an increasing in drainage of pancreatic fluid collections. A variety of studies has been conducted and the opinion of experts has been analyzed searching for the answer to the question: the endoscopic drainage is superior to surgical or radiological intervention? However, to date no randomized, controlled, multicentric, and prospective study was performed. Anyway, endoscopic approach is minimally invasive, eliminating the morbidity associated with postoperative healing of surgical drainage and the possibility of fistula after percutaneous drainage.

The advantages of EUS-guided drainage include: the ability to accurately define the characteristics of pancreatic fluid collections, the exclusion of other possible diagnoses and determine the presence of vascular structures which at least hypothetically could reduce one of the complications of endoscopic drainage. From a therapeutic standpoint, we can access collections without bulging in sites of difficult access. The biggest disadvantage of endoscopic treatment is that it is not available in all institutions, and the general time is over for its implementation, especially if we decided to use EUS. Placing nasocystic drainage is associated with patient discomfort when the daily necrosectomy is required. The development of new accessories and stents can make it more effective and safe.

## Author details

José Celso Ardengh[1,2*], Eder Rios de Lima Filho[3], Rafael Kemp[4] and José Sebastião dos Santos[3]

*Address all correspondence to: jcelso@uol.com.br

1 Endoscopy Unit, Hospital 9 de Julho, São Paulo, Brazil

2 Endoscopy Unity, Division of Surgery and Anatomy, Ribeirão Preto School of Medicine – University of São Paulo, Brazil

3 Department of Surgery, Hospital Federal dos Servidores do Estado, Rio de Janeiro, Brazil

4 Endoscopy Unity, Division of Surgery and Anatomy, Ribeirão Preto School of Medicine – University of São Paulo, Brazil

## References

[1] Marshall JB. Acute pancreatitis. A review with an emphasis on new developments. Arch Intern Med. 1993 May 24;153(10):1185-98. PubMed PMID: 8494472.

[2] Mehdi M, Deutsch JP, Arrive L, Ayadi K, Ladeb MF, Tubiana JM. [Acute pancreatitis]. Ann Radiol (Paris). 1996;39(1):37-44. PubMed PMID: 8794575.

[3] United Kingdom guidelines for the management of acute pancreatitis. British Society of Gastroenterology. Gut. 1998 Jun;42 Suppl 2:S1-13. PubMed PMID: 9764029.

[4]   Dalzell DP, Scharling ES, Ott DJ, Wolfman NT. Acute pancreatitis: the role of diagnostic imaging. Crit Rev Diagn Imaging. 1998 Sep;39(5):339-63. PubMed PMID: 9791748.

[5]   Pandol SJ. Acute pancreatitis. Curr Opin Gastroenterol. 2006 Sep;22(5):481-6. PubMed PMID: 16891878.

[6]   Bittner R, Block S, Buchler M, Beger HG. Pancreatic abscess and infected pancreatic necrosis. Different local septic complications in acute pancreatitis. Dig Dis Sci. 1987 Oct;32(10):1082-7. PubMed PMID: 3308374.

[7]   Bradley EL, 3rd, Allen K. A prospective longitudinal study of observation versus surgical intervention in the management of necrotizing pancreatitis. Am J Surg. 1991 Jan;161(1):19-24; discussion -5. PubMed PMID: 1987854.

[8]   Calleja GA, Barkin JS. Acute pancreatitis. Med Clin North Am. 1993 Sep;77(5): 1037-56. PubMed PMID: 7690443.

[9]   Grendell JH. Idiopathic acute pancreatitis. Gastroenterol Clin North Am. 1990 Dec; 19(4):843-8. PubMed PMID: 2269520.

[10]  Levy MJ, Geenen JE. Idiopathic acute recurrent pancreatitis. The American journal of gastroenterology. 2001 Sep;96(9):2540-55. PubMed PMID: 11569674.

[11]  Steinberg WM. Predictors of severity of acute pancreatitis. Gastroenterol Clin North Am. 1990 Dec;19(4):849-61. PubMed PMID: 2269521.

[12]  Glasbrenner B, Adler G. [Acute pancreatitis: diagnosis]. Ther Umsch. 1996 May;53(5): 333-41. PubMed PMID: 8685850.

[13]  Acosta JM, Ledesma CL. Gallstone migration as a cause of acute pancreatitis. N Engl J Med. 1974 Feb 28;290(9):484-7. PubMed PMID: 4810815.

[14]  Dayan L, Cherif-Zahar K, Lepage B, Bories-Azeau A. [Diagnostic traps and procedure to follow in radio-invisible biliary calculi]. J Chir (Paris). 1976 Apr;111(4):431-42. PubMed PMID: 956297.

[15]  Lankisch PG, Schirren CA, Schmidt H, Schonfelder G, Creutzfeldt W. Etiology and incidence of acute pancreatitis: a 20-year study in a single institution. Digestion. 1989;44(1):20-5. PubMed PMID: 2599279.

[16]  Patti MG, Pellegrini CA. Gallstone pancreatitis. Surg Clin North Am. 1990 Dec;70(6): 1277-95. PubMed PMID: 2247815.

[17]  Thomson SR, Hendry WS, McFarlane GA, Davidson AI. Epidemiology and outcome of acute pancreatitis. Br J Surg. 1987 May;74(5):398-401. PubMed PMID: 3594136.

[18]  Goodman AJ, Neoptolemos JP, Carr-Locke DL, Finlay DB, Fossard DP. Detection of gall stones after acute pancreatitis. Gut. 1985 Feb;26(2):125-32. PubMed PMID: 2578422.

[19] Lee SP, Nicholls JF. Nature and composition of biliary sludge. Gastroenterology. 1986 Mar;90(3):677-86. PubMed PMID: 3943697.

[20] Aube C, Delorme B, Yzet T, Burtin P, Lebigot J, Pessaux P, et al. MR cholangiopancreatography versus endoscopic sonography in suspected common bile duct lithiasis: a prospective, comparative study. AJR Am J Roentgenol. 2005 Jan;184(1):55-62. PubMed PMID: 15615951.

[21] Moon JH, Cho YD, Cha SW, Cheon YK, Ahn HC, Kim YS, et al. The detection of bile duct stones in suspected biliary pancreatitis: comparison of MRCP, ERCP, and intraductal US. The American journal of gastroenterology. 2005 May;100(5):1051-7. PubMed PMID: 15842578.

[22] De Bolla AR, Obeid ML. Mortality in acute pancreatitis. Ann R Coll Surg Engl. 1984 May;66(3):184-6. PubMed PMID: 6721405.

[23] McMahon MJ, Shefta JR. Physical characteristics of gallstones and the calibre of the cystic duct in patients with acute pancreatitis. Br J Surg. 1980 Jan;67(1):6-9. PubMed PMID: 7357248.

[24] Armstrong CP, Taylor TV, Jeacock J, Lucas S. The biliary tract in patients with acute gallstone pancreatitis. Br J Surg. 1985 Jul;72(7):551-5. PubMed PMID: 4016539.

[25] Houssin D, Castaing D, Lemoine J, Bismuth H. Microlithiasis of the gallbladder. Surg Gynecol Obstet. 1983 Jul;157(1):20-4. PubMed PMID: 6857468.

[26] Tarnasky PR, Hawes RH. Endoscopic diagnosis and therapy of unexplained (idiopathic) acute pancreatitis. Gastrointest Endosc Clin N Am. 1998 Jan;8(1):13-37. PubMed PMID: 9405749.

[27] Sugiyama M, Wada N, Atomi Y, Kuroda A, Muto T. Diagnosis of acute pancreatitis: value of endoscopic sonography. AJR Am J Roentgenol. 1995 Oct;165(4):867-72. PubMed PMID: 7676983.

[28] Levy MJ. The hunt for microlithiasis in idiopathic acute recurrent pancreatitis: should we abandon the search or intensify our efforts? Gastrointestinal endoscopy. 2002 Feb;55(2):286-93. PubMed PMID: 11818945.

[29] Liu CL, Lo CM, Chan JK, Poon RT, Lam CM, Fan ST, et al. Detection of choledocholithiasis by EUS in acute pancreatitis: a prospective evaluation in 100 consecutive patients. Gastrointestinal endoscopy. 2001 Sep;54(3):325-30. PubMed PMID: 11522972.

[30] Tandon M, Topazian M. Endoscopic ultrasound in idiopathic acute pancreatitis. The American journal of gastroenterology. 2001 Mar;96(3):705-9. PubMed PMID: 11280538.

[31] Khalid A, Slivka A. Approach to idiopathic recurrent pancreatitis. Gastrointest Endosc Clin N Am. 2003 Oct;13(4):695-716, x. PubMed PMID: 14986794.

[32] Steinberg WM. Acute pancreatitis--never leave a stone unturned. N Engl J Med. 1992 Feb 27;326(9):635-7. PubMed PMID: 1734255.

[33] Lee SP, Nicholls JF, Park HZ. Biliary sludge as a cause of acute pancreatitis. N Engl J Med. 1992 Feb 27;326(9):589-93. PubMed PMID: 1734248.

[34] Ros E, Navarro S, Bru C, Garcia-Puges A, Valderrama R. Occult microlithiasis in 'idiopathic' acute pancreatitis: prevention of relapses by cholecystectomy or ursodeoxycholic acid therapy. Gastroenterology. 1991 Dec;101(6):1701-9. PubMed PMID: 1955135.

[35] Millat B, Guillon F. [Prognostic indices in acute pancreatitis. Practical implications]. Gastroenterol Clin Biol. 1995;19(5 Pt 2):B33-40. PubMed PMID: 8522100.

[36] Neoptolemos JP, Carr-Locke DL, London NJ, Bailey IA, James D, Fossard DP. Controlled trial of urgent endoscopic retrograde cholangiopancreatography and endoscopic sphincterotomy versus conservative treatment for acute pancreatitis due to gallstones. Lancet. 1988 Oct 29;2(8618):979-83. PubMed PMID: 2902491.

[37] Ranson JH. Acute pancreatitis: pathogenesis, outcome and treatment. Clin Gastroenterol. 1984 Sep;13(3):843-63. PubMed PMID: 6386241.

[38] Miquel JF, Rollan A, Guzman S, Nervi F. Microlithiasis and cholesterolosis in 'idiopathic' acute pancreatitis. Gastroenterology. 1992 Jun;102(6):2188-90. PubMed PMID: 1587452.

[39] Seror J, Rives J, Stoppa R. [Importance of the concept of microlithiasis in biliary pathology; sphincteral and choledochal incidences.]. Afr Francaise Chir. 1961 3d Trimest; 19:166-9. PubMed PMID: 13910846.

[40] Moskovitz M, Min TC, Gavaler JS. The microscopic examination of bile in patients with biliary pain and negative imaging tests. The American journal of gastroenterology. 1986 May;81(5):329-33. PubMed PMID: 3706246.

[41] Pfefferman R, Luttwak EM. Gallstone pancreatitis. Exploration of the biliary system in pancreatitis of undetermined origin. Arch Surg. 1971 Oct;103(4):484-6. PubMed PMID: 5094553.

[42] Bertrand L, Lamarque JL. [Biliary microlithiasis. Medico-radiological observations]. Nouv Presse Med. 1975 Dec 20;4(44):3135-8. PubMed PMID: 1219621.

[43] Filly RA, Allen B, Minton MJ, Bernhoft R, Way LW. In vitro investigation of the origin of echoes with biliary sludge. J Clin Ultrasound. 1980 Jun;8(3):193-200. PubMed PMID: 6769957.

[44] Lee SP, Hayashi A, Kim YS. Biliary sludge: curiosity or culprit? Hepatology. 1994 Aug;20(2):523-5. PubMed PMID: 8045512.

[45] Barraya L, Pujol Soler R, Yvergneaux JP. [The region of Oddi's sphincter: millimetric anatomy]. Presse Med. 1971 Dec 25;79(55):2527-34. PubMed PMID: 5157911.

[46] Ardengh JC, Malheiros CA, Ganc AJ, Ferrari A. Endoscopic ultrasound (EUS) in the diagnosis of gallbladder microlithiasis in patients with idiopathic acute pancreatitis. Digestion. 1998;59(3):40(136).

[47] Chak A, Hawes RH, Cooper GS, Hoffman B, Catalano MF, Wong RC, et al. Prospective assessment of the utility of EUS in the evaluation of gallstone pancreatitis. Gastrointestinal endoscopy. 1999 May;49(5):599-604. PubMed PMID: 10228258.

[48] Norton SA, Alderson D. Endoscopic ultrasonography in the evaluation of idiopathic acute pancreatitis. Br J Surg. 2000 Dec;87(12):1650-5. PubMed PMID: 11122178.

[49] Amouyal P, Amouyal G, Levy P, Tuzet S, Palazzo L, Vilgrain V, et al. Diagnosis of choledocholithiasis by endoscopic ultrasonography. Gastroenterology. 1994 Apr; 106(4):1062-7. PubMed PMID: 8143973.

[50] Sugiyama M, Atomi Y. Endoscopic ultrasonography for diagnosing choledocholithiasis: a prospective comparative study with ultrasonography and computed tomography. Gastrointestinal endoscopy. 1997 Feb;45(2):143-6. PubMed PMID: 9040999.

[51] Sugiyama M, Atomi Y. Acute biliary pancreatitis: the roles of endoscopic ultrasonography and endoscopic retrograde cholangiopancreatography. Surgery. 1998 Jul; 124(1):14-21. PubMed PMID: 9663246.

[52] Ardengh JC, Ganc AJ, Ferrari A, Malheiros CA, Rahal F. Accuracy of endoscopic ultrasonography (EUS) for diagnosis of microcholedocholithiasis in patients with acute pancreatitis. Endoscopy. 2000;32:A27(P68).

[53] Norton SA, Cheruvu CV, Collins J, Dix FP, Eyre-Brook IA. An assessment of clinical guidelines for the management of acute pancreatitis. Ann R Coll Surg Engl. 2001 Nov;83(6):399-405. PubMed PMID: 11777135.

[54] Uomo G, Visconti M, Manes G, Calise F, Laccetti M, Rabitti PG. Nonsurgical treatment of acute necrotizing pancreatitis. Pancreas. 1996 Mar;12(2):142-8. PubMed PMID: 8720660.

[55] Neoptolemos JP, Davidson BR, Winder AF, Vallance D. Role of duodenal bile crystal analysis in the investigation of 'idiopathic' pancreatitis. Br J Surg. 1988 May;75(5): 450-3. PubMed PMID: 3390676.

[56] Shimpi RA, Ho S, Branch MS, Jowell PS, Baillie J, Gress FG. The Diagnostic Utility of Endoscopic Ultrasound (EUS) and ERCP in Evaluating Patients with Idiopathic Acute Recurrent Pancreatitis (IARP): An Update. Gastrointestinal endoscopy. 2006;63(5):AB262 (W1304).

[57] Feller ER. Endoscopic retrograde cholangiopancreatography in the diagnosis of unexplained pancreatitis. Arch Intern Med. 1984 Sep;144(9):1797-9. PubMed PMID: 6476999.

[58] Frossard JL, Sosa-Valencia L, Amouyal G, Marty O, Hadengue A, Amouyal P. Usefulness of endoscopic ultrasonography in patients with "idiopathic" acute pancreatitis. Am J Med. 2000 Aug 15;109(3):196-200. PubMed PMID: 10974181.

[59] Gregor JC, Ponich TP, Detsky AS. Should ERCP be routine after an episode of "idiopathic" pancreatitis? A cost-utility analysis. Gastrointestinal endoscopy. 1996 Aug; 44(2):118-23. PubMed PMID: 8858315.

[60] Scapa E. To do or not to do an endoscopic retrograde cholangiopancreatography in acute biliary pancreatitis? Surg Laparosc Endosc. 1995 Dec;5(6):453-4. PubMed PMID: 8611991.

[61] Scholmerich J, Lausen M, Lay L, Salm R, Ruckauer K, Gross V, et al. Value of endoscopic retrograde cholangiopancreatography in determining the cause but not course of acute pancreatitis. Endoscopy. 1992 May;24(4):244-7. PubMed PMID: 1612037.

[62] Siegel JH, Veerappan A, Cohen SA, Kasmin FE. Endoscopic sphincterotomy for biliary pancreatitis: an alternative to cholecystectomy in high-risk patients. Gastrointestinal endoscopy. 1994 Sep-Oct;40(5):573-5. PubMed PMID: 7988821.

[63] Block MA, Priest RJ. Acute pancreatitis related to grossly minute stones in a radiographically normal gallbladder. Am J Dig Dis. 1967 Sep;12(9):934-8. PubMed PMID: 6039573.

[64] Good LI, Edell SL, Soloway RD, Trotman BW, Mulhern C, Arger PA. Ultrasonic properties of gallstones. Effect of stone size and composition. Gastroenterology. 1979 Aug;77(2):258-63. PubMed PMID: 447040.

[65] Simeone JF, Mueller PR, Ferruci JT, Jr., Harbin WP, Wittenberg J. Significance of nonshadowing focal opacities at cholecystosonography. Radiology. 1980 Oct;137(1 Pt 1): 181-5. PubMed PMID: 7422843.

[66] Farrar JT. Underdiagnosis of biliary tract disorders? Gastroenterology. 1966 Dec; 51(6):1074-5. PubMed PMID: 5958606.

[67] Goinard P, Pelissier G. [Biliary micro-lithiasis.]. Presse Med. 1962 Feb 3;70:260-1. PubMed PMID: 13899584.

[68] Venu RP, Geenen JE, Toouli J, Stewart E, Hogan WJ. Endoscopic retrograde cholangiopancreatography. Diagnosis of cholelithiasis in patients with normal gallbladder x-ray and ultrasound studies. Jama. 1983 Feb 11;249(6):758-61. PubMed PMID: 6185702.

[69] Aliperti G. Complications related to diagnostic and therapeutic endoscopic retrograde cholangiopancreatography. Gastrointest Endosc Clin N Am. 1996 Apr;6(2): 379-407. PubMed PMID: 8673333.

[70] Thoeni RF, Fell SC, Goldberg HI. CT detection of asymptomatic pancreatitis following ERCP. Gastrointest Radiol. 1990 Fall;15(4):291-5. PubMed PMID: 2210197.

[71] Dahan P, Andant C, Levy P, Amouyal P, Amouyal G, Dumont M, et al. Prospective evaluation of endoscopic ultrasonography and microscopic examination of duodenal bile in the diagnosis of cholecystolithiasis in 45 patients with normal conventional ultrasonography. Gut. 1996 Feb;38(2):277-81. PubMed PMID: 8801211.

[72] Ardengh JC, Malheiros CA, Rahal F, Pereira V, Ganc AJ. Microlithiasis of the gallbladder: role of endoscopic ultrasonography in patients with idiopathic acute pancreatitis. Rev Assoc Med Bras. 2010 Jan-Feb;56(1):27-31. PubMed PMID: 20339782. Epub 2010/03/27. eng.

[73] Liu CL, Lo CM, Chan JK, Poon RT, Fan ST. EUS for detection of occult cholelithiasis in patients with idiopathic pancreatitis. Gastrointestinal endoscopy. 2000 Jan;51(1): 28-32. PubMed PMID: 10625791.

[74] Baron TH, Harewood GC, Morgan DE, Yates MR. Outcome differences after endoscopic drainage of pancreatic necrosis, acute pancreatic pseudocysts, and chronic pancreatic pseudocysts. Gastrointest Endosc. 2002 Jul;56(1):7-17. PubMed PMID: 12085029.

[75] Pitchumoni CS, Agarwal N. Pancreatic pseudocysts. When and how should drainage be performed? Gastroenterol Clin North Am. 1999 Sep;28(3):615-39. PubMed PMID: 10503140.

[76] Hawes RH. Endoscopic management of pseudocysts. Rev Gastroenterol Disord. 2003 Summer;3(3):135-41. PubMed PMID: 14502117.

[77] Howell DA, Elton E, Parsons WG. Endoscopic management of pseudocysts of the pancreas. Gastrointest Endosc Clin N Am. 1998 Jan;8(1):143-62. PubMed PMID: 9405756.

[78] Kloppel G. Pseudocysts and other non-neoplastic cysts of the pancreas. Semin Diagn Pathol. 2000 Feb;17(1):7-15. PubMed PMID: 10721803.

[79] Kloppel G, Kosmahl M. Cystic lesions and neoplasms of the pancreas. The features are becoming clearer. Pancreatology. 2001;1(6):648-55. PubMed PMID: 12120249.

[80] Wade JW. Twenty-five year experience with pancreatic pseudocysts. Are we making progress? Am J Surg. 1985 Jun;149(6):705-8. PubMed PMID: 3925799.

[81] Etzkorn KP, DeGuzman LJ, Holderman WH, Abu-Hammour A, Schlesinger PK, Harig JM, et al. Endoscopic drainage of pancreatic pseudocysts: patient selection and evaluation of the outcome by endoscopic ultrasonography. Endoscopy. 1995 May; 27(4):329-33. PubMed PMID: 7555940.

[82] Imrie CW, Buist LJ, Shearer MG. Importance of cause in the outcome of pancreatic pseudocysts. Am J Surg. 1988 Sep;156(3 Pt 1):159-62. PubMed PMID: 2458684.

[83] Lawson JM, Baillie J. Endoscopic therapy for pancreatic pseudocysts. Gastrointest Endosc Clin N Am. 1995 Jan;5(1):181-93. PubMed PMID: 7728343.

[84]  Walt AJ, Bouwman DL, Weaver DW, Sachs RJ. The impact of technology on the management of pancreatic pseudocyst. Fifth annual Samuel Jason Mixter Lecture. Arch Surg. 1990 Jun;125(6):759-63. PubMed PMID: 2189377.

[85]  Sand J, Nordback I. The differentiation between pancreatic neoplastic cysts and pancreatic pseudocyst. Scand J Surg. 2005;94(2):161-4. PubMed PMID: 16111099.

[86]  Warshaw AL, Compton CC, Lewandrowski K, Cardenosa G, Mueller PR. Cystic tumors of the pancreas. New clinical, radiologic, and pathologic observations in 67 patients. Ann Surg. 1990 Oct;212(4):432-43; discussion 44-5. PubMed PMID: 2171441.

[87]  Ardengh JC, Lopes CV, de Lima-Filho ER, Kemp R, Dos Santos JS. Impact of endoscopic ultrasound-guided fine-needle aspiration on incidental pancreatic cysts. A prospective study. Scand J Gastroenterol. 2014 Jan;49(1):114-20. PubMed PMID: 24188361.

[88]  Brugge WR. Approach to cystic pancreatic lesions. Gastrointest Endosc Clin N Am. 2005 Jul;15(3):485-96, viii. PubMed PMID: 15990053.

[89]  Brugge WR, Lewandrowski K, Lee-Lewandrowski E, Centeno BA, Szydlo T, Regan S, et al. Diagnosis of pancreatic cystic neoplasms: a report of the cooperative pancreatic cyst study. Gastroenterology. 2004 May;126(5):1330-6. PubMed PMID: 15131794.

[90]  Sarr MG, Kendrick ML, Nagorney DM, Thompson GB, Farley DR, Farnell MB. Cystic neoplasms of the pancreas: benign to malignant epithelial neoplasms. Surg Clin North Am. 2001 Jun;81(3):497-509. PubMed PMID: 11459267.

[91]  Bhutani MS. Endoscopic ultrasound in pancreatic diseases. Indications, limitations, and the future. Gastroenterol Clin North Am. 1999 Sep;28(3):747-70, xi. PubMed PMID: 10503148.

[92]  Wiersema MJ, Vilmann P, Giovannini M, Chang KJ, Wiersema LM. Endosonography-guided fine-needle aspiration biopsy: diagnostic accuracy and complication assessment. Gastroenterology. 1997 Apr;112(4):1087-95. PubMed PMID: 9097990.

[93]  Andren-Sandberg A, Dervenis C. Pancreatic pseudocysts in the 21st century. Part I: classification, pathophysiology, anatomic considerations and treatment. Jop. 2004 Jan;5(1):8-24. PubMed PMID: 14730118.

[94]  Bradley EL, Clements JL, Jr., Gonzalez AC. The natural history of pancreatic pseudocysts: a unified concept of management. Am J Surg. 1979 Jan;137(1):135-41. PubMed PMID: 758840.

[95]  Vitas GJ, Sarr MG. Selected management of pancreatic pseudocysts: operative versus expectant management. Surgery. 1992 Feb;111(2):123-30. PubMed PMID: 1736380.

[96]  Maringhini A, Uomo G, Patti R, Rabitti P, Termini A, Cavallera A, et al. Pseudocysts in acute nonalcoholic pancreatitis: incidence and natural history. Dig Dis Sci. 1999 Aug;44(8):1669-73. PubMed PMID: 10492151.

[97]   Aranha GV, Prinz RA, Esguerra AC, Greenlee HB. The nature and course of cystic pancreatic lesions diagnosed by ultrasound. Arch Surg. 1983 Apr;118(4):486-8. PubMed PMID: 6830440.

[98]   Beckingham IJ, Krige JE, Bornman PC, Terblanche J. Long term outcome of endoscopic drainage of pancreatic pseudocysts. Am J Gastroenterol. 1999 Jan;94(1):71-4. PubMed PMID: 9934733.

[99]   Weckman L, Kylanpaa ML, Puolakkainen P, Halttunen J. Endoscopic treatment of pancreatic pseudocysts. Surg Endosc. 2006 Apr;20(4):603-7. PubMed PMID: 16424988.

[100]  Chan AT, Heller SJ, Van Dam J, Carr-Locke DL, Banks PA. Endoscopic cystgastrostomy: role of endoscopic ultrasonography. Am J Gastroenterol. 1996 Aug;91(8):1622-5. PubMed PMID: 8759673.

[101]  Lo SK, Rowe A. Endoscopic management of pancreatic pseudocysts. Gastroenterologist. 1997 Mar;5(1):10-25. PubMed PMID: 9074916.

[102]  Binmoeller KF, Seifert H, Walter A, Soehendra N. Transpapillary and transmural drainage of pancreatic pseudocysts. Gastrointest Endosc. 1995 Sep;42(3):219-24. PubMed PMID: 7498686.

[103]  Kozarek RA, Ball TJ, Patterson DJ, Raltz SL, Traverso LW, Ryan JA, et al. Transpapillary stenting for pancreaticocutaneous fistulas. J Gastrointest Surg. 1997 Jul-Aug;1(4): 357-61. PubMed PMID: 9834370.

[104]  Libera ED, Siqueira ES, Morais M, Rohr MR, Brant CQ, Ardengh JC, et al. Pancreatic pseudocysts transpapillary and transmural drainage. HPB Surg. 2000;11(5):333-8. PubMed PMID: 10674749.

[105]  Will U, Wegener C, Graf KI, Wanzar I, Manger T, Meyer F. Differential treatment and early outcome in the interventional endoscopic management of pancreatic pseudocysts in 27 patients. World J Gastroenterol. 2006 Jul 14;12(26):4175-8. PubMed PMID: 16830368.

[106]  Yusuf TE, Baron TH. Endoscopic transmural drainage of pancreatic pseudocysts: results of a national and an international survey of ASGE members. Gastrointest Endosc. 2006 Feb;63(2):223-7. PubMed PMID: 16427925.

[107]  Ardengh JC, Coelho DE, Coelho JF, de Lima LF, dos Santos JS, Modena JL. Single-step EUS-guided endoscopic treatment for sterile pancreatic collections: a single-center experience. Dig Dis. 2008;26(4):370-6. PubMed PMID: 19188730.

[108]  Andersson B, Nilsson E, Willner J, Andersson R. Treatment and outcome in pancreatic pseudocysts. Scand J Gastroenterol. 2006 Jun;41(6):751-6. PubMed PMID: 16716977.

[109]   Shah RJ, Martin SP. Endoscopic retrograde cholangiopancreatography in the diagnosis and management of pancreatic diseases. Curr Gastroenterol Rep. 2000 Apr;2(2): 133-45. PubMed PMID: 10981015.

[110]   Cremer M, Deviere J, Engelholm L. Endoscopic management of cysts and pseudocysts in chronic pancreatitis: long-term follow-up after 7 years of experience. Gastrointest Endosc. 1989 Jan-Feb;35(1):1-9. PubMed PMID: 2920879.

[111]   Chak A. Endosonographic-guided therapy of pancreatic pseudocysts. Gastrointest Endosc. 2000 Dec;52(6 Suppl):S23-7. PubMed PMID: 11115944.

[112]   Froeschle G, Meyer-Pannwitt U, Brueckner M, Henne-Bruns D. A comparison between surgical, endoscopic and percutaneous management of pancreatic pseudocysts--long term results. Acta Chir Belg. 1993 May-Jun;93(3):102-6. PubMed PMID: 8372580.

[113]   Barthet M, Bugallo M, Moreira LS, Bastid C, Sastre B, Sahel J. Management of cysts and pseudocysts complicating chronic pancreatitis. A retrospective study of 143 patients. Gastroenterol Clin Biol. 1993;17(4):270-6. PubMed PMID: 8339886.

[114]   Wiersema MJ. Endosonography-guided cystoduodenostomy with a therapeutic ultrasound endoscope. Gastrointest Endosc. 1996 Nov;44(5):614-7. PubMed PMID: 8934175.

[115]   Vilmann P, Hancke S, Pless T, Schell-Hincke JD, Henriksen FW. One-step endosonography-guided drainage of a pancreatic pseudocyst: a new technique of stent delivery through the echo endoscope. Endoscopy. 1998 Oct;30(8):730-3. PubMed PMID: 9865567.

[116]   Giovannini M, Pesenti C, Rolland AL, Moutardier V, Delpero JR. Endoscopic ultrasound-guided drainage of pancreatic pseudocysts or pancreatic abscesses using a therapeutic echo endoscope. Endoscopy. 2001 Jun;33(6):473-7. PubMed PMID: 11437038.

[117]   Ardengh JC, Ferrari A, Libera ED. Endosonography-guided treatment of pancreatic pseudocysts. Endoscopy. 2000;32(2):A38(P100).

[118]   Poley JW, Haringsma J, Murad SD, Dees J, Van Eijck CHJ, Kuipers EJ. Endoscopic Ultrasound (EUS) Guided Drainage of Pseudocysts: Safer and More Effective Compared to Standard Endoscopic Drainage. Gastroint Endosc. 2006;63:AB266(1320).

[119]   Lopes CV, Pesenti C, Bories E, Caillol F, Giovannini M. Endoscopic-ultrasound-guided endoscopic transmural drainage of pancreatic pseudocysts and abscesses. Scand J Gastroenterol. 2007;42:1-6.

[120]   Bradley EL, 3rd. A clinically based classification system for acute pancreatitis. Summary of the International Symposium on Acute Pancreatitis, Atlanta, Ga, September 11 through 13, 1992. Arch Surg. 1993 May;128(5):586-90. PubMed PMID: 8489394.

[121] Frey CF. Surgical management of pancreatic abscess. In: Bradley ELI, editor. Acute Pancreatits Diagnosis and therapy. New York: Raven Press; 1994. p. Ch.21.

[122] Beger HG. Surgery in acute pancreatitis. Hepatogastroenterology. 1991 Apr;38(2): 92-6. PubMed PMID: 1855779.

[123] Das SL, Singh PP, Phillips AR, Murphy R, Windsor JA, Petrov MS. Newly diagnosed diabetes mellitus after acute pancreatitis: a systematic review and meta-analysis. Gut. 2014 May;63(5):818-31. PubMed PMID: 23929695.

[124] Lumsden A, Bradley EL, 3rd. Secondary pancreatic infections. Surg Gynecol Obstet. 1990 May;170(5):459-67. PubMed PMID: 2183376.

[125] Widdison AL, Alvarez C, Reber HA. Surgical intervention in acute pancreatitis: when and how. Pancreas. 1991;6 Suppl 1:S44-51. PubMed PMID: 1788252.

[126] Kaushik SP, Vohra R, Verma GR, Kaushik S, Sabharwal A. Pancreatic abscess: a review of seventeen cases. Br J Surg. 1984 Feb;71(2):141-3. PubMed PMID: 6692108.

[127] Warshaw AL, Jin GL. Improved survival in 45 patients with pancreatic abscess. Ann Surg. 1985 Oct;202(4):408-17. PubMed PMID: 4051596.

[128] Sunday ML, Schuricht AL, Barbot DJ, Rosato FE. Management of infected pancreatic fluid collections. Am Surg. 1994 Jan;60(1):63-7. PubMed PMID: 8273976.

[129] Steiner E, Mueller PR, Hahn PF, Saini S, Simeone JF, Wittenberg J, et al. Complicated pancreatic abscesses: problems in interventional management. Radiology. 1988 May; 167(2):443-6. PubMed PMID: 3357953.

[130] Baril NB, Ralls PW, Wren SM, Selby RR, Radin R, Parekh D, et al. Does an infected peripancreatic fluid collection or abscess mandate operation? Ann Surg. 2000 Mar; 231(3):361-7. PubMed PMID: 10714629.

[131] vanSonnenberg E, Wittich GR, Chon KS, D'Agostino HB, Casola G, Easter D, et al. Percutaneous radiologic drainage of pancreatic abscesses. AJR Am J Roentgenol. 1997 Apr;168(4):979-84. PubMed PMID: 9124154.

[132] Park JJ, Kim SS, Koo YS, Choi DJ, Park HC, Kim JH, et al. Definitive treatment of pancreatic abscess by endoscopic transmural drainage. Gastrointest Endosc. 2002 Feb;55(2):256-62. PubMed PMID: 11818936.

[133] Seewald S, Groth S, Omar S, Imazu H, Seitz U, de Weerth A, et al. Aggressive endoscopic therapy for pancreatic necrosis and pancreatic abscess: a new safe and effective treatment algorithm (videos). Gastrointest Endosc. 2005 Jul;62(1):92-100. PubMed PMID: 15990825.

[134] Maravi-Poma E, Patchen Dellinger E, Forsmark CE, Layer P, Levy P, Shimosegawa T, et al. [International multidisciplinary classification of acute pancreatitis severity: the 2013 Spanish edition]. Medicina intensiva / Sociedad Espanola de Medicina Intensiva y Unidades Coronarias. 2014 May;38(4):211-7. PubMed PMID: 23747189. Clasifica-

cion Internacional y Multidisciplinaria de la Pancreatitis Aguda: Edicion Espanola 2013.

[135] Coelho D, Ardengh JC, Eulalio JM, Manso JE, Monkemuller K, Coelho JF. Management of infected and sterile pancreatic necrosis by programmed endoscopic necrosectomy. Dig Dis. 2008;26(4):364-9. PubMed PMID: 19188729.

[136] Baron TH. Endoscopic pancreatic necrosectomy. Gastroenterology & hepatology. 2008 Sep;4(9):617-20. PubMed PMID: 22798744. Pubmed Central PMCID: 3394485.

[137] Seewald S, Ang TL, Richter H, Teng KY, Zhong Y, Groth S, et al. Long-term results after endoscopic drainage and necrosectomy of symptomatic pancreatic fluid collections. Digestive endoscopy : official journal of the Japan Gastroenterological Endoscopy Society. 2012 Jan;24(1):36-41. PubMed PMID: 22211410.

[138] Venu RP, Brown RD, Marrero JA, Pastika BJ, Frakes JT. Endoscopic transpapillary drainage of pancreatic abscess: technique and results. Gastrointest Endosc. 2000 Apr; 51(4 Pt 1):391-5. PubMed PMID: 10744807.

[139] Seifert H, Dietrich C, Schmitt T, Caspary W, Wehrmann T. Endoscopic ultrasound-guided one-step transmural drainage of cystic abdominal lesions with a large-channel echo endoscope. Endoscopy. 2000 Mar;32(3):255-9. PubMed PMID: 10718392.

[140] Hookey LC, Debroux S, Delhaye M, Arvanitakis M, Le Moine O, Deviere J. Endoscopic drainage of pancreatic-fluid collections in 116 patients: a comparison of etiologies, drainage techniques, and outcomes. Gastrointest Endosc. 2006 Apr;63(4):635-43. PubMed PMID: 16564865.

[141] Papachristou GI, Takahashi N, Chahal P, Sarr MG, Baron TH. Peroral endoscopic drainage/debridement of walled-off pancreatic necrosis. Ann Surg. 2007 Jun;245(6): 943-51. PubMed PMID: 17522520. Pubmed Central PMCID: 1876949.

[142] Ardengh JC, Baron TH, Taglieri E, Micelli-Neto O, Orsini ET, Mota GA, et al. Programmed EUS-Guided Necrosectomy for Infected Walled-off Pancreatic Necrosis After Severe Acute Pancreatitis. Gastrointest Endosc. 2013;77.

[143] Antillon MR, Shah RJ, Stiegmann G, Chen YK. Single-step EUS-guided transmural drainage of simple and complicated pancreatic pseudocysts. Gastrointest Endosc. 2006 May;63(6):797-803. PubMed PMID: 16650541.

# 9

# Chronic Pancreatitis as an Inductor of Pancreatic Cancer — Correlations With Inflammatory Pathways

Simona Olimpia Dima, Dana Cucu,
Nicolae  Bacalbasa and Irinel Popescu

## 1. Introduction

The immune system and inflammation are processes with dual roles in cancer development. Firstly, immunity responds to the presence of a tumour by producing anti-inflammatory agents with the role of restoring the homeostasis and improving adverse health effects. On the other hand, immune cells create a tumoural microenvironment which supports angiogenesis, cell proliferation and migration, being thus correlated with cancer initiation and progression. In the same vein, recent studies show correlations between pancreatic inflammation and pancreatic cancer *(reviewed in [1])*. The most common causative agents of both conditions are generally considered alcoholism, smoking, toxic-metabolic and genetic factors. Because chronic pancreatitis is taken into account as an etiological issue of pancreatic cancer progress, this review aims to explain the molecular pathways from inflammation to pancreatic carcino-genesis, in support of the prevention, diagnosis and therapies of this dreadful disease. Moreover, inflammatory mediators are connected to pain and cachexia, the associated conditions that dramatically affect quality of life in pancreatic cancer. In this context, it is clear that the evaluation of the cellular pathways from inflammation to cancer is an important step in revealing the mechanisms underlying cancer development and opening new avenues for possible therapies. In this chapter, the common features of chronic pancreatitis and pancreatic cancer linked by the inflammatory process will be presented along with some of the anti-inflammatory therapies proposed so far.

## 2. Incidence of chronic pancreatitis and pancreatic cancer

Over the last years, many studies have reported an increased burden of pancreatic disorders that is expected to amplify even more over time. Acute, chronic pancreatitis and pancreatic cancer are the major disorders described which affect the exocrine pancreas. Acute pancreatitis is the condition with the higher incidence, between five and 80/ 100,000 people annually being reported worldwide [2], and it is considered as one of the most frequent gastrointestinal diseases for admission in hospitals in the US [3]. The annual incidence of chronic pancreatic (CP) is much lower. In Europe and other regions six to seven/ 100,000 persons are affected [4] with a slight increase in China and India [5]. Despite its lower incidence as compared to acute pancreatitis and because of disease exacerbation and secondary endocrine deficiencies, it dramatically impacts quality of life [6]. Although in industrialized countries, CP cases are associated with long alcohol consumption, about 10-30% of them were attributed to unknown causes. In these instances, the term idiopathic CP is used. An important change in the understanding of the disease comes from genetic studies which show that idiopathic CP mainly has a genetic background [7].

## 3. The role of inflammatory modulators in chronic pancreatitis and the development of pancreatic cancer

Pancreatic cancer is a cancer with a lower incidence, but with one of the worst prognoses. From among the many types of pancreatic tumours, 75% of pancreatic cancers refer to pancreatic ductal adenocarcinoma (PDA). In an attempt to describe and cure these pancreatic diseases (CP and PDA) the insightful question raised is whether there is a continuum of events among them or whether each should be considered as an independent condition. The hypothesis of CP-PDA interplay is based on the connection between chronic inflammation and the increased risk of cancer of the organ affected [8].

Moreover, in the last years, it has become clear that inflammation may be, at least in part, responsible for fibrosis of the pancreatic tissue. Chronic pancreatitis is characterized by progressive, recurrent pancreatic injury leading to fibrosis, ductal and exocrine atrophy and inflammatory response. In the last years, pancreatic stellate cells (PaSCs) have caught the attention of the scientific community, being described as a principal source of fibrosis [9]. During the course of chronic pancreatitis, the fibrotic response depends on the activation of PaSCs, which produce the extracellular matrix (ECM) proteins from the pancreatic tumour stroma [10]. PDA is also characterized by a strong desmoplastic reaction, such that ~90% of the tumour volume is represented by stromal content, a feature specific to PDA. Activated PaSCs were also observed in the vicinity of pancreatic epithelial lesions [11]. Therefore, over the last years many studies have concentrated on the signalling pathways and bidirectional influence between PaSCs, PDA and chronic pancreatitis. Molecular studies showed that ECM synthesis is mediated by the transforming growth factor β1 (TGF-β1) and the fibroblast growth factor (FGF), whereas PaSCs proliferation is supported by ciclooxygenase-2 [11]. In addition to fibrosis, PaSCs may mediate PDA-associated inflammation via intricate paracrine interactions with inflammatory cells, acinar cells and PDA cells. During the development of chronic pancreatitis or PDA acinar pancreatic cells, immune cells and endothelial cells produce cytokines and growth factors which have the ability to activate PaSCs. Stellate cells also may secrete cytokines and growth factors.

Despite these recent data, the exact link between the long-standing process of CP and pancreatic carcinogenesis remains an open question.

As mentioned above, many inflammatory mediators that exist in CP have also been linked to PDA [12]. Inflammatory processes consecutive to ductal or acinary injury represent the activation of the immune system that releases pro-inflammatory factors in order to prevent the harmful effect. These factors include cytokines (tumour necrosis factor (TNF-$\alpha$), transforming growth factor (TGF) $\beta$ interleukins (IL-1, IL-6, and IL-8), chemokines (e.g., monocyte chemoattractant protein-1, macrophage inflammatory protein-1, monocyte chemoattractant protein-1, and growth-related oncogenes), adhesion molecules, reactive-oxygen and reactive-nitrogen species. Many of these inflammatory products could also be involved in tumourigenesis. In the digestive system, inflammation has been described in gastric carcinoma subsequent to persistent Helicobacter pylori [13], colorectal cancer associated with inflammatory bowel disease [14, 15] and oesophageal adenocarcinoma following reflux esophagitis [16]. When treated inadequately, chronic inflammation may increase the risk of cancer, both processes sharing the same signalling pathways in increased proliferation rate, apoptosis, angiogenesis.

One mechanism that enhances the risk of cancer and strongly relates to the inflammatory process is the infiltration of immune products into the tumour microenvironment. There is also abundant evidence that pro-inflammatory cytokines and their receptors are expressed in pancreatic cells and infiltrating immune cells within inflamed pancreatic tissues [17, 18]. We review in the next paragraphs the best described pro-inflammatory mediators and their participation in chronic pancreatitis and PDA.

### 3.1. Tumour Necrosis Factor (TNF-$\alpha$)

Tumour necrosis factor (TNF-$\alpha$) is a cytokine produced especially by activated macrophages but also by other cells (e.g., fibroblasts, keratinocytes) as a pro-inflammatory cytokine. and in concequence participates in regulating the cellular homeostasis and the defence of the harmed organisms. In the immune systems, TNF-$\alpha$ contributes to the correct functioning of NK cells, B cells and T cells. Other results suggest that besides these important roles, TNF-$\alpha$ is associated with chronic inflammatory diseases and ultimate tumourigenesis. [19].

TNF-$\alpha$ was first describe by Carswell et al. [20] and many following studies have shown that immune cells produce two types of tumour necrosis factors: TNF-$\alpha$ produced by activated macrophages and TNF-$\beta$ produced by mitogen stimulated lymphocytes. Pioneering studies by Balkin et al. [21] showed that TNF-$\alpha$ is a tumour promoter of skin cancer. An anti-tumour necrosis factor-alpha antibody inhibits the development of experimental skin tumours [22]. Thereafter, many studies have pointed out that this cytokine has a role in autoimmune diseases, chronic inflammatory processes and, despite its name, in malignancy. Systemic levels of TNF-$\alpha$ together with various cytokines such as IL-6, Il-8, IL-10 were found to be significantly higher in patients with PDA compared to healthy subjects [23, 24]. PDA cells are exposed to TNF-$\alpha$ secreted by the infiltrated macrophages but also to their own endogenous TNF-$\alpha$.

The major role of this cytokine is to switch between inflammatory and tumourigenic processes thus stimulating the ability of cancer cells to undergo migration and invasion. The detailed signalling pathways through which TNF-$\alpha$ exerts this role are yet to be revealed. However, the TNF-$\alpha$ receptors are well-described (TNF-R1 and TNF-R2). While TNF-R2 is expressed only in endothelial and immune cells, TNF-R1 was described in many tumoural tissues including PDA. After binding to its ligands, TNF-$\alpha$ receptors suffer a conformational change leading to a stable trimeric form and subsequent activation of various signalling pathways. On the one hand, the NF-$\kappa$b pathway may be activated and this will trigger the inflammatory response, anti-apoptotic processes and cell survival. On the other hand, TNF-$\alpha$ may induce the activation of the mitogen- activated protein kinase (MAPK) signalling pathway with subsequent effects on proliferation, differentiation, and apoptosis of cells. These rather conflicting signals raised even more questions whether TNF-$\alpha$ may be used as a PDA therapeutic target. Following the anti-apoptotic signalling inhibitors of TNF-$\alpha$ infliximab and etanercept were proposed as possible therapeutic agents in PDA, especially after pancreaticoduodenectomy [25]. Interestingly, both anti-TNF compounds are currently used for the treatment of chronic inflammation. However, this study and others were not able to prove that TNF-$\alpha$ is the missing link between chronic pancreatitis and PDA, but the results obtained so far using inhibitors of this cytokine support this assumption.

### 3.2. Interleukine-6 (IL-6)

Many other interleukins have increased levels in PDA as well as in CP. Among them, Interleukine-6 was systematically described in many studies as a pro-inflammatory cytokine overexpressed in PDA tumours and in the systemic circulation of patients. Moreover, high levels of IL-6 in the serum of diseased persons directly correlate with increased mortality [26, 27]. IL-6 binds to its specific receptor formed by two subunits; one ligand-specific IL-6R$\alpha$ and one signal transducer gp130. The intracellular domain of gp130 activates the Junus Kinase (JAK) and MAPK pathways. JAK activates the transcription factor STAT3 involved in invasion and metastasis, and identified in many tumours including PDA [28]. The inhibition of the STAT3 phosphorylation pathway was considered a good therapeutic approach in previous studies [29]. Although IL-6 has shown high levels in chronic pancreatitis, a genetic analysis failed to prove a correlation with the prognosis for this condition [30].

The role of IL-6 and the signalling pathway has yet to be investigated because it is clear that CP is a factor in the development of PDA.

### 3.3. Cyclooxygenases

Cyclooxygenases (COX-1 and COX-2), also known as prostaglandin (PG) endoperoxide synthases, are isoenzymes required for in the conversion of arachidonic acid to prostaglandins. COX-1 and-2 share ~65 structural similarities and have almost identical catalytic domains.

COX-1 is a constitutive enzyme and is produced by almost all cells in normal physiological processes, whereas COX-2 is an inducible enzyme with almost undetectable levels in normal cells and with a high expression in many cancer types including PDA [31]. Importantly, COX-2 is induced by inflammatory factors, therefore, it may be one of the mediators between chronic pancreatitis and PDA. The strongest evidence that favours this link comes from a mouse model (BK5.COX-2) in which the over-expression of COX-2 induces pancreatic acinar to ductal metaplasia progression to severe dysplasia [32]. In this model the authors have shown that all transgenic mice develop pancreatic inflammation and metaplasia specific to human CP. Afterward, the initiation of dysplastic lesions featuring PDA was observed. This is one of the most convincing models that favour COX-2 as a key modulator of a tumour microenvironment in response to inflammatory stimuli.

### 3.4. Transforming Growth Factor (TGF)-β

Transforming growth factor (TGF)-β is a cytokine which inhibits cell proliferation and modulates the immune response. In normal pancreas it blocks the G1/S phase cell cycle progression, whereas in pancreatic cancer it decreases suppressive activity through an impairment of the signalling pathway [33]. It was shown that (TGF)-β is involved in pancreatic fibrosis, because collagen synthesis was augmented secondary to exogenous cytokine treatment. Moreover, in a rat model of caerulein-induced pancreatitis the levels of (TGF)-β were upregulated [34].

The above presented results match the hypothesis that inflammatory products are the hallmarks of pancreatic cancer and that they can bridge the conceptual gap between idiopathic CP and PDA. The inflammatory products operate by shifting this pathway into a tumourigenic one and promote cellular proliferation, invasion and migration. To do so they have to activate oncogenic networks of transcription factors throughout the regulation of specific genes.

## 4. Oncogenes and tumour suppressor genes common in chronic pancreatitis and pancreatic adenocarcinoma

In the last years, many studies have reported the detection of proto-oncogenes and tumour suppressor gene mutations in the pathogenesis of CP and PDA. Developments in molecular biology and biotechnologies such as ADN microarrays for genome-wide chromosomal localization enable the detection of genetic causes in both conditions. Oncogenes are genes that when mutated have the potential to cause cancer, whereas transcription factors represent a group of proteins that regulate gene transcription by binding to specific DNA sequences and modulate mRNA synthesis.

## 4.1. K-Ras proto-oncogene

One of the genes involved in CP may be the K-Ras proto-oncogene. The product of K-Ras gene is a small GTPase protein and a key player in many intracellular signalling processes. As all GTPase molecules, K-Ras has an enzymatic activity that relies on the conversion of GTP to GDP, consistent with the active state of the protein. The switch from the active to the inactivate state is mediated by GTPase-activating proteins (GAP), whereas the activation of K-Ras is promoted by guanine nucleotide exchange proteins (GEFs). In pancreatic cancer one point mutation of the encoding K-Ras gene at codon G12 impairs the inactivation of K-Ras, placing the protein in a permanent active state. All the downstream signalling pathways are subsequently perturbed and thus drive the processes characteristic to cancer [35]. The main process generated by the K-Ras mutation is the activation of the inflammatory microenvironment and subsequent fibrosis. Without any doubt, K-Ras mutation is observed in most PDA. However, a new concept has come out, centred around the mutation level that K-Ras has to reach in order to initiate PDA. This new idea is based on studies showing that healthy people have high levels of K-Ras oncogens at rates exceeding cancer patients. In other words, expression of the oncogenic K-Ras from its endogenous locus is insufficient to activate downstream signaling pathways, so that a pathological threshold is necessary for K-Ras mutation to be reached in order to initiate PDA. When non-endogenous levels are reached, CP and not PDA will develop, at least in one mouse model [36]. These results became extremely important in showing that K-Ras mutation is not important per se in PDA, but rather the level of the subsequent activated signalling pathway. This discrete modulation may be the reason why attempts to inhibit this molecule as a cancer therapy, failed.

Moreover, the same studies suggest the oncogenic K-Ras accelerates tumour development only in an inflammatory milieu in the sense that inflammatory mediators activate the oncogenic K-Ras, which in turn stimulates the desmoplastic reaction. These results are consistent with data obtained from patients showing that 30% of CP persons bear a K-Ras mutation. Therefore, the idea that the K-Ras mutation is a PDA marker should be reconsidered in the context of the inflammatory environment.

## 4.2. Notch

Notch is another well described oncogene in PDA and experimental CP in mice is connected to the upregulation of Notch and acinar to ductal metaplasia. The Notch gene encodes for transmembrane proteins that regulate the mechanism of lateral inhibition during embryogenesis. Using mice with induced Notch activity, it was shown that only upon coactivation with K-Ras, Notch initiates the promotion of pancreatic lesions [37]. Moreover, using cDNA microarray technology, deregulated Notch pathways were found in CP [38]. This study showed that Notch receptors, Notch1 and Notch2, as well as Notch targets such as HES-related repressor protein, were upregulated in CP. Another study showed how crosstalk between TNF-α and Notch sustains the intrinsic inflammatory profile of pancreatic cancer cells [39]. TNF-α stimulates the transcription factor NF-κB signalling and, together with Notch signals, induced the optimal expression of Notch targets. The enhancement of these target genes suppresses the anti-inflammatory protein expression and creates a feedback loop that keeps the cells in an inflammatory state.

### 4.3. Transcription factor Nf-κB

The transcription factor Nf-κB was initially described in activated B lymphocytes and there-after characterised in almost every cell. It controls the activity of ~ 150 genes and the biological answers to various external stimuli. Nf-κB is a heterodimeric protein sequestered in the cytoplasm by IκB protein. In response to different stimuli (including those of inflammatory origin), IκB is phosphorylated and then degraded. The IκB proteolysis permits the release of Nf-κB and translocation to the nucleus where it binds to specific promoter regions and initiates gene transcription. Several studies indicate that Nf-κB is constitutively expressed in PDA cell lines, in humans and animal models of pancreatic cancer with functions in proliferation, resistance to apoptosis and inflammation-induced cancer development [40, 41]. Importantly, active Nf-κB was determined in experimental models of pancreatitis and was asserted as an early response to inflammation [42]. Other experiments sustain a model in which Nf-κB positively links the oncogenic Ras signalling and the inflammatory process [43]. Augmented values of Nf-κB mRNA favour pro-apoptotic pathways in acinar cells, whereas the islets are not affected. From these results, the authors concluded that in CP only the endocrine cells may be subjected to cell reprogramming by evading immune attack, whereas exocrine cells exibit an altered state resulting from Nf-κB transcriptional activity [44].

In a caerulein-induced pancreatitis mouse model NF-κB activation was described [45]. NF-κB activation promotes inflammation and the milieu that favours cancer development [46].

Other transcription factors with oncogenic potential activated by inflammation and described in pancreatic cancer are: i) Nuclear factor of activated T-cells (NFATc1) that belongs to the same family as NF-κB and regulates genes participating in cell growth and differentiation, and ii) the GLI1 family important for tumour microenvironment modulation, cell apoptosis, autophagy and proliferation.

# 5. Other molecular markers for PDA and/or CP involved in inflammation

## 5.1. The fibroblast-specific protein 1

A factor that may mediate the cross talk between PDA cells and inflammation is the fibroblast-specific protein 1 or S100A4. S100A4 is an important player in metastatic dissemination, and increased expression of the protein has been associated with poor prognosis in various human cancer types [47]. The metastasis-promoting protein S100A4 belongs to the S100 family of calcium-binding proteins, but its function has not yet been well described. The protein seems to exert dual, intracellular and extracellular functions that may contribute to its pro-metastatic effects [48, 49]. S100A4 is expressed in many cancer cells [50, 51] and in several types of stromal cells, e.g., fibroblasts, lymphocytes, macrophages [52-54]. Previous studies showed that in PDA patients, S100A4 together with S100A2 are associated with more aggressive tumours and predict worse survival after surgery. These two markers are proposed to stratify resectable pancreatic cancer into different phenotypes of prognosis and response to therapy. S100A4 is also secreted by PDA cell lines in vitro [51, 55] and can be detected in the tumour interstitial fluid [52], suggesting a role for S100A4 in the tumour-stroma interplay.

## 5.2. Transforming Growth Factor (TGF)-$\alpha$

Transforming growth factor (TGF)-$\alpha$ is a polypeptide that induces mitogenic and cell differentiation responses. The specific receptor is the tyrosine kinase EGF receptor (EGFR) common for (TGF)-$\alpha$ and epidermal growth factor. The overexpression of both TGF-$\alpha$ and EGFR were upregulated in CP and in pancreatic cancer. Apparently,TGF-$\alpha$ excessively stimulates EGFR contributing in this way to the pathology of these diseases [56].

# 6. Prophylactic and therapeutic use of the anti-inflammatory agents in CP and PC

Chronic inflammation connected to CP triggers the progression to cancer through the occurrence of the following precancerous lesions: pancreatic intraepithelial neoplasia (PanINs), intraductal papillary mucinous neoplasms (IPMN), and mucinous cystic neoplasms (MCN). The progression of these lesions into pancreatic ductal adenocarcinoma (PDA) involves many diverse molecular pathways.

Many studies published so far have shown increased incidence of pancreatic cancer in CP patients [57]. The cumulative risk of PC in subjects with CP is 1.8% after 10 years and 4% after 20 years, with an incidence ratio of 1.8% [58]. Over the last few years a major breakthrough towards understanding PDA patho-biology was made by deciphering the molecular events responsible for the development of PDA [59, 60].

New chemo-therapeutic drugs are needed in PC. Targeting inflammatory pathways with anti-inflammatory drugs may be of benefit for a combined, multi-target approach to PDA therapy. Anti-inflammatory agents may potentiate the tumoural growth's inhibitory effect of chemo-therapeutic agents, such as Gemcitabine.

## 6.1. Cyclooxygenase-2 (COX-2) inhibitors (specific and non-specific)

The selective inhibition of the Cox-2 gene expression and of its enzymatic activity may have chemoprotective potential in high-risk patients for PC. Similar to familial adenomatous polyposis (FAP) treated with sulindac, COX-2 inhibitor therapy may delay pancreatic cancer precursor lesion progression and reduce the incidence of pancreatic cancers.

Experimental studies using a genetically modified mouse model of pancreatic cancer development (K-Ras[G12D]; PDX-1-Cre mice, BOP treated hamster) and cell lines have shown efficacy in reducing the development of high-grade pancreatic intraepithelial neoplasias (PanIN) and ductal adenocarcinoma [61]. Cox-2 inhibitors such as etodolac, sulindac, celocoxib and nimesulide inhibited the proliferation of pancreatic cancer cells [62, 63]. The antitumoural activity of aspirin, a nonsteroidal anti-inflammatory drug (NSAID), involves numerous molecular targets, including Cox-2. Sclabas et al. showed that aspirin inhibits the activation of the NF-kB pathway in cultured cells and decreased the expression of the COX-2 gene [42, 64]. Moreover, aspirin may activate adenosine monophosphate-activated protein kinase (AMPK), and may affect Notch, Wnt/β-catenin, and other signalling pathways [65]. Nimesulide (4-nitro-2 phenoxymethanesulfonanilide), another NSAID, significantly decreases PDA in mice treated during the postinitiation phase of pancreatic carcinogenesis [66]. Moreover, the progression of later stage PanIN was lowered by this drug [62]. While experimental data are highly available, only a few clinical trials of pancreatic cancer using COX-2 inhibitors as chemopreventive agents have shown a possible clinical benefit. A randomized phase II study (Apricot-P) evaluated Apricoxib in combination with Gemcitabine and Erlotinib (Modiano M. et al., personal communication). Similarly, celocoxib was also evaluated in combination with Gemcitabine and Cisplatin in patients with metastatic PC or combined with Gemcitabin [67]. In both studies, the primary endpoint was a survival rate at six months, although no improvement in Gemcitabine activity has been observed.

## 6.2. TGF-β inhibitors

Traberdersen, a specific inhibitor of TGF-b2, was used as a 2nd line treatment in a phase I/II study of 37 patients with PDA. The median survival was 13.4 months and one patient showed a complete response [68]. Although the study is in an incipient phase, TGF-β shows to be a promising clinical target.

## 6.3. Aspirin

In vitro findings suggest that aspirin might inhibit pancreatic carcinogenesis, but epidemiological data are inconsistent. There are studies indicating that nonsteroidal anti-inflammatory drugs (NSAIDs) reduce the risk of gastrointestinal (GI) cancers and pancreatic cancer, but other results indicate that there is no significant association between aspirin use and pancreatic cancer risk. A limited number of populational-based studies are available. According to Streicher SA et al., significant relationships between aspirin use and decreased pancreas-cancer incidence and mortality have been shown in four out of 13 studies [69]. In some studies the benefit was positively correlated with the frequency of aspirin intake [70]. In a systematic review and meta-analysis, Cui X et al. analysed the association between aspirin intake and its effect for the chemoprevention of pancreatic cancer. They carried out a total of 10 studies (four case-control studies, five prospective cohort studies, and one randomized controlled trial) published between 2002 to 2011 with 7,252 cases of pancreatic cancer and more than 120,0000 healthy control subjects enrolled in the studies. The conclusion of the study was that high-dose, rather than low-dose, aspirin intake was associated with an 0.88-fold decreased risk for pancreatic cancer compared with non-use [71]. Table 1 overviews the information from studies that analysed the association of the aspirin or NSAID intake with pancreatic cancer.

| Study design | No of patients | Period | Drug type | Dose and duration of NSAID use | Conclusions |
|---|---|---|---|---|---|
| Prospective cohort study [72] | 28,283 postmenopausal women- 80 incident cases of pancreatic cancer | 1992 to 1999 | Aspirin and other NSAIDs | Not collected | Aspirin might be chemopreventive for pancreatic cancer |
| Case-control Surveillance Study [73] | 149 patients with pancreatic cancer ($n = 504$), stomach ($n = 254$), oesophagus ($n = 215$), gallbladder ($n = 125$), or liver ($n = 51$) and Controls were 5,952 ( non tumoral diseases) | 1977 to 1998 | Salicylates (e.g., aspirin), indoles (e.g., indomethacin), propionic acids (e.g., ibuprofen), fenamates (e.g., mefenamic acid), and/or oxicams (e.g., piroxicam). | At least four days/week for at least three months, initiated at least one year before admission. | No effect of NSAID use |
| Case-control study [74] | 12,174 incident cancer cases (396 pancreatic cancer) and 34,934 controls | 1993 to 1995 | 13–36 months before cancer diagnosis | 13-36 months before cancer diagnosis | The increased risks of pancreatic cancer could be due to chance or to undetected biases |
| Clinic-based case-control study [75] | 904 cases and 1,224 controls | April 2004 to September 2010 | Aspirin, NSAID and acetaminophen | Aspirin use ≥ 1 day/month | Aspirin use, but not non-aspirin NSAID use, is associated with a lowered risk of developing pancreatic cancer |
| Hospital-based case-control study ( Roswell Park Cancer Institute) [76] | 194 patients with pancreatic cancer were compared to 582 age and sex-matched patients with non-neoplastic condition | 1982 to 1998 | Aspirin | At least one tablet per week for at least six months was classified as regular aspirin use. | Regular aspirin use may not be associated with a lower risk of pancreatic cancer |
| Multicentric hospital-based case-control study in Italy [77] | 308 patients with incident pancreatic cancer and controls were 477 with acute conditions | 1991 and 2008 | 22 cases (7%) and 37 controls (8%) - regular aspirin | Nonregular use | No association between regular aspirin use and pancreatic cancer risk, although our results suggested a possible protective effect for long-term current users |

| Study design | No of patients | Period | Drug type | Dose and duration of NSAID use | Conclusions |
|---|---|---|---|---|---|
| Prospective cohort study [78] | 161 cases with pancreatic cancer ( 88,378 women without cancer at the baseline) | 1980 to 1998 | Aspirin | Two or more standard tablets per week | Extended periods of regular aspirin use appear to be associated with a statistically significantly increased risk of pancreatic cancer among women |
| Population-based cohort study [79] | 11,683 patients with rheumathoid arthritis, 840 patients with cancer, 32 with pancreatic cancer | 1965 to 1983 | NSAID | No information regarding doses | Slightly reduced risk for pancreatic cancer |
| Population-based Connecticut study [69] | 362 pancreas-cancer cases frequency matched to 690 randomly sampled controls. | 2005 to 2009 | Aspirin ( low dose, regular dose) | Daily | Daily aspirin regimen may reduce risk of developing pancreatic cancer |
| Prospective cohort study [80] | Cancer Prevention Study II (CPS-II) cohort- 98,7590 4,577 deaths from pancreatic cancer | 1982 to 2000 | Aspirin | Frequent aspirin use (> or =30 times per month) | Aspirin use was not associated with pancreatic cancer mortality |

## 7. The "therapeutic" role of surgical treatment in the progression of chronic pancreatitis to PDA

Pancreas resection is indicated in CP patients who have small-duct disease or those in whom endoscopic drainage fails.

There are experimental and clinical studies that take into consideration the fact that the surgical treatment of chronic pancreatitis may reduce the risk of the development of PDA. Even though the mechanism of the protective role of surgery remains unknown, possible explanations could be linked to the fact that through the endoscopic drainage procedures or resection procedures of the CP, pancreatic tissue and the inflamed tissue are removed or diminished. Ueda J et al. have found that patients who underwent surgical treatment for chronic pancreatitis had a significantly lower incidence of pancreatic cancer. According to this study, 5.1% of patients who had not received surgical treatment for CP developed pancreatic cancer, whereas PDA was observed in 0.7% of patients who had undergone surgery for chronic pancreatitis [81]. G.H. Sakorafas et al. reviewed the experience of 484 consecutive patients who underwent surgery for chronic pancreatitis; pancreatic cancer was diagnosed after a mean of 3.4 years after the initial operation for chronic pancreatitis in 2.9% of the 484 patients [82]. Even though the percentage of patients who underwent pancreatic resection for CP and subsequently developed PDA is higher than in the study by Ueda J et al., it is smaller than in the studies that analyse patients with CP without surgical treatment.

# 8. Conclusions

The tumour microenvironment is a critical determinant of PDA progression and treatment outcome. From the above presented studies, it is clear that CP may be considered as a prerequisite of the PDA condition. The major evidence supporting this assumption is based on studies revealing that the tumour microenvironment of the ductal epithelium increases the risk of neoplastic transformation. In the onset of CP, the pathways and molecules described so far are activated and promote the transformation from normal epithelium to metaplasmic, early neoplasmic lesions (PanIN) and finally pancreatic cancer. Despite the fact that many studies determined that inflammatory components and downstream effectors are present in both CP and pancreatic cancers, there is not a clear common pathway for pancreatic cancer development which includes chronic inflammatory processes and finally stroma formation. When revealed, these findings may guide us to novel strategies for pancreatic cancer therapy.

# Acknowledgements

The production of this paper was financially supported by the research grant PNII-PT-PCCA 90/2012.

# Author details

Simona Olimpia Dima[1*], Dana Cucu[2], Nicolae  Bacalbasa[3] and Irinel Popescu[1]

*Address all correspondence to: dima.simona@gmail.com

1 Center of General Surgery and Liver Transplantation "Dan Setlacec", Fundeni Clinical Institute, Bucharest, Romania

2 Department of Anatomy, Physiology and Biophysics, Faculty of Biology, University of Bucharest, Bucharest, Romania

3 Carol Davila University of Medicine and Pharmacy, Bucharest, Romania

# References

[1] Ling, S., et al., *Inflammation to cancer: The molecular biology in the pancreas (Review)*. Oncol Lett, 2014. 7(6) 1747-1754.

[2] Sekimoto, M., et al., *JPN Guidelines for the management of acute pancreatitis: epidemiology, etiology, natural history, and outcome predictors in acute pancreatitis*. J Hepatobiliary Pancreat Surg, 2006. 13(1) 10-24.

[3] Yadav, D. and A.B. Lowenfels, *The epidemiology of pancreatitis and pancreatic cancer*. Gastroenterology, 2013. 144(6) 1252-1261.

[4] Jupp, J., D. Fine, and C.D. Johnson, *The epidemiology and socioeconomic impact of chronic pancreatitis*. Best Pract Res Clin Gastroenterol, 2010. 24(3) 219-231.

[5] Garg, P.K., *Chronic pancreatitis in India and Asia*. Curr Gastroenterol Rep, 2012. 14(2) 118-124.

[6] Oza, V.M. and M. Kahaleh, *Endoscopic management of chronic pancreatitis*. World J Gastrointest Endosc, 2013. 5(1) 19-28.

[7] Bhanot, U.K. and P. Moller, *Mechanisms of parenchymal injury and signaling pathways in ectatic ducts of chronic pancreatitis: implications for pancreatic carcinogenesis*. Lab Invest, 2009. 89(5) 489-497.

[8] Talamini, G., et al., *Chronic pancreatitis: relationship to acute pancreatitis and pancreatic cancer*. JOP, 2000. 1(3 Suppl) 69-76.

[9] Zimnoch, L., B. Szynaka, and Z. Puchalski, *Mast cells and pancreatic stellate cells in chronic pancreatitis with differently intensified fibrosis*. Hepatogastroenterology, 2002. 49(46) 1135-1138.

[10] Haber, P.S., et al., *Activation of pancreatic stellate cells in human and experimental pancreatic fibrosis*. Am J Pathol, 1999. 155(4) 1087-1095.

[11] Apte, M.V., et al., *A starring role for stellate cells in the pancreatic cancer microenvironment*. Gastroenterology, 2013. 144(6) 1210-1219.

[12] Tong, G.X., et al., *Association between pancreatitis and subsequent risk of pancreatic cancer: a systematic review of epidemiological studies*. Asian Pac J Cancer Prev, 2014. 15(12) 5029-5034.

[13] Peek, R.M., Jr. and J.E. Crabtree, *Helicobacter infection and gastric neoplasia*. J Pathol, 2006. 208(2) 233-248.

[14] Eaden, J.A., K.R. Abrams, and J.F. Mayberry, *The risk of colorectal cancer in ulcerative colitis: a meta-analysis*. Gut, 2001. 48(4) 526-535.

[15] Canavan, C., K.R. Abrams, and J. Mayberry, *Meta-analysis: colorectal and small bowel cancer risk in patients with Crohn's disease.* Aliment Pharmacol Ther, 2006. 23(8) 1097-1104.

[16] Solaymani-Dodaran, M., et al., *Risk of oesophageal cancer in Barrett's oesophagus and gastro-oesophageal reflux.* Gut, 2004. 53(8) 1070-1074.

[17] Duell, E.J., et al., *Inflammation, genetic polymorphisms in proinflammatory genes TNF-A, RANTES, and CCR5, and risk of pancreatic adenocarcinoma.* Cancer Epidemiol Biomarkers Prev, 2006. 15(4) 726-731.

[18] Ryu, B., et al., *Invasion-specific genes in malignancy: serial analysis of gene expression comparisons of primary and passaged cancers.* Cancer Res, 2001. 61(5) 1833-1838.

[19] Landskron, G., et al., *Chronic inflammation and cytokines in the tumor microenvironment.* J Immunol Res, 2014. 2014 149185.

[20] Carswell, E.A., et al., *An endotoxin-induced serum factor that causes necrosis of tumors.* Proc Natl Acad Sci U S A, 1975. 72(9) 3666-3670.

[21] Szlosarek, P.W. and F.R. Balkwill, *Tumour necrosis factor alpha: a potential target for the therapy of solid tumours.* Lancet Oncol, 2003. 4(9) 565-573.

[22] Arnott, C.H., et al., *Expression of both TNF-alpha receptor subtypes is essential for optimal skin tumour development.* Oncogene, 2004. 23(10) 1902-1910.

[23] Dima, S.O., et al., *An exploratory study of inflammatory cytokines as prognostic biomarkers in patients with ductal pancreatic adenocarcinoma.* Pancreas, 2012. 41(7) 1001-1007.

[24] Blogowski, W., et al., *Selected cytokines in patients with pancreatic cancer: a preliminary report.* PLoS One, 2014. 9(5) e97613.

[25] Egberts, J.H., et al., *Anti-tumor necrosis factor therapy inhibits pancreatic tumor growth and metastasis.* Cancer Res, 2008. 68(5) 1443-1450.

[26] Okitsu, K., et al., *Involvement of interleukin-6 and androgen receptor signaling in pancreatic cancer.* Genes Cancer, 2010. 1(8) 859-867.

[27] Noh, K.W., et al., *Do cytokine concentrations in pancreatic juice predict the presence of pancreatic diseases?* Clin Gastroenterol Hepatol, 2006. 4(6) 782-789.

[28] Coppola, D., *Molecular prognostic markers in pancreatic cancer.* Cancer Control, 2000. 7(5) 421-427.

[29] Liu, A., et al., *LLL12 inhibits endogenous and exogenous interleukin-6-induced STAT3 phosphorylation in human pancreatic cancer cells.* Anticancer Res, 2011. 31(6) 2029-2035.

[30] Mroczko, B., et al., *Diagnostic usefulness of serum interleukin 6 (IL-6) and C-reactive protein (CRP) in the differentiation between pancreatic cancer and chronic pancreatitis.* J Clin Lab Anal, 2010. 24(4) 256-261.

[31] Hill, R., et al., *Cell intrinsic role of COX-2 in pancreatic cancer development.* Mol Cancer Ther, 2012. 11(10) 2127-2137.

[32] Colby, J.K., et al., *Progressive metaplastic and dysplastic changes in mouse pancreas induced by cyclooxygenase-2 overexpression.* Neoplasia, 2008. 10(8) 782-796.

[33] Birnbaum, D.J., E. Mamessier, and D. Birnbaum, *The emerging role of the TGFbeta tumor suppressor pathway in pancreatic cancer.* Cell Cycle, 2012. 11(4) 683-686.

[34] Gress, T., et al., *Enhancement of transforming growth factor beta 1 expression in the rat pancreas during regeneration from caerulein-induced pancreatitis.* Eur J Clin Invest, 1994. 24(10) 679-685.

[35] Eser, S., et al., *Oncogenic KRAS signalling in pancreatic cancer.* Br J Cancer, 2014.

[36] Guerra, C., et al., *Chronic pancreatitis is essential for induction of pancreatic ductal adenocarcinoma by K-Ras oncogenes in adult mice.* Cancer Cell, 2007. 11(3) 291-302.

[37] De La, O.J. and L.C. Murtaugh, *Notch and Kras in pancreatic cancer: at the crossroads of mutation, differentiation and signaling.* Cell Cycle, 2009. 8(12) 1860-1864.

[38] Bhanot, U., et al., *Evidence of Notch pathway activation in the ectatic ducts of chronic pancreatitis.* J Pathol, 2008. 214(3) 312-319.

[39] Maniati, E., et al., *Crosstalk between the canonical NF-kappaB and Notch signaling pathways inhibits Ppargamma expression and promotes pancreatic cancer progression in mice.* J Clin Invest, 2011. 121(12) 4685-4699.

[40] Liu, L., et al., *Triptolide reverses hypoxia-induced epithelial-mesenchymal transition and stem-like features in pancreatic cancer by NF-kappaB downregulation.* Int J Cancer, 2014. 134(10) 2489-2503.

[41] Johnson, J.L. and E.G. de Mejia, *Flavonoid apigenin modified gene expression associated with inflammation and cancer and induced apoptosis in human pancreatic cancer cells through inhibition of GSK-3beta/NF-kappaB signaling cascade.* Mol Nutr Food Res, 2013. 57(12) 2112-2127.

[42] Zhang, Z. and B. Rigas, *NF-kappaB, inflammation and pancreatic carcinogenesis: NF-kappaB as a chemoprevention target (review).* Int J Oncol, 2006. 29(1) 185-192.

[43] Hosokawa, Y., et al., *API2-MALT1 fusion protein induces transcriptional activation of the API2 gene through NF-kappaB binding elements: evidence for a positive feed-back loop pathway resulting in unremitting NF-kappaB activation.* Biochem Biophys Res Commun, 2005. 334(1) 51-60.

[44] Hasel, C., et al., *Parenchymal regression in chronic pancreatitis spares islets reprogrammed for the expression of NFkappaB and IAPs.* Lab Invest, 2005. 85(10) 1263-1275.

[45] Sah, R.P., et al., *Cerulein-induced chronic pancreatitis does not require intra-acinar activation of trypsinogen in mice.* Gastroenterology, 2013. 144(5) 1076-1085 e1072.

[46]  Grivennikov, S.I., F.R. Greten, and M. Karin, *Immunity, inflammation, and cancer.* Cell, 2010. 140(6) 883-899.

[47]  Garrett, S.C., et al., S100A4, a mediator of metastasis. J Biol Chem, 2006. 281(2) 677-680.

[48]  Sherbet, G.V., *Metastasis promoter S100A4 is a potentially valuable molecular target for cancer therapy.* Cancer Lett, 2009. 280(1) 15-30.

[49]  Boye, K. and G.M. Maelandsmo, *S100A4 and metastasis: a small actor playing many roles.* Am J Pathol, 2010. 176(2) 528-535.

[50]  Ebralidze, A., et al., *Isolation and characterization of a gene specifically expressed in different metastatic cells and whose deduced gene product has a high degree of homology to a Ca2+-binding protein family.* Genes Dev, 1989. 3(7) 1086-1093.

[51]  Kikuchi, N., et al., *Nuclear expression of S100A4 is associated with aggressive behavior of epithelial ovarian carcinoma: an important autocrine/paracrine factor in tumor progression.* Cancer Sci, 2006. 97(10) 1061-1069.

[52]  Cabezon, T., et al., *Expression of S100A4 by a variety of cell types present in the tumor microenvironment of human breast cancer.* Int J Cancer, 2007. 121(7) 1433-1444.

[53]  Schmidt-Hansen, B., et al., *Functional significance of metastasis-inducing S100A4(Mts1) in tumor-stroma interplay.* J Biol Chem, 2004. 279(23) 24498-24504.

[54]  Wetting, H.L., et al., *S100A4 expression in xenograft tumors of human carcinoma cell lines is induced by the tumor microenvironment.* Am J Pathol, 2011. 178(5) 2389-2396.

[55]  Grum-Schwensen, B., et al., *Suppression of tumor development and metastasis formation in mice lacking the S100A4(mts1) gene.* Cancer Res, 2005. 65(9) 3772-3780.

[56]  Korc, M., et al., *Chronic pancreatitis is associated with increased concentrations of epidermal growth factor receptor, transforming growth factor alpha, and phospholipase C gamma.* Gut, 1994. 35(10) 1468-1473.

[57]  Whitcomb, D.C., *Inflammation and Cancer V. Chronic pancreatitis and pancreatic cancer.* Am J Physiol Gastrointest Liver Physiol, 2004. 287(2) G315-319.

[58]  Lowenfels, A.B., et al., *Cigarette smoking as a risk factor for pancreatic cancer in patients with hereditary pancreatitis.* JAMA, 2001. 286(2) 169-170.

[59]  Hruban, R.H. and N.V. Adsay, *Molecular classification of neoplasms of the pancreas.* Hum Pathol, 2009. 40(5) 612-623.

[60]  Farrow, B., D. Albo, and D.H. Berger, *The role of the tumor microenvironment in the progression of pancreatic cancer.* J Surg Res, 2008. 149(2) 319-328.

[61]  Guerra, C., et al., *Pancreatitis-induced inflammation contributes to pancreatic cancer by inhibiting oncogene-induced senescence.* Cancer Cell, 2011. 19(6) 728-739.

[62]  Funahashi, H., et al., *Delayed progression of pancreatic intraepithelial neoplasia in a conditional Kras(G12D) mouse model by a selective cyclooxygenase-2 inhibitor.* Cancer Res, 2007. 67(15) 7068-7071.

[63]  Merati, K., et al., *Expression of inflammatory modulator COX-2 in pancreatic ductal adenocarcinoma and its relationship to pathologic and clinical parameters.* Am J Clin Oncol, 2001. 24(5) 447-452.

[64]  Sclabas, G.M., et al., *Nuclear factor kappa B activation is a potential target for preventing pancreatic carcinoma by aspirin.* Cancer, 2005. 103(12) 2485-2490.

[65]  Yue, W., et al., *Repurposing of metformin and aspirin by targeting AMPK-mTOR and inflammation for pancreatic cancer prevention and treatment.* Cancer Prev Res (Phila), 2014. 7(4) 388-397.

[66]  Furukawa, F., et al., *A cyclooxygenase-2 inhibitor, nimesulide, inhibits postinitiation phase of N-nitrosobis(2-oxopropyl)amine-induced pancreatic carcinogenesis in hamsters.* Int J Cancer, 2003. 104(3) 269-273.

[67]  El-Rayes, B.F., et al., *A phase II study of celecoxib, gemcitabine, and cisplatin in advanced pancreatic cancer.* Invest New Drugs, 2005. 23(6) 583-590.

[68]  Schlingensiepen, K.H., et al., *Transforming growth factor-beta 2 gene silencing with trabedersen (AP 12009) in pancreatic cancer.* Cancer Sci, 2011. 102(6) 1193-1200.

[69]  Streicher, S.A., et al., *Case-control study of aspirin use and risk of pancreatic cancer.* Cancer Epidemiol Biomarkers Prev, 2014. 23(7) 1254-1263.

[70]  Sahin, I.H., M.M. Hassan, and C.R. Garrett, *Impact of non-steroidal anti-inflammatory drugs on gastrointestinal cancers: current state-of-the science.* Cancer Lett, 2014. 345(2) 249-257.

[71]  Cui, X.J., et al., *High-dose aspirin consumption contributes to decreased risk for pancreatic cancer in a systematic review and meta-analysis.* Pancreas, 2014. 43(1) 135-140.

[72]  Anderson, K.E., et al., *Association between nonsteroidal anti-inflammatory drug use and the incidence of pancreatic cancer.* J Natl Cancer Inst, 2002. 94(15) 1168-1171.

[73]  Coogan, P.F., et al., *Nonsteroidal anti-inflammatory drugs and risk of digestive cancers at sites other than the large bowel.* Cancer Epidemiol Biomarkers Prev, 2000. 9(1) 119-123.

[74]  Langman, M.J., et al., *Effect of anti-inflammatory drugs on overall risk of common cancer: case-control study in general practice research database.* BMJ, 2000. 320(7250) 1642-1646.

[75]  Tan, X.L., et al., *Aspirin, nonsteroidal anti-inflammatory drugs, acetaminophen, and pancreatic cancer risk: a clinic-based case-control study.* Cancer Prev Res (Phila), 2011. 4(11) 1835-1841.

[76]  Menezes, R.J., et al., *Regular use of aspirin and pancreatic cancer risk.* BMC Public Health, 2002. 2 18.

[77]  Bonifazi, M., et al., *Aspirin use and pancreatic cancer risk.* Eur J Cancer Prev, 2010. 19(5) 352-354.

[78]  Schernhammer, E.S., et al., *A prospective study of aspirin use and the risk of pancreatic cancer in women.* J Natl Cancer Inst, 2004. 96(1) 22-28.

[79]  Gridley, G., et al., *Incidence of cancer among patients with rheumatoid arthritis.* J Natl Cancer Inst, 1993. 85(4) 307-311.

[80]  Jacobs, E.J., et al., *Aspirin use and pancreatic cancer mortality in a large United States cohort.* J Natl Cancer Inst, 2004. 96(7) 524-528.

[81]  Ueda, J., et al., *Surgery for chronic pancreatitis decreases the risk for pancreatic cancer: a multicenter retrospective analysis.* Surgery, 2013. 153(3) 357-364.

[82]  Sakorafas, G.H. and M.G. Sarr, Pancreatic cancer after surgery for chronic pancreatitis. Dig Liver Dis, 2003. 35(7) 482-485.

# Intra-abdominal Hypertension and Abdominal Compartment Syndrome in Acute Pancreatitis

Carla Mancilla Asencio and Zoltán Berger Fleiszig

## 1. Introduction

Intra-abdominal Hypertension (IAH) is an entity that was described in the 19th century but which importance has been recognized in the last two decades. IAH is caused by persistent elevation in intra-abdominal pressure that is associated with multiple physiological derangements in almost all systems. In the setting of intensive care, this condition is considered as an organ failure that negatively impacts the prognosis and requires specific treatment. The most severe form of IAH is called Abdominal Compartment Syndrome (ACS) and is a high mortality entity [1].

Severe acute pancreatitis (SAP) is almost always accompanied by certain degree of IAH with an incidence of approximately 70%. Underlying conditions such as ileus, retroperitoneal edema, presence of fluid collections and fluid overload explain this phenomenon. IAH increases morbidity and mortality in acute pancreatitis (AP) and has become an issue of concern [2].

The aim of this chapter is to review basic pathophysyology and clinical concepts about prevention, diagnosis and medical-surgical management of IAH in the setting of AP.

First we will review some basic concepts about definitions and pathophysiology of IAH and then we will present a detailed analysis of IAH in the setting of AP.

## 2. Definitions

The abdomen is a closed compartment. The interaction between solid organs, hollow viscera, gas, fluids and the cavity generates a pressure known as intra-abdominal pressure (IAP).

Normal levels of IAP range from subatmospheric to 5-7 mm de Hg. Sustained elevation of IAP is associated with multiple physiologic alterations (Intra-abdominal Hypertension) and may be life threatening when exceeds certain levels (Abdominal Compartment Syndrome).

According to the consensus document by the World Society of the Abdominal Compartment Syndrome (WSACS), updated on 2013, **Intra-abdominal Hypertension** is defined by a persistent or repeated elevation of IAP over 12 mmHg [3].

IAH can be graded as follows:

Grade I:IAP 12-15 mmHg

Grade II:IAP 16-20 mmHg

Grade III:IAP 21-25 mmHg

Grade IV:IAP > 25 mmHg

A sustained increase of IAP over 20 mmHg associated with a new organ failure is recognized as the **Abdominal Compartment Syndrome** (ACS).

The **Abdominal Perfusion Pressure** (APP) is considered a resuscitation endpoint.

APP=Mean Arterial Pressure (PAM)-IAP

## 3. Measuring IAP

IAP can be measured in any abdominal organ but the standardized technique is via the bladder. By means of a Foley urinary catheter, a volume of no more than 25 mL of sterile saline is instilled into the empty bladder. After 60 seconds (to avoid detrusor contractil activity), at end-expiration, IAP is registered in a monitor. The patient must be in the complete supine position, and the transducer must be zeroed at the level of the midaxillary line (figure 1). IAP should be expressed in mm Hg [4]. 1 mmHg = 1,36 cmH$_2$O

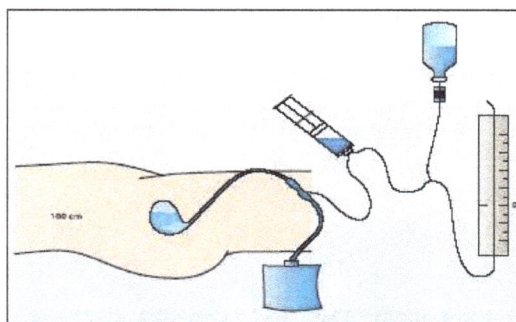

**Figure 1.** Intra-abdominal pressure recording via the bladder technique

# 4. Pathophysyology of IAH

## 4.1. Cardiovascular effects

IAH, by compression of porto-caval bed, diminishes venous return and cardiac pre-load. On the other hand, IAH increases systemic vascular resistance and left ventricular afterload. Both conditions lead to a decrease in cardiac output which is accompanied by an elevation of central venous pressure that reflects, in an imperfect fashion, the real status of intravascular volume in this scenario [5].Stasis in deep venous circulation puts the patient in an increased risk for thromboemolism.

## 4.2. Respiratory effects

Cephalic displacement of diaphragm results in pulmonary basal atelectases with alveolar collapse. Patients develop respiratory insufficiency due to ventilation/perfusion mismatch and sometimes require positive pressure mechanical ventilation with need of positive end expiration pressure (PEEP) at levels that relate to the amount of IAH. Maximal, mean and plateau pressures will increase. Hypoxemia and hypercarbia are late signs [6].

## 4.3. Renal effects

Kidney is a very sensitive organ to elevations in IAP. IAH alters renal perfusion and decreases venous outflow. These phenomena, associated with lower cardiac output lead to activation of renin, angiotensin and aldosterone, resulting in oliguria and can progress to anuria. Urinary sodium is low, reflecting a "pseudo pre-renal" condition.

## 4.4. Gastrointestinal effects

Splachnic territory is the most susceptible to augmented IAP. Over 10 mmHg, it is possible to demonstrate a decrease in mesenteric flow leading to intestinal hypoperfusion and increasing the risk of bacterial translocation. It is likely that the decrease in abdominal perfusion pressure, by compromising perfusion of the pancreas, furthers contributes to pancreatic damage, necrosis, and local infection. In grade IV IAH necrosis of the gut can occur.

Otto et al, in a porcine model, showed that experimentally induced intra-abdominal hypertension provoked histological pancreatic findings similar to those of acute pancreatitis [7].In another animal model of acute pancreatitis with and without IAH, IAH worsened evolution of severe experimental pancreatitis. No difference was found as concerns the pancreatic damage which was extremely severe in every experimental group [8]. Obviously, there are no data on the effect of IAH on the pancreas in human pancreatitis. However, these experimental data seem to be sufficient to affirm, that IAH is not only a consequence of SAP, but may contribute in the progressive pancreatic injury. It means, the more severe is AP, it is more likely that IAH develops, which in turn increases destruction of the already damaged pancreatic tissue.

Portal and hepatic artery blood flow are also altered and can explain ischemic hepatic insufficiency and lactic acidosis [9].

### 4.5. Central nervous systems effects

Transmission of IAP to the thorax can difficult brain venous return increasing intra-craneal pressure and eventually compromising cerebral perfusion pressure or leading to cerebral edema.

## 5. Risk factors for IAH in acute pancreatitis

The WSACS suggest to measure IAP in every patient who presents any risk factor for development of IAH (Table 1).

---

1. Factors that decrease abdominal wall distensibility

Acute respiratory failure

Abdominal surgery with primary tight fascial closure

Major trauma/ burns

Prone positioning

Obesity

---

2. Factors that increase intra-abdominal contents

Gastroparesis

Ileus

Colonic pseudo-obstruction

Hemoperitoneum/ pneumoperitoneum

Ascites

---

3. Factors that increase capillary leak/ fluid overload

Acidosis (pH<7,2)

Hypotension

Hypothermia (<33°C)

Polytransfusion (> 10 U packed red blood/24 h)

Coagulopathy

(platelets< 55000, KPTT> 2times normal, INR> 1,5)

Massive fluid resuscitation

(> 5 L/24 h) or positive fluid balance > 3,5 L/24 h

Peritoneal dialysis

Sepsis/ bacteremia

Major trauma / burns

Damage control laparotomy

---

**Table 1.** Risk factors for IAH

It is clear that AP may present various of these conditions. Furthermore, in AP, it is necessary to add local factors that contribute to increase IAP (Table 2).

| |
|---|
| Retroperitoneal inflammation |
| Peripancreatic inflammation and edema |
| Ascites formation |
| Retroperitoneal hemorrhage |
| Ileus |
| Fluid collections |
| Edema of abdominal wall |

Table 2. Local factors that increase IAP in Acute Pancreatitis

Some studies have explored specific risk factors for development of IAH in AP. Ke et al found a significant correlation between the serum calcium level, 24 h fluid balance and number of fluid collections in computed tomography and the risk of IAH. Patients who developed IAH had lower calcium levels, higher fluid balance and major number of collections [10].

Dambrauskas et al showed clinical scores APACHE II >7, MODS > 2 and Glasgow-Imrie > 3 were predictive of development of ACS, thus suggesting that IAP should be recorded in these patients [11].

Bezmarevic et al investigated the role of procalcitonin (PCT) as predictor of IAH in acute pancreatitis. They found a significant correlation between PCT values and IAP levels at 24 h of admission and between maximum PCT and IAP levels [12].

# 6. Clinical relevance of IAH and ACS in acute pancreatitis

Since recognition of IAH/ACS as a frequent complication in AP, various clinical case series have been published. Even though different criteria have been used to define severity of AP, all reports show IAH/ACS as a complication of SAP. It is possible that exists some bias in estimating the incidence of IAH in AP given that patients who present with mild clinical features are not subjects for urinary catheterization and record of IAP. Incidence of IAH is estimated between 60-80%, whereas incidence of ACS has been reported in 10-56% [13,14].

As systematically reported, IAH/ACS are early complications of SAP that present in the first week of the illness and are usually accompanied by other organic failures. Up to 70% of patients present IAH at ICU admission.

Evolution of IAP in the subsequent days is also important. Survivors evolve with progressive decrease of IAP during the first days meanwhile nonsurvivors maintain high IAP values during the first week. A decrease in IAP could be considered as a good prognostic factor in

SAP. On the other hand, it is likely that part of early mortality, typically attributed to multi-organ failure in setting of inflammatory response, is related to ACS. ACS should be considered as a tentative cause underlying fulminant presentation because it requires a very different approach.

Morbidity and mortality are clearly affected by the presence of IAH/ACS. Mortality related to IAH in AP has been reported 30-40% and 50-75% for ACS [15,16]. Hospital stay is longer in patients affected by IAH and the risk of infection of pancreatic necrosis is also greater in this patients may be due to increased bacterial translocation [17].

In our experience (partially communicated at The European Pancreas Club Meeting 2009) in a group of 28 patients with SAP (mean APACHE II score 16,6), 22 (78%) developed IAH. In this subset, 5 patients evolved with ACS. All the patients received medical treatment to lower IAP. 15 patients underwent percutaneous drainage of collections. One patient with IAP 33mmHg and anuria required decompressive laparotomy with immediate relief of IAH and recovery of renal function. 2 patients died later, not related to IAH/ACS [18].

# 7. Prevention

It is likely that prevention is the most important issue to consider, given that therapeutic interventions may increase IAP. As previously mentioned, fluid overload is a very important cause of IAH in any setting, and particularly in AP. Management of fluids represents a real challenge, since patients severely ill, usually require resuscitation in the first hours and the appropriate amount and rate of infusion has not been clearly defined.

Circulatory abnormalities in AP, similar to septic shock, can lead to oxygen debt that compromises organ perfusion, mainly in splachnic territory, leading to multiorgan disfunction. Local microthrombosis further impaires oxygen supply to the pancreas, contributing to necrosis and release of cytokines. Randomized trials have shown that patients who receive more than 4L fluids in the first 24 h have an increased risk of respiratory failure and IAH/ACS. The same consequences have been reported in patients that receive rapid fluid expansion, defined as 10-15ml/kg/h compared to 5-10 ml/kg/h [19,20].

Another issue is the type of fluid used to restore intravascular volume. Zhao et al showed that patients with SAP treated with a combination of normal saline with hydroxyethylstarch and glutamine reached hemodynamic stability more quickly, with less fluid volume and less risk of ACS [21] and the trial by Du et al revealed that patients randomized to hydroxyethylstarch versus Ringer lactate, also received less volume and had lower IAP levels [22]. Recently, a randomized trial by Bu et al compared normal saline with Ringer lactate resulting that patients in the Ringer group had less systemic inflammation assessed by C-reactive protein levels. The authors suggested that Ringer lactate offers better local pH homeostasis [23].

The American College of Gastroenterology Guidelines suggest that aggressive hydration, defined as 250 – 500 ml per hour of isotonic crystalloid solution, should be provided to all patients in the first 12 – 24 h. After that, fluid requirements should be periodically reassessed.

Clinical end points should be restorage of diuresis, normalization of BUN and correction of hemoconcentration [24].

Enteral nutrition has systematically shown to improve evolution in acute pancreatitis. Enteral nutrition was tested as a measure to prevent development of IAH. Patients who received early enteral nutrition (in the first 48 hours from admission) had a significantly lower risk of IAH than patients fed after 8th day [25].

## 8. Management of IAH/ACS

General interventions that are useful to diminish IAP can be classified according to their mechanism of action. These therapies are recommended for the WSACS with different levels of strength according to the quality of the evidence (Table 3). All this measures can be applied in patients with AP in order to prevent development of IAH or progression of IAH to ACS and even to treat ACS.

---

**Therapies to improve abdominal wall compliance**

Sedation and analgesia

Neuromuscular blockade

Consider supine position < 20º- Avoid prone position

Remove constrictive dressings and abdominal eschars

---

**Therapies to evacuate intraluminal contents**

Nasogastric/colonic decompression

Promotility agents

Enemas

Colonoscopic decompression

---

**Evacuation of abdominal collections**

Percutaneous drainage

Paracentesis

---

**Management of fluids**

Restriction of fluids/ permissive hypotension in trauma

Negative fluid balance

Use of diuretics/albumin

Hemodialysis/ultrafiltration

---

**Maintain APP > 60 mmHg**

Fluids/Vasoactive drugs

---

**Table 3.** Medical treatment of IAH/ACS

Cytokines released from immune cells are fundamental in the pathophysiology of systemic inflammatory response that leads to multiorgan disfunction in AP. Continuous hemofiltration and hemodiafiltration have been evaluated in SAP to test if diminishing blood cytokine levels improves evolution and reduces the risk of IAH.

Xu et al treated a group of patients with SAP and IAH and elevated levels of TNF-$\alpha$ at admission with continuous veno-venous hemofiltration (CVVH). 24 hours after initiating CVVH they noted a significant decrease in TNF-$\alpha$ levels and IAP. There was a positive correlation between levels of TNF-$\alpha$ and IAP [26]. Oda et al obtained similar results with early continuous venous hemodiafiltration in SAP. Hemodiafiltration decreased levels of IL-6 accompanied by a reduction in IAP [27]. A retrospective analysis of 10 years experience by Pupelis et al, shows that continuous hemofiltration/hemodiafiltration improves fluid balance, reduces cytokine plasma levels and reduces IAP, without changes in mortality [28].

Finally ACS not responding to medical interventions is an indication for decompressive laparotomy. In the last decades it has been clear that surgery should be avoided or at least delayed in AP, since this approach offers a better prognosis and reduces mortality. Nevertheless, one of the few remaining indications for surgery is refractory ACS, given that natural evolution in this situation is almost always fatal.

A retrospective review of 12 patients who were treated with decompressive laparotomy for ACS in the setting of SAP showed a mortality of 50%. Median time to decompression was 4,5 days and five patients underwent exploration of lesser sac in this group. However it is relevant to consider that these patients were treated between 2000 and 2009 and critical care in AP has evolved substantially in recent years [29].

Robin-Lersundi et al presented 5 patients with SAP complicated with ACS who underwent decompressive laparotomy with a mean IAP of 28 mmHg. A bilateral subcostal laparotomy was done with a temporary abdominal closure with a polytetrafluoroethylene mesh. The abdominal wall defect was repaired later. Four of five patients survived [30].

An intermediate alternative to surgical decompression is percutaneous drainage of fluid collections. In our series, 15 of 22 SAP patients with IAH were treated successfully in this way.

With existing information it is not possible to issue an emphatic recommendation about abdominal decompression in pancreatitis related ACS. It is not expected that randomized trials will come up and this decision-making will always suppose a big challenge where multidisciplinary confrontation of the patient is warrantied.

In conclusion IAH/ACS are very frecquent complications in patients with SAP. They represent a factor that worsens prognosis and complicates management. It is clear that we must increase our awareness to detect IAH, including in our clinical praxis algorithms to prevent, diagnose and treat this life threatening complication.

# Author details

Carla Mancilla Asencio[1*] and Zoltán Berger Fleiszig[2]

*Address all correspondence to: carlitamancilla@yahoo.com

1 Critical Care Unit, Department of Medicine, University of Chile`s Hospital and Las Lilas Clinic, Santiago, Chile

2 Gastroenterology, Department of Medicine, University of Chile`s Hospital and Dávila Clinic, Santiago, Chile

# References

[1] Malbrain ML, Deeren D, De Potter TJ.Intra-abdominal hypertension in the critically ill: it is time to pay attention. Curr Opin Crit Care. 2005; 11(2): 156-71.

[2] De Waele JJ, Leppäniemi AK. Intra-abdominal hypertension in acute pancreatitis.World J Surg. 2009; 33(6): 1128-33.

[3] Kirkpatrick AW, Roberts DJ, De Waele J, Jaeschke R, Malbrain ML, De Keulenaer B, Duchesne J, Bjorck M, Leppaniemi A, Ejike JC, Sugrue M, Cheatham M, Ivatury R, Ball CG, Reintam Blaser A, Regli A, Balogh ZJ, D'Amours S, Debergh D, Kaplan M, Kimball E, Olvera C; Pediatric Guidelines Sub-Committee for the World Society of the Abdominal Compartment Syndrome.Intra-abdominal hypertension and the abdominal compartment syndrome: updated consensus definitions and clinical practice guidelines from the World Society of the Abdominal Compartment Syndrome. Intensive Care Med. 2013;39(7):1190-206.

[4] De Keulenaer BL, Regli A, Malbrain ML. Intra-abdominal measurement techniques: is there anything new? Am Surg. 2011;77 Suppl 1:S17-22.

[5] Malbrain ML.Is it wise not to think about intraabdominal hypertension in the ICU? Curr Opin Crit Care. 2004 ;10(2):132-45.

[6] Pelosi P, Quintel M, Malbrain ML.Effect of intra-abdominal pressure on respiratory mechanics.Acta Clin Belg Suppl. 2007;(1):78-88.

[7] Otto J1, Afify M, Jautz U, Schumpelick V, Tolba R, Schachtrupp A. Histomorphologic and ultrastructural lesions of the pancreas in a porcine model of intra-abdominal hypertension.Shock. 2010;33(6):639-45.

[8] Ke L, Tong ZH, Ni HB, Ding WW, Sun JK, Li WQ, Li N, Li JS. The effect of intra-abdominal hypertension incorporating severe acute pancreatitis in a porcine model. PLoS One. 2012;7(3):e33125.

[9] Sánchez-Miralles A, Castellanos G, Badenes R, Conejero R.Abdominal compartment syndrome and acute intestinal distress syndrome.Med Intensiva. 2013;37 (2) :99-109.

[10] Ke L, Ni HB, Sun JK, Tong ZH, Li WQ, Li N, Li JS. Risk factors and outcome of intra-abdominal hypertension in patients with severe acute pancreatitis. World J Surg. 2012 ; 36(1):171-8.

[11] Dambrauskas Z, Parseliunas A, Gulbinas A, Pundzius J, Barauskas G. Early recognition of abdominal compartment syndrome in patients with acute pancreatitis. World J Gastroenterol. 2009;15(6):717-21.

[12] Bezmarevic M, Mirkovic D, Soldatovic I, Stamenkovic D, Mitrovic N, Perisic N, Marjanovic I, Mickovic S, Karanikolas M. Correlation between procalcitonin and intra-abdominal pressure and their role in prediction of the severity of acute pancreatitis. Pancreatology. 2012 ; 12(4):337-43.

[13] De Waele JJ, Leppäniemi AK.Intra-abdominal hypertension in acute pancreatitis.World J Surg. 2009; 33(6):1128-33.

[14] Al-Bahrani AZ, Abid GH, Holt A, McCloy RF, Benson J, Eddleston J, Ammori BJ. Clinical relevance of intra-abdominal hypertension in patients with severe acute pancreatitis. Pancreas. 2008; 36(1):39-43.

[15] Leppäniemi A, Johansson K, De Waele JJ. Abdominal compartment syndrome and acute pancreatitis. Acta Clin Belg Suppl. 2007; (1):131-5.

[16] Aitken EL, Gough V, Jones A, Macdonald A. Observational study of intra-abdominal pressure monitoring in acute pancreatitis. Surgery. 2014; 155(5):910-8.

[17] Mifkovic A, Skultety J, Sykora P, Prochotsky A, Okolicany R. Intra-abdominal hypertension and acute pancreatitis.Bratisl Lek Listy. 2013; 114(3):166-71.

[18] Arancibia JP, Mancilla C, Palavecino P, Berger Z. Intra-abdominal hypertension and abdominal compartment syndrome in severe acute pancreatitis. Pancreatology 2009; 9: 505.

[19] de-Madaria E, Soler-Sala G, Sánchez-Payá J, Lopez-Font I, Martínez J, Gómez-Escolar L, Sempere L, Sánchez-Fortún C, Pérez-Mateo M.Influence of fluid therapy on the prognosis of acute pancreatitis: a prospective cohort study.Am J Gastroenterol. 2011;106(10):1843-50.

[20] MAO En-qiang, TANG Yao-qing, FEI Jian, QIN Shuai, WU Jun, LI Lei, MIN Dong and ZHANG Sheng-dao. Fluid therapy for severe acute pancreatitis in acute response stage. Chinese Medical Journal 2009; 122(2):169-173

[21] Zhao G, Zhang JG, Wu HS, Tao J, Qin Q, Deng SC, Liu Y, Liu L, Wang B, Tian K, Li X, Zhu S, Wang CY. Effects of different resuscitation fluid on severe acute pancreatitis. World J Gastroenterol. 2013; 19(13):2044-52.

[22] Xiao-Jiong Du, Wei-Ming Hu, Qing Xia, Zhong-Wen Huang, Guang-Yuan Chen, Xiao-Dong Jin, Ping Xue, Hui-Min Lu, Neng-wen Ke, Zhao-Da Zhang and Quan-

Sheng Li.Hydroxyethyl Starch Resuscitation Reduces the Risk of Intra-Abdominal Hypertension in Severe Acute Pancreatitis. Pancreas 2011; 40: 1220-1225.

[23] Wu BU, Hwang JQ, Gardner TH, Repas K, Delee R, Yu S, Smith B, Banks PA, Conwell DL. Lactated Ringer's solution reduces systemic inflammation compared with saline in patients with acute pancreatitis. Clin Gastroenterol Hepatol. 2011; 9(8): 710-717.

[24] Tenner S, Baillie J, DeWitt J, Vege SS; American College of Gastroenterology.American College of Gastroenterology guideline: management of acute pancreatitis. Am J Gastroenterol. 2013 Sep; 108(9):1400-15.

[25] Sun JK, Li WQ, Ke L, Tong ZH, Ni HB, Li G, Zhang LY, Nie Y, Wang XY, Ye XH, Li N, Li JS. Early enteral nutrition prevents intra-abdominal hypertension and reduces the severity of severe acute pancreatitis compared with delayed enteral nutrition: a prospective pilot study. World J Surg. 2013; 37(9):2053-60.

[26] Xu J, Tian X, Zhang C, Wang M, Li Y. Management of abdominal compartment syndrome in severe acute pancreatitis patients with early continuous veno-venous hemofiltration. Hepatogastroenterology. 2013; 60(127):1749-52.

[27] Oda S, Hirasawa H, Shiga H, Matsuda K, Nakamura M, Watanabe E, Moriguchi T. Management of intra-abdominal hypertension in patients with severe acute pancreatitis with continuous hemodiafiltration using a polymethyl methacrylate membrane hemofilter. Ther Apher Dial. 2005; 9(4):355-61

[28] Pupelis G, Plaudis H, Zeiza K, Drozdova N, Mukans M, Kazaka I. Early continuous veno-venous haemofiltration in the management of severe acute pancreatitis complicated with intra-abdominal hypertension: retrospective review of 10 years' experience. Ann Intensive Care. 2012; 2 Suppl 1:S21.

[29] Boone B, Zureikat A, Hughes SJ, Moser AJ, Yadav D, Zeh HJ, Lee KK. Am Surg. 2013; 79(6):601-7.Abdominal compartment syndrome is an early, lethal complication of acute pancreatitis.

[30] Robin-Lersundi A, Abella Álvarez A, Cruz Cidoncha A, López-Monclús J, Gordo Vidal F, García-Ureña MA. Severe acute pancreatitis and abdominal compartment syndrome: treatment in the form of decompressive laparotomy and temporary abdominal closure with a expanded polytetrafluoroethylene mesh. Med Intensiva. 2013; 37(4):301-2.

# Pancreatic Acinar and Island Vascular Apparatus Associated with Acute and Chronic Inflammatory Processes

Garofita-Olivia Mateescu, Bogdan Oprea,
Liliana Stanca, Mihaela Hincu, Malina Coman,
Stelian Mogoanta, Dragos Voicu, Relu Stanescu and
Ion Rogoveanu

## 1. Introduction

Pancreatitis is the inflammation of the pancreas parenchyma with alterations of the stroma and acinar structures. It may be classified as either acute or chronic. Acute pancreatitis is the reversible injury to the pancreatic parenchyma associated with inflammation. Its reversibility depends on the degree and surface of the lesions and eventually on the co-existent morbidities.

Etio-pathogenesis of acute pancreatitis begins by the activation of pancreatic enzymes. Acute pancreatitis has as main physiopathological event the destruction of the parenchymal architecture. The parenchymal changes induce matrix alteration accompanied by vascular and nervous destruction. All these events have as main cause enzymatic mechanisms [1].

The mechanism behind this activation may be pancreatic duct obstruction, primary acinar cell injury, hyperstimulation of pancreas, reflux of bile, defective intracellular transport of proenzymes within acinar cells. Among the numerous causes, two factors which account for about 70-80% of cases of acute pancreatitis are biliary tract disease and alcoholism [1].

The acute inflammatory process associate with acute pancreatitis induces lesions due to the activation of immunity involved cell that produce TNF, nuclear factor kB and STAT1, that may lead to the overexpression of the pancreatic lesions and to the possibility of secondary infections. All the described events may lead in the end to SIRS, MOD or even death [2,3].

Pancreatic Acinar and Island Vascular Apparatus Associated with Acute and Chronic Inflammatory...

203

Recent studies have proposed chronic pancreatitis to develop through stimulation of stellate cells into myofibroblasts, which are responsible for the production of collagen and parenchymal fibrosis [4-7]. However, a molecular study has referred to important role of genetic polymorphism in the pathobiology of pancreatic diseases. [8]

Several studies proved that the prevalence of chronic pancreatitis tends toward 0.6% in several countries of Europe and United States [8,9], with an annual incidence of 10 cases for 100000 persons [10]. The most frequent factors that may lead to the appearance of chronic pancreatitis are: the obstruction of main excretory ducts, autoimmunity or individual risk factors (working and life conditions, alcohol consumption, smoking, different drugs, etc.) [11]. Chronic pancreatitis is characterized by the replacement of the secretory and endocrine parenchyma by the matrix elements with the predominance of fibrillar collagen structures, associated with the atrophy of the secretory and endocrine units. The fibrotic scar is triggered by the activation of the pancreatic stellate cells which appear in parenchyma destruction areas. These lesions induce severe disorganization of the architecture of the pancreatic lobules, associated with atrophic processes and dilations of the remaining intra and extra lobular excretory ducts. These aspects constitute the bases of multiple associated diseases as malnutrition or more frequently diabetes [12-14].

The lesions of acute and chronic pancreatitis and are especially related to chronic alcoholism. The alcohol may act directly as a parenchyma toxic through blood vessel wall absoption activating the stellate cells. They may be indirectly activated by alcohol metabolites and by cytokines and growth factors. The growth factors may also initiate angio and vasculo-genesis.

Necrosis and hemorrhage in acute pancreatitis are initiated by intracapillary leucocyte accumulation that adheres to capillary endothelium leading to capillary occlusion and lysis. This aspect may be observed in larger vessels with tunica media present. Leucocytes can substantially plug capillaries under pathological conditions leading to disturbances in microvascular blood flow which induces a so-called "no-reflow" condition with subsequent tissue damage [15-17].

Vascular lesions in chronic pancreatitis are different that in the case of acute pancreatitis, being characterized by vascular occlusion due to fibrosis.

In acute pancreatitis, the vessel destruction is due to the elastic fibers digestion by elastases [18]. In chronic pancreatitis the reticular network is ruptured by endothelial cells function and fibrosis in the tunica media.

## 2. Material and methods

We used 20 tissue samples from deceased patients diagnosed during necropsy with either chronic or acute pancreatitis. The inclusion criterion was the macroscopic examination of harvested samples. Thus the sclerotic pancreas was microscopically confirmed as chronic pancreatitis in 6 cases. The visible increasing of the gland's volume with pale aspect and diffuse edema or fatty necrosis with hemorrhage areas was diagnosed as acute pancreatitis in 14 cases.

The samples were fixed in 10% buffered formalin solution for 3-4 days depending of their size, and were paraffin-wax processed. The 10% buffered formaline solution is a soft fixative that preserves the antigen expression of various cells, thus being suitable for immunohistochemistry. It also maintains the morphology of the tissue without alteration of the histo-architecture of the pancreas. A higher fixative volume compared with the volume of the sample insures the optimization of the fixation process. The paraffin blocks were cut using the microtome to 5μm thick sections. The sections were harvested on poli-L-lisyne slides in order to have better adherence and to exclude the eventual cross reactions.

For the histological evaluation we used the standard hematoxylin-eosin staining, Goldner-Szeckelly trichrome staining and Gőmőri silver staining.

The immunohistochemical procedure was carried out after previous heat mediated antigen retrieval in the microwave oven, using the Mouse anti Human CD34 and Col IV (Dako) primary antibody in 1:50 dillution each. For detection we used Dako's EnVision system, and DAB *(3,3'-diaminobenzidine)* as chromogen substrate. The nuclei were counterstained using Mayer hematoxylin.

The obtained slides were examined using the Nikon Eclipse 90i microscope.

## 3. Results and discussion

Acinar and isle lesions in acute and chronic pancreatitis with blood vessel alterations differ regarding the etiologic agent of the disease. As it is already known the etiology of pancreatitis may be metabolic, genetic, mechanic, infectious or vascular. No matter which etiology the characteristic lesions in acute pancreatitis with parenchyma and stroma involvement imply inflammatory processes, edema, focal hemorrhage and severe necrotic lesions [4] (figure 1).

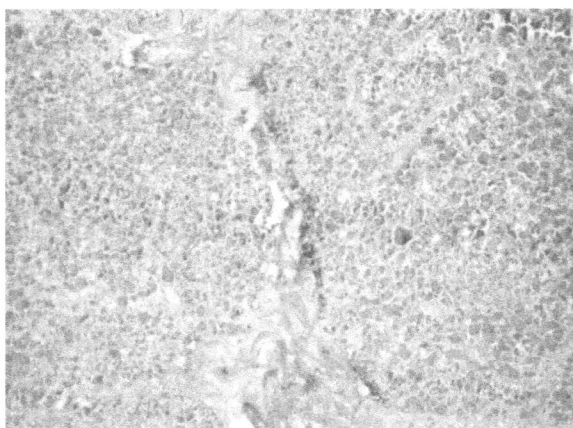

**Figure 1.** Histo-architecture changes of stroma and parenchyma-acute pancreatitis. HE x100

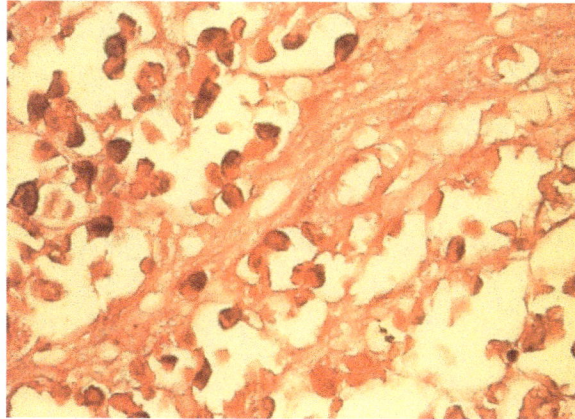

**Figure 2.** Isolated exocrine parenchymal cells surrounded by necrotic lesions and incipient fibril-genesis. HE x200

In the vicinity of the necrosis areas we observed the presence of isolated cells remained in the formed acinar and ductal structures zones. These cells may be involved in the initiation of partial remodeling processes or in the initiation of fibril-genesis along with already known myofibroblasts [19-21] (figure 2). In these areas the vascular apparatus lacks. We consider that necrotic lesions involve the capillaries with the appearance of parenchymal focal micro-hemorrhages.

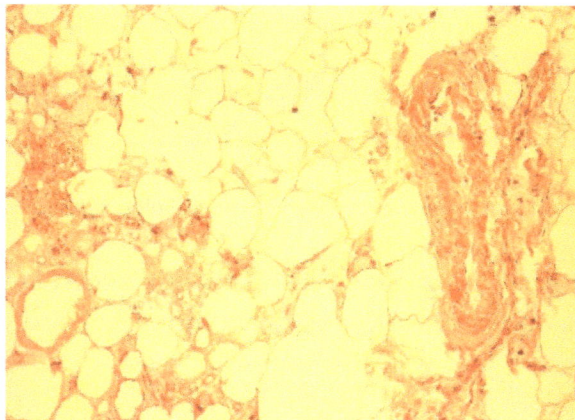

**Figure 3.** Reminiscent vascullar apparatus in an area of fat necrosis. HE x100

In areas of necrosis or fatty necrosis the remained vessels are of venular or arteriolar type. This aspect leads to the idea that pancreatic enzymes first target the reticular febrile network (this being the reason for capillary disappearance) and then the collagen and elastic network in the tunica media of arterioles or small veins (figure 3).

In acinar and isle dystrophic lesions areas we frequently observed with or without micro-thrombosis. We consider that these "gemini" vessels in acinar-isle transition zones may provide the vascular support for acino-isle reconversion (figure 4).

These aspects were not observed in areas of pure exocrine parenchyma.

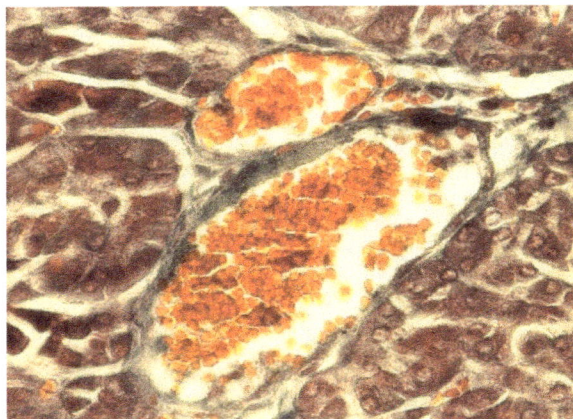

**Figure 4.** Micro-thrombosis of "gemini" vessels in an area of acinar and isle architecture partially unaltered. Goldner Szeckelly trichrome x200

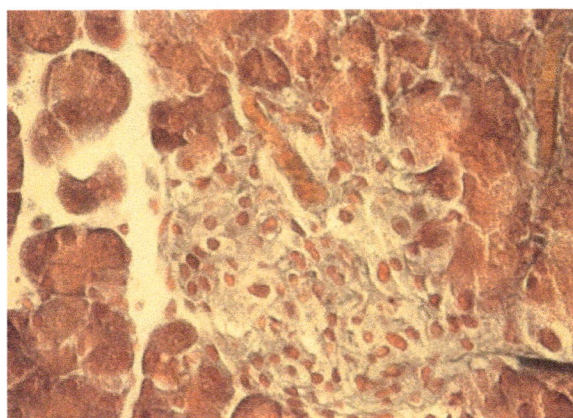

**Figure 5.** Peripheral vascularization of a Langerhans isle. Goldner Szeckelly trichrome x200

The characteristic of dystrophic Langerhans isles is the presence of capillaries in the periphery under the pseudo-capsule and their disappearance in medial and central areas. This aspect supports the above mentioned theory of the "gemini" vessels.

Recent studies [22] have reported that Langergans isles maintain their structure despite the necrotic surrounding, due to two main factors: the resistant collagen pseudo-capsule and the peripheral vascularization (figure 5).

Isle lesions associated to the acino-ductal ones are represented by focal accumulation of sclerotic islets of variable size; occasional neoformation of islets by ductoinsular proliferation (neosidioblastosis); and peri-capillary fibrosis in atrophic islets.

At the periphery of the pseuo-isle structures consequent to necrotic lesions, the pericytes are activated and develop myo-fibroblastic like characteristics, initiating the perivascular fibrosis.

The alterations of the vascular wall (endothelium and basement membrane of the capillary), focal ischemia, induce important dystrophic lesions of the endocrine and exocrine parenchy-

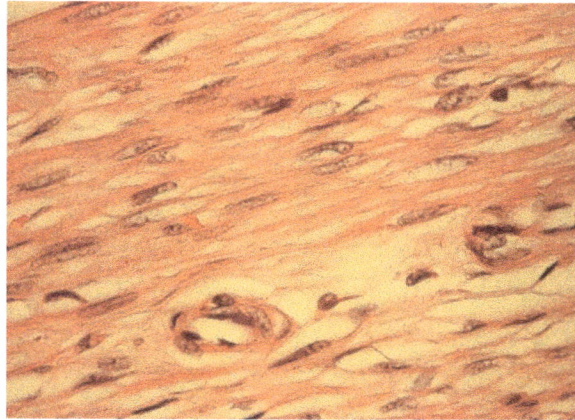

**Figure 6.** Capillary in a fibrosis area. HE x200

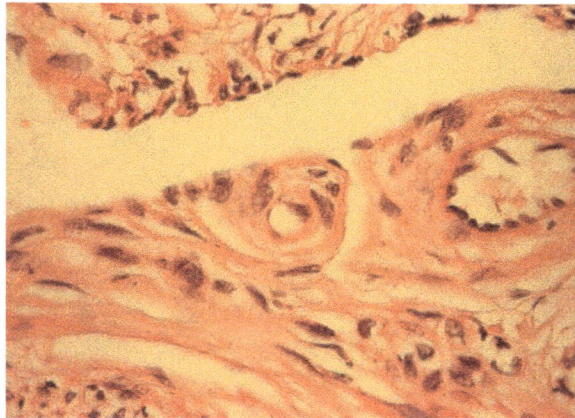

**Figure 7.** Vascular apparatus in a fibrosis area. HE x200

ma. This may have the pathologic support the alterations of endothelial and lysosome dynamics (figure 6 and 7).

In fibrosis areas characteristic to chronic pancreatitis, we observed capillaries with turgescent endothelia, nuclear hypertrophy of the pericytes. These may be the beginning of angio and vasculo-genesis with later differentiation into veins and arteries.

The fibroblastic, myo-fibroblastic-like cells in the fibrosis areas support the above mentions, being involved in collagen secretion and matrix remodeling as well as angioblastic cyto-formation substrate (figure 8).

Medium caliber vessels presented discontinuous endothelium with edema and myo-lytic lesions in the tunica media, the adventitia being completely modified by edema (figure 9). The myocytes or endothelial cell apoptosis may lead to the appearance of focal micro-hemorrhages.

In the inter-acinar spaces there are some CD34 positive groups of cells without lumen, possibly as angio genesis precursors (figure 10).

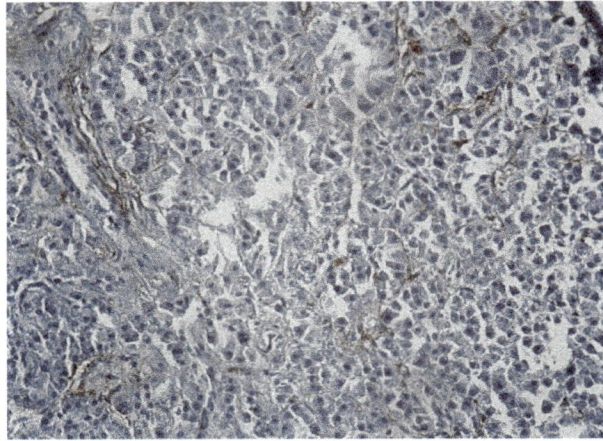

**Figure 8.** Immunostaining for Col IV, Collagen sinthesys at the periphery of the Langeshans isle. DAB x200

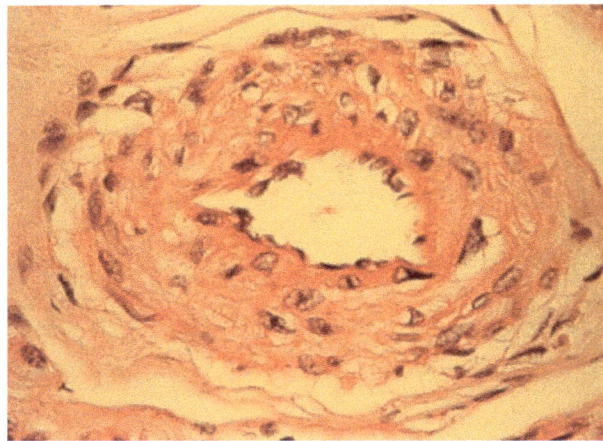

**Figure 9.** Myocytes lysis and edema in tunica media of the arteriole. HE x200

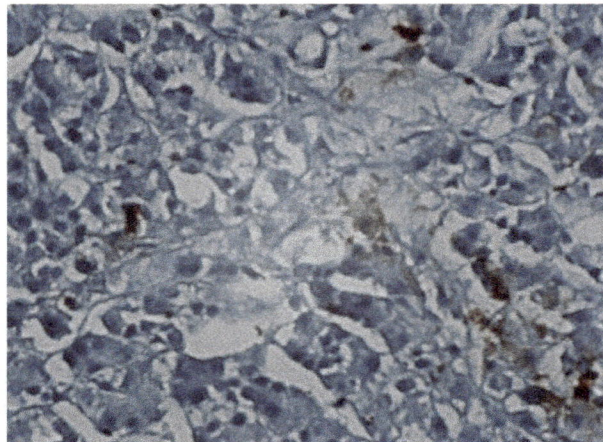

**Figure 10.** Issolated inter-acinar cells positive to CD34 immunostaining. DAB x400

The appearance of some fibrosis areas initiated in the peri-lobular septum, and the replacement of the parenchyma may lead to vessel "suffocation" (the fusion of the extracellular matrix with the vessels' adventitia and media with vascular collapse).

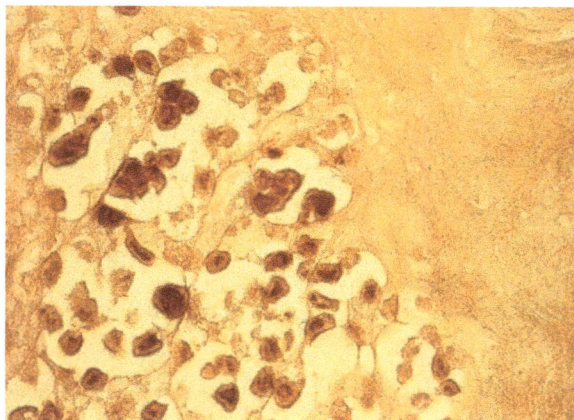

**Figure 11.** Argirophil cells anchored to the basement membrane in the neighboring of a fibrosis area. Silver staining x200

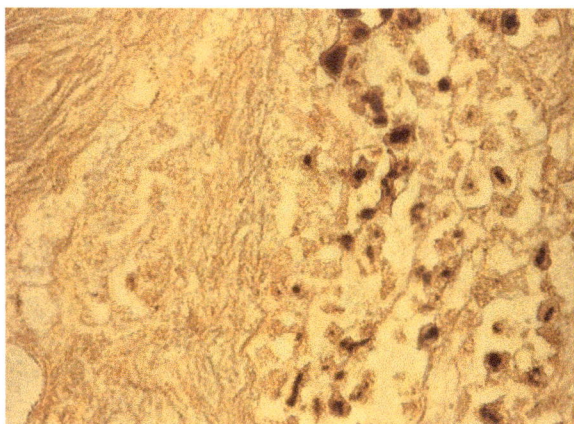

**Figure 12.** Argirophil stellate cells anchored to the basement membrane in the neighboring of a fibrosis area. Silver staining x200

In case of acute pancreatitis we observed isolated cells in the vicinity of intense necrotic lesions, this aspect being maintained in the vicinity of fibrosis zones in chronic pancreatitis (figure 11 and 12). These argirophils may provide the reticular fibril-genesis for vascular apparatus of the parenchyma [23].

The inhibition of MMP-3 and MMP-9 reduce the collagen degradation having as consequence the enhancement of fibriologenesis. This process is mediated by the pancreatic stellate cells in the matrix that produces regulatory cytokines involved in matrix remodeling [24].

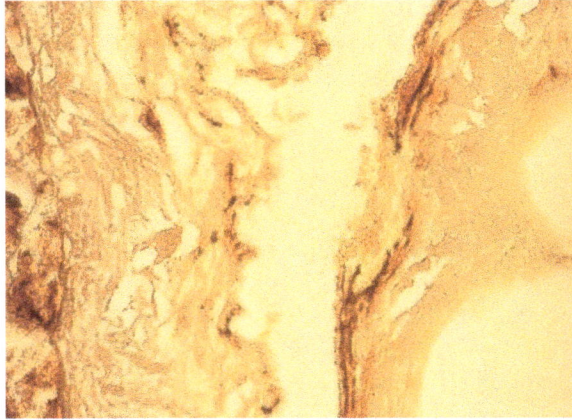

**Figure 13.** Ruptured reticular network in vessel's wall. Silver staining x200

In chronic pancreatitis fragmentations of the reticular fibers appear (figure 13). The fusion of the fibrosis area with the adventitia and media of the vessels lead to the maintenance of the vascular shape, this being the reason for the lack of hematic extravasations. The continuous of reticular network may lead to intravascular micro-thrombosis.

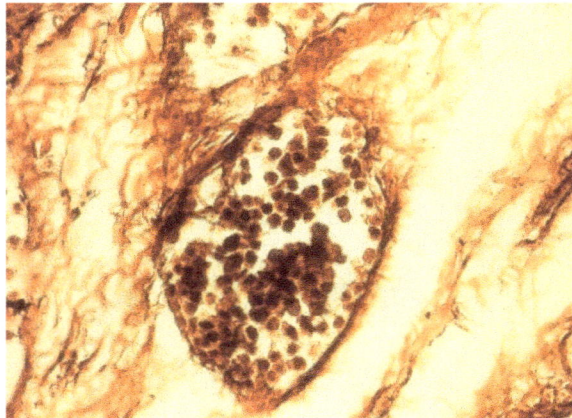

**Figure 14.** Partially kept reticular network with micro-thrombosis. Silver staining x200

The partial or total invasion of the fibrotic process in the tunica media of the arteriole may lead to the formation of high resistivity pseudo-fibrotic vascular apparatus (figure 14 and 15). This may be the pathogenic mechanism of low peripheral irrigation and eventually ischemia that may lead to a new acute pancreatic episode.

The described aspect is confirmed by collagen IV immunohistochemistry, that proves the accumulation of uni-directional fibers surrounding a former arteriole (figure 16).

In acute pancreatitis the characteristic dystrophic and necrotic lesions involved especially the intra-lobular vasculo-parenchymatous possibly due to aggressive protolithic attack. In chronic pancreatitis due to oxidative lesions there is an "activation" of the peri-lobular areas (stroma-

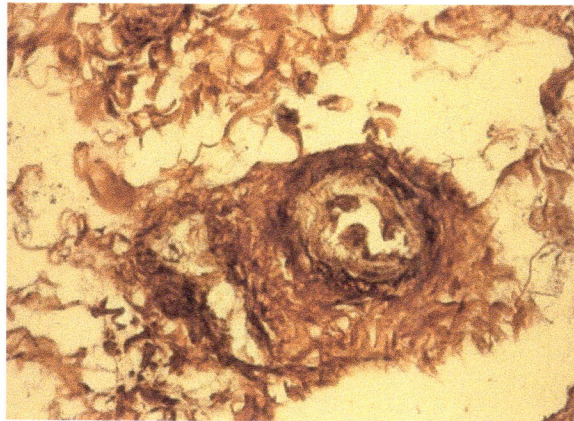

**Figure 15.** Blood vessels in a fibrosis area. Silver staining x200

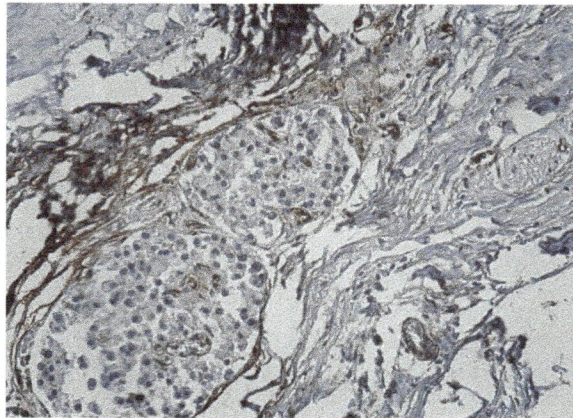

**Figure 16.** Unidirrectional collagen fibers surrounding blood vessels. Immunostaining for Col IV, DAB x200

septum) that lead to the "suffocation" of the blood vessels in some areas and to the appearance of pseudo-fibrotic arterioles as a compensation mechanism.

The endothelial and pericytar apoptosis may be the reason for the initial destruction of capillaries in acute pancreatitis, while in chronic pancreatitis there is a endothelial and pericyte hypertrophy is found as part of angio and vasculo genesis, Due to the non-typical aspect of the isle's capillaries, they disappear in isle involvement of acute pancreatitis, the vascularization being provided by the "gemini" vessels in the periphery of the Langerhans isle.

Vascular endothelial discontinuities and stasis associated to hemolysis, are typical lesion that occur in the small blood vessels areas that subsequently evolves into thrombosis. It it possible for this micro-thrombosis to be the key vascular event in acute necrotic pancreatitis [25-29]. These lesions may be observed in the early stages when stromal edema appears and there is no necrosis as yet. The thrombosis does not produce occlusion, only partial stenosis that leads to distal ischemia. This leasions often associate myo-lysis in the tunica media of and endothelial apoptosis. The necrosis appears as a consequence of vascular occlusion. Studies report as main vascular changes in chronic pancreatitis, the tortuosity and liminal irregularities of the

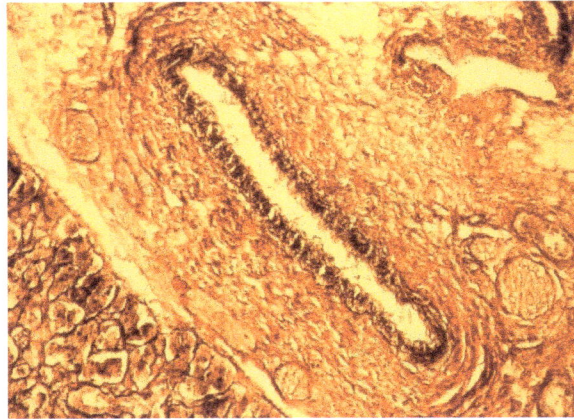

**Figure 17.** Blood vessels and nerves in a necrosis area. Silver staining x200

pancreatic arteries [30]. Those changes observed by angiography and micro-angiography [31-33] are confirmed by the microscopic aspect described in our study.

The argyrophilic structures of the pancreatic parenchyma is partially maintained even in necrosis areas, compared with the argyrophilic architecture of the small or large vesse Early or late acino-isle changes associated with stromal alterations do not usually involve the nerves, which are resistant to destruction [34-36] (figure 17). Pancreatic pain is characteristically described as a constant, severe, dull, epigastric pain that often radiates to the back and typically worsens after high-fat meals. However, many different pain patterns have been described, ranging from no pain to recurrent episodes of pain and pain free intervals, to constant pain with clusters of severe exacerbations [35-37].

Nerve structure of the nerve remains intact in fields of total necrosis, this being reflected in the noisy clinical symptoms associated to pancreatitis.

Pancreatic acinar cells seem to be especially vulnerable to endoplasmatic reticulum (ER) dysfunction owing to their dependence on high ER volume and functionality [38]. Pancreatic acinar cells, which are specialized in synthesis, storage and secretion of digestive enzymes, have the highest rate of protein synthesis among human tissues [39-41] and possess characteristically rich volume of ER. Thus, owing to the dependence on high ER volume and functionality, pancreatic acinar cells might be especially susceptible to perturbations in ER homeostasis. Indeed, ER stress has been previously described in pancreatic acinar cells during L-arginine induced experimental acute pancreatitis [42]. ER stress is newly considered to be a trypsinogen independent causing factor of pancrestitis.

## 4. Conclusions

Vascular dynamics differs in acute versus chronic pancreatitis.

In acute pancreatitis, areas of necrosis lack the vascular apparatus of capillary type with the appearance of focal intra-parenchymatous hemorrhages. In border zone, peri-necrotic, arterio-venullar apparatus remains.

In areas with acinar and isle architecture partially maintained, we identified "gemini" vessels with double involvement. They represent the starting point of the exocrine, respectively endocrine vascularization of the pen-umbra, with dystrophic Langerhans isles. The presence of capillaries in the periphery of the isle under the pseudo-capsule is a phenomenon frequently observed.

Partial lesions of capillary wall induce the activation of pericytes which acquire myo-fibroblast-like proprieties, initiating the perivascular fibrosis in the vicinity of necrotic areas.

In the fibrosis-necrosis border, we identified isolated argirophilic stellate cells presumably initiating the fibrosis. Due to their anchoring in the basement membrane of the former acinus we may assume the involvement of stellate cells in post-necrotic phagocytosis generating optically-void spaces.

In acute pancreatitis edema and myocytolysis was observed in the tunica media of large caliber vessels, while in chronic pancreatitis the fibrotic process of the media dominates leading to vessel "suffocation".

In chronic pancreatitis the hemorrhages are rare or absent due to the fusion of partially fragmented reticular network with the collagen fibers of the fibrosis areas.

We observed that in chronic pancreatitis, the nerva vasorum remains intact, leading to the idea of their resistance to the characteristic lesions of the acute event.

The most important difference, in our opinion, between chronic and acute pancreatitis is that the physiopathologic cascade is induced by the vascular apparatus. Thus in acute pancreatitis the lesions have a centrifuge evolution, while in chronic pancreatitis the centripetal evolution is characteristic.

# Author details

Garofita-Olivia Mateescu[1], Bogdan Oprea[1], Liliana Stanca[2], Mihaela Hincu[3], Malina Coman[4], Stelian Mogoanta[5], Dragos Voicu[4], Relu Stanescu[6] and Ion Rogoveanu[7]

1 University of Medicine and Pharmacy Craiova, Histology Department, Romania

2 University of Medicine and Pharmacy Craiova, Forensic Department, Romania

3 University "Ovidius" Constanta, Histology Department, Romania

4 "Dunarea de Jos" University Galati, Morphology Department, Romania

5 University of Medicine and Pharmacy Craiova, General surgery Department, Romania

6 University of Medicine and Pharmacy Craiova, Anatomy Department, Romania

7 University of Medicine and Pharmacy Craiova, Gastroenterology Department, Romania

# References

[1] Glasbrenner B., Adler G. Pathophysiology of acute pancreatitis. Hepatogastroenterology 1993;40(6) 517-521.

[2] A. Izakson, T. Ezri, Dana Weiner, Diana Litmanovich, E.V. Khankin New developments in understanding of pathophysiology, diagnosis and treatment of severe acute pancreatitis. Jurnalul Roman de Anestezie Terapie Intensiva 2012;19(1) 39-50.

[3] Oiva J, Mustonen H Patients with acute pancreatitis complicated by organ failure show highly aberrant monocyte signaling profiles assessed by phospho-specific flow cytometry. Crit Care Med 2010;38 1702-1708.

[4] B. Suresh Kumar Shetty, Ramdas Naik, Adithi S. Shetty, Sharadha Rai, Ritesh G. Menezes and Tanuj Kanchan. Acute Pancreatitis-The Current Concept in Ethiopathogenesis, Morphology and Complications, Pancreatitis-Treatment and Complications, Prof. Luis Rodrigo (Ed.), ISBN: 978-953-51-0109-3: InTech; 2012.

[5] Apte MV, Wilson JS. Stellate cell activation in alcoholic pancreatitis. Pancreas 2003;27 316-320.

[6] Bachem MG, Zhou Z, Zhou S, Siech M. Role of stellate cells in pancreatic fibrogenesis associated with acute and chronic pancreatitis. J Gastroenterol Hepatol 2006;21Suppl 3 92-96.

[7] Friedman SL. Mechanisms of hepatic fibrogenesis. Gastroenterology 2008;134 1655-1669.

[8] Christina Brock, Lecia Moller Nielsen, Dina Lelic, and Asbjørn Mohr Drewes, Pathophysiology of chronic pancreatitis. World J Gastroenterol. 2013;19(42) 7231-7240.

[9] Lévy P, Barthet M, Mollard BR, Amouretti M, Marion-Audibert AM, Dyard F. Estimation of the prevalence and incidence of chronic pancreatitis and its complications. Gastroenterol Clin Biol. 2006;30 838-844.

[10] Andersen BN, Pedersen NT, Scheel J, Worning H. Incidence of alcoholic chronic pancreatitis in Copenhagen. Scand J Gastroenterol. 1982;17 247-252.

[11] Schneider A, Löhr JM, Singer MV. The M-ANNHEIM classification of chronic pancreatitis: introduction of a unifying classification system based on a review of previous classifications of the disease. J Gastroenterol. 2007;42 101-119.

[12] Klöppel G, Detlefsen S, Feyerabend B. Fibrosis of the pancreas: the initial tissue damage and the resulting pattern. Virchows Arch. 2004;445 1-8.

[13] Etemad B, Whitcomb DC. Chronic pancreatitis: diagnosis, classification, and new genetic developments. Gastroenterology. 2001;120 682-707.

[14] Andrén-Sandberg A, Hoem D, Gislason H. Pain management in chronic pancreatitis. Eur J Gastroenterol Hepatol. 2002;14 957-970.

[15] Pace A, Weerth AD, Berna M, Hillbricht K, Tsokos M, Bläker M, et al. Pancreas and liver injury are associated in individuals with increased alcohol consumption. Clin Gastroenterol Hepatol 2009;7 1241-1246.

[16] Whitcomb DC. Genetic polymorphisms in alcoholic pancreatitis. Dig Dis 2005;23 247-254.

[17] E Ryschich, V Kerkadze, O Deduchovas, O Salnikova, A Parseliunas, A Marten,W Hartwig, M Sperandio, J Schmidt, Intracapillary leucocyte accumulation as a novel antihaemorrhagic mechanism in acute pancreatitis in mice. Gut 2009;58 1508-1516.

[18] Schmid-Schonbein GW. The damaging potential of leukocyte activation in the microcirculation. Angiology 1993;44 45–56.

[19] Fitzal F, Delano FA, Young C, et al. Early capillary no-reflow during low-flow reperfusion after hind limb ischemia in the rat. Ann Plast Surg 2002;49 170-180.

[20] Helin H, Mero M, Helin M, Markkula H., Elastic tissue injury in human acute pancreatitis, Pathol Res Pract. 1981;172(1-2) 170-175.

[21] Garofita-Olivia Mateescu, Contribution to the histological study of the pancreas in ethanol consummators, PhD thesis. University of Medicine and Pharmacy of Craiova;

[22] Hu W, Fu L., Simultaneous characterization of pancreatic stellate cells and other pancreatic components within three-dimensional tissue environment during chronic pancreatitis, J Biomed Opt. 2013;18(5) 56002.

[23] Apte M V, Pirola RC, Wilson JS. Mechanisms of alcoholic pancreatitis. J Gastroenterol Hepatol 2010;25 1816-26.

[24] Shek FW, Benyon RC, Walker FM, McCrudden PR, Pender SL, Williams EJ, Johnson PA, Johnson CD, Bateman AC, Fine DR. Expression of transforming growth factor-beta 1 by pancreatic stellate cells and its implications for matrix secretion and turnover in chronic pancreatitis. Am J Pathol. 2002;160 1787–1798.

[25] I. Kovalska, O. Dronov, S. Zemskov, E. Deneka, M. Zemskova, Patterns of Pathomorphological Changes in Acute Necrotizing Pancreatitis, International Journal of Inflammation, 2012 1-4.

[26] Mann DA, Mann J. Epigenetic regulation of hepatic stellate cell activation. J Gastroenterol Hepatol 2008;23Suppl 1 108-111.

[27] D. Uhlmann, H. Lauer, F. Serr, and H. Witzigmann, Pathophysiological role of platelets and platelet system in acute pancreatitis. Microvascular Research. 2008;76(2) 114-123

[28] C. M. Cuthbertson and C. Christophi, Disturbances of the microcirculation in acute pancreatitis, British Journal of Surgery. 2006;93(5) 518–530.

[29]  T.Hackert,D. Pfeil,W.Hartwig Platelet function in acute experimental pancreatitis. Journal of Gastrointestinal Surgery. 2007;11(4), 439–444.

[30]  Pekka Pítkäranta, Leena Kivisaari, Stig Nordling, Pekka Nuutinen, Torn Schröder, Vascular changes of pancreatic ducts and vessels in acute necrotizing, and in chronic pancreatitis in humans. International Journal of Pancreatology. 1991;8(1) 13-22

[31]  Reuter SR, Redman HC, Joseph RR. Angiographic findings in pancreatitis. Amer. J. Roentgenol. 1969;107 56–64.

[32]  Boijsen E, Tylen U. Vascular changes in chronic pancreatitis. Acta Radiol. Diagn. 1972; 12 34–48.

[33]  Tylen U, Arnesjö B. Angiographic diagnosis of inflammatory disease of the pancreas. Acta Radiol. Diagn. 1973;14 215–240.

[34]  T. Kerner, B. Vollmar, M. D. Menger, H. Waldner, and K. Messmer. Determinants of pancreatic microcirculation in acute pancreatitis in rats. Journal of Surgical Research. 1996;62(2) 165–171.

[35]  E. Malecka-Panas, A. Gasiorowska, A. Kropiwnicka, A. Zlobinska, and J. Drzewoski, Endocrine pancreatic function in patients after acute pancreatitis, Hepato-gastroenterology. 2002;49(48) 1707–1712.

[36]  Kumar V., Abbas A.K., Fausto N., Aster J.C., Robins and Cotran Pathologic Basis of Disease, 8th Edition, Philadelphia, Elsevier, 2010, 850.

[37]  Poulsen JL1, Olesen SS, Malver LP, Frøkjær JB, Drewes AM. Pain and chronic pancreatitis: a complex interplay of multiple mechanisms. World J Gastroenterol. 2013;19(42) 7282-7291.

[38]  Fasanella KE, Davis B, Lyons J, Chen Z, Lee KK, Slivka A, Whitcomb DC. Pain in chronic pancreatitis and pancreatic cancer. Gastroenterol Clin North Am. 2007;36 335-364.

[39]  Ammann RW, Muellhaupt B. The natural history of pain in alcoholic chronic pancreatitis. Gastroenterology. 1999;116 1132–1140.

[40]  Sah RP, Garg SK, Dixit AK, Dudeja V, Dawra RK, Saluja AK2. Endoplasmic Reticulum stress is chronically activated in chronic pancreatitis. J Biol Chem. 2014.

[41]  Case, R. M. Synthesis, intracellular transport and discharge of exportable proteins in the pancreatic acinar cell and other cells. Biol Rev Camb Philos Soc. 1978;53 211-354.

[42]  Kubisch, C. H., Sans, M. D., Arumugam, T., Ernst, S. A., Williams, J. A., and Logsdon, C. D. Early activation of endoplasmic reticulum stress is associated with arginine-induced acute pancreatitis. Am J Physiol Gastrointest Liver Physiol 2006;291 238-245.

# Permissions

The contributors of this book come from diverse backgrounds, making this book a truly international effort. This book will bring forth new frontiers with its revolutionizing research information and detailed analysis of the nascent developments around the world.

We would like to thank all the contributing authors for lending their expertise to make the book truly unique. They have played a crucial role in the development of this book. Without their invaluable contributions this book wouldn't have been possible. They have made vital efforts to compile up to date information on the varied aspects of this subject to make this book a valuable addition to the collection of many professionals and students.

This book was conceptualized with the vision of imparting up-to-date information and advanced data in this field. To ensure the same, a matchless editorial board was set up. Every individual on the board went through rigorous rounds of assessment to prove their worth. After which they invested a large part of their time researching and compiling the most relevant data for our readers.

The editorial board has been involved in producing this book since its inception. They have spent rigorous hours researching and exploring the diverse topics which have resulted in the successful publishing of this book. They have passed on their knowledge of decades through this book. To expedite this challenging task, the publisher supported the team at every step. A small team of assistant editors was also appointed to further simplify the editing procedure and attain best results for the readers.

Apart from the editorial board, the designing team has also invested a significant amount of their time in understanding the subject and creating the most relevant covers. They scrutinized every image to scout for the most suitable representation of the subject and create an appropriate cover for the book.

The publishing team has been an ardent support to the editorial, designing and production team. Their endless efforts to recruit the best for this project, has resulted in the accomplishment of this book. They are a veteran in the field of academics and their pool of knowledge is as vast as their experience in printing. Their expertise and guidance has proved useful at every step. Their uncompromising quality standards have made this book an exceptional effort. Their encouragement from time to time has been an inspiration for everyone.

The publisher and the editorial board hope that this book will prove to be a valuable piece of knowledge for researchers, students, practitioners and scholars across the globe.

# List of Contributors

**Marcel Cerqueira César Machado, Fabiano Pinheiro da Silva and Ana Maria Mendonça Coelho**
Emergency Medicine Department, University of São Paulo, Brazil

**Mukaddes Esrefoglu**
Bezmialem Vakif University, Medical Faculty, Dept. of Histology and Embryology, Fatih, Istanbul, Turkey

**Rone Antônio Alves de Abreu**
Faculty of Medicine ITPAC-Araguaína – Tocantins, Brazil
Federal University of São Paulo – UNIFESP, Brazil
General Surgery of Hospital Reference Araguaína – Tocantins, Brazil

**Manlio Basilio Speranzini**
Department of Gastroenterology, Faculty of Medicine, University of São Paulo (retired), Brazil
Hospital Complex of Mandaqui-São Paulo, Brazil

**Eugenia Lauret, María Rodríguez-Peláez and Luis Rodrigo Sáez**
Gastroenterology Unit, Central University Hospital of Asturias, Asturias, Spain

**Charing Ching Ning Chong, Anthony Yuen Bun Teoh and Paul Bo San Lai**
Department of Surgery, Prince of Wales Hospital, the Chinese University of Hong Kong, SAR

**Francis Ka Leung Chan**
Institute of Digestive Disease, Prince of Wales Hospital, the Chinese University of Hong Kong, SAR

**James Yun Wong Lau**
Department of Surgery, Prince of Wales Hospital, the Chinese University of Hong Kong, SAR
Institute of Digestive Disease, Prince of Wales Hospital, the Chinese University of Hong Kong, SAR

**Vincenzo Neri**
General Surgery-Dept. of Medical and Surgical Sciences-University of Foggia, Italy

**Hirotaka Okamoto**
Department of Surgery, Tsuru Municipal Hospital, Japan
Department of Gastrointestinal, Breast & Endocrine Surgery, Faculty of Medicine, University of Yamanashi, Japan

**Hideki Fujii**
Department of Gastrointestinal, Breast & Endocrine Surgery, Faculty of Medicine, University of Yamanashi, Japan

**José Celso Ardengh**
Endoscopy Unit, Hospital 9 de Julho, São Paulo, Brazil
Endoscopy Unity, Division of Surgery and Anatomy, Ribeirão Preto School of Medicine – University of São Paulo, Brazil

**Eder Rios de Lima Filho and José Sebastião dos Santos**
Department of Surgery, Hospital Federal dos Servidores do Estado, Rio de Janeiro, Brazil

**Rafael Kemp**
Endoscopy Unity, Division of Surgery and Anatomy, Ribeirão Preto School of Medicine – University of São Paulo, Brazil

**Simona Olimpia Dima and Irinel Popescu**
Center of General Surgery and Liver Transplantation "Dan Setlacec", Fundeni Clinical Institute, Bucharest, Romania

**Dana Cucu**
Department of Anatomy, Physiology and Biophysics, Faculty of Biology, University of Bucharest, Bucharest, Romania

**Nicolae Bacalbasa**
Carol Davila University of Medicine and Pharmacy, Bucharest, Romania

**Carla Mancilla Asencio**
Critical Care Unit, Department of Medicine, University of Chile`s Hospital and Las Lilas Clinic, Santiago, Chile

**Zoltán Berger Fleiszig**
Gastroenterology, Department of Medicine, University of Chile`s Hospital and Dávila Clinic, Santiago, Chile

**Garofita-Olivia Mateescu and Bogdan Oprea**
University of Medicine and Pharmacy Craiova, Histology Department, Romania

**Liliana Stanca**
University of Medicine and Pharmacy Craiova, Forensic Department, Romania

**Mihaela Hincu**
University "Ovidius" Constanta, Histology Department, Romania

**Malina Coman and, Dragos Voicu**
"Dunarea de Jos" University Galati, Morphology Department, Romania

**Stelian Mogoanta**
University of Medicine and Pharmacy Craiova, General surgery Department, Romania

**Relu Stanescu**
University of Medicine and Pharmacy Craiova, Anatomy Department, Romania

**Ion Rogoveanu**
University of Medicine and Pharmacy Craiova, Gastroenterology Department, Romania

# Index